Theory and Diagnosis of Osteoporosis

Theory and Diagnosis of Osteoporosis

Edited by **Dan Heller**

FOSTER
ACADEMICS

New Jersey

Published by Foster Academics,
61 Van Reypen Street,
Jersey City, NJ 07306, USA
www.fosteracademics.com

Theory and Diagnosis of Osteoporosis
Edited by Dan Heller

International Standard Book Number: 978-1-63242-399-3 (Hardback)

Printed in the United States of America.

Contents

Preface

Osteoporosis is a serious health problem across the globe. In the last few years, growth has been seen in the knowledge of the pathophysiological mechanism of the disease. Modern technologies have added significant information in bone mineral density measurements and, furthermore, mechanical and geometrical properties of bone. Novel bone indices have been formulated from hormonal and biochemical measurements for the investigation of bone metabolism. Although, it is evident that drugs are a crucial part of the therapy. Beyond medication, there are other mediations in the management of the disease. Prevention of this disease begins at young age and goes on with the process of aging for the purpose of prevention of fractures related to the impaired quality of life, mortality, physical decline, and high cost for the health system. Several distinct specialties are holding the scientific knowledge in this disease. In this book, information from scientific departments from across the world has been compiled. Updated information regarding the fundamentals of bone, diagnosis and evaluation of osteoporosis, and public health data of osteoporosis have been compiled in this all-inclusive book.

After months of intensive research and writing, this book is the end result of all who devoted their time and efforts in the initiation and progress of this book. It will surely be a source of reference in enhancing the required knowledge of the new developments in the area. During the course of developing this book, certain measures such as accuracy, authenticity and research focused analytical studies were given preference in order to produce a comprehensive book in the area of study.

This book would not have been possible without the efforts of the authors and the publisher. I extend my sincere thanks to them. Secondly, I express my gratitude to my family and well-wishers. And most importantly, I thank my students for constantly expressing their willingness and curiosity in enhancing their knowledge in the field, which encourages me to take up further research projects for the advancement of the area.

Editor

Part 1

The Basics of Bone

Genetics and Osteoporosis

Margarita Valdés-Flores, Leonora Casas-Avila,
Valeria Ponce de León-Suárez and Edith Falcón-Ramírez
Instituto Nacional de Rehabilitación, Secretaría de Salud, México, D.F.
México

1. Introduction

Osteoporosis is a multifactorial disease influenced by multiple factors and characterized by an imbalance in the regulation of bone remodeling that cause microarchitectural deterioration which compromises the bone strength and leads to bone fragility increasing the fracture risk. Since several years ago, the World Health Organization has considered osteoporosis as one of the most important public health issues worldwide, with a great repercussion in patients' life quality and in their familiar, social and work environments. Osteoporosis is an important problem in Latin America, currently its prevalence is similar to that in South Europe and slightly lower than in North Europe and among white population in the USA; World Health Organization estimates that in the forthcoming 50 years, osteoporosis prevalence will increase in Latin America until reach those of the currently observable in Europe and USA (World Health Organization [WHO], 1994; National Institute of Health [NIH], 2001 Consensus Development Panel on Osteoporosis Prevention, Diagnosis and Therapy; Cole ZA et al., 2008). During the last decades, the life expectancy has been increased notoriously and the number of subjects older than 60 years old has been increased. This situation in combination with the adverse environmental conditions and the life style, will cause a notorious increment in the incidence of chronic-degenerative diseases in the next decades, as will occur with osteoporosis. Certainly, primary osteoporosis use to be more frequent in posmenopausal women (Greespan et al., 1993); however occasionally it appears in premenopausal women which present several risk factors and even males may be affected by this disorder. It is important to mention that the actual life style favours the inadequate bone quality of children and young people (Asociación Mexicana de Metabolismo Óseo y Mineral, 2001). There are two forms of osteoporosis; primary OP, named posmenopausal or senile form and secondary OP, which is related to diverse endocrine, renal, rheumatic and genetic diseases, and with the prolonged administration of some drugs which induce bone loss (Riggs et al., 1986; Elliot-Gibson et al., 2004).

Discussing about osteoporosis it is necessary to mention the term "peak bone mass" (PBM), which refers to the maximum bone mass that an individual reaches in his life and it occurs between 20-30 years old approximately. PBM is the result of the interaction of multiple genetic and environmental factors; upon the PBM is reached, progressive loss of bone mass occurs naturally, depending on the magnitude and speed of subsequent bone loss (Burclar et al., 1989; Kanis et al., 1994; Guéguen et al., 1995.). The annual average bone loss in posmenopausal women is estimated in 1-2%, and 0.2.-0.5 % in males. It is considered that about 30% of women at this phase shows an accelerated bone loss (approximately 5% per year) during the first 5 years after menopause, which represents higher risk to suffer osteoporotic fractures at this moment of their lives (Elliot –Gibson V et al., 2004).

Osteoporosis has been characterized for having a very discrete clinic behavior; it is practically "silent" remaining latent for years or could get worsen without causing significant symptoms. Nevertheless, one of the most frequent clinic manifestations is the back chronic pain, which may be attributed to the presence of vertebral micro-fractures, frequently it can be noted progressive height loss due to vertebral compression and/or slimming; this anomalies can be heterogeneous and cause loss of the spine natural conformation causing abnormal curvatures and scoliosis (Ismail et al., 1999). Fractures are the most frequent and dangerous complication of osteoporosis and may occur practically in all bones, even with a discrete trauma and spontaneously. As has been documented in LAVOS (*Latín American Vertebral Osteoporosis Study*) (Clark et al., 2009). and EVOS (European Vertebral Osteoporosis Study) (Raspe et al., 1998) studies, the spine is the most common site in which fracture occur. Booth studies showed that, the frequency of these fractures are related to gender and age, but also to races geographic distribution. Apparently they are more common in Scandinavian and North American population, whereas they are less frequent in South of Europe. Interestingly, the frequency is higher in urban areas than in rural ones, which outstands the importance of environmental factors in this disease besides of the genetic predisposition. After vertebral fractures, hip fractures occur, followed by forearm. It is estimated that about 25% of individuals showing this kind of fractures die due to complications, and other 25% (even the after the surgery), never recover the life quality they have before the fracture. On the other hand, patients who have suffered one or more fractures (in any place) predispose to have new fractures, independently of their bone mineral density (BMD). The risk for new fractures is higher in individuals who have suffered first fractures at early age and in those who have higher number of previous fractures.

2. Genetic susceptibility in osteoporosis

There are several elements that suggest that bone phenotype is under of an important genetic influence. The first observation is the familial aggregation detected in the clinical practice, in which can be observed the segregation of some phenotypic characteristics, like family history of bad bone quality of osteoporotic fractures (Guéguez et al 1995; Fox et al., 1998; Kannus et al., 1999). On the other hand, description in literature of several diseases of genetic origin with monogenetic inheritance, which phenotype includes the loss or gain of mineral bone density, supports the hypothesis that bone phenotype has an important genetic component. Some of the most studied diseases are the different forms of osteogenesis imperfecta, the diverse varieties of osteopetrosis, pyknodisostosis, sclerostenosis and osteoporosis syndrome accompanied by pseudoglioma (Barros et al., 2007), among others. Besides, there are reports of severe osteoporosis cases in which mutations have been detected in genes which have been previously associated with the genetic control of mineral bone density, as the genes for estrogens receptors 1 and 2 (ESR1, ESR2), androgens receptor (AR) and vitamin D receptor (VDR). Changes in the normal sequence of those genes could cause osteoporosis. However, the primary osteoporosis represents the most common form in all populations (Duncan et al., 2005, 2008, 2010). Primary osteoporosis has a multi-factorial and polygenic origin and the evidences that it shows clearly genetic susceptibility are family history of bad bone quality and fractures, familial or demographic similarity during the natural history development of the disease or even differences in the pharmacological management response. In accordance to National Osteoporosis Foundation (IOF) 2008 statements, fractures family history represents an important risk factor independently of the bone mineral density and the presence of osteoporosis in first degree relatives has been related to the decrease in peak bone mass.

The analysis of genetic susceptibility to osteoporosis has been complicated because it is caused by the effect of multiple genes that exert their effect on the bone phenotype, taking in account that a great number of environmental factors acting on BMD are involved; however, despite all these difficulties, a large amount and variety of worldwide investigations suggest that BMD heritability ranges between 40-70% in spine, between 70-85% in hip and between 50-60% in wrist (Andrew et al., 2005; Michaelsson et al 2005; Deng et al., 2002). Densitometric studies in monozygotic twins (MC) and dicygotic twins (DC) have revealed that spine and femoral neck BMD consistency is higher (6-8:1) in MC twins than in DC twins. Family studies have estimated that fractures heritability ranges between 20-60%, depending on the anatomic region where those occur (Michaelsson et al 2005; MacGregor et al., 2000; Deng et al., 2002). In these cases, classic segregation studies have facilitated identifying new genes related to the BMD genetic control.

In the other hand, association studies have also been very helpful to associate particular phenotypic characteristics, such as bone mineral density or the occurrence of fractures, with very specific genetic variants (gene polymorphisms, specially single nucleotide variants). Besides, there are other bones characteristics with evident heritable component, among them are: geometry and length of the femoral neck, bone ultrasonic properties (which represent the trabecular interconnectivity degree), growth and speed of bone remodeling, bone dimensions and other conditions that have an impact on bone quality (Slemenda et al., 1996; Arden et al., 1996); for example body mass index and age at which menopause occurs. It is convenient to mention that family history of hip fractures has consistently been shown to be a risk factor for osteoporosis(Andrew et al., 2005).

The functioning of osteoarticular system is extremely dynamic and complex, it is constantly under remodeling and it have multiple and varied mechanisms to maintain homeostasis; therefore, its genetic regulation mechanisms are also complex to understand and integrate. Genes that have been linked with BMD genetic control are distributed along all the human genome and, they are in practically all chromosomes, each of them fulfills different functions and contributes in a different way to the genetic control of bone phenotype (Stewart et al., 2006; Xiong et al., 2006; Marini et al., 2010). There are some genes with important roles in bone homeostasis because their products are involved in elemental functions related to bone structure and metabolism (formation, growth, differentiation, resorption, maintenance, etc.) (Ralston et al., 2002; Williams et al., 2006).

Since long time ago, we know that bone metabolism has a great hormonal influence; therefore, genes that encode for its receptors are elemental in bone metabolism genetic regulation, among them we have genes ESR1 and ESR2 which encode for estrogens α and β receptors and are expressed in various bone cells types (osteoblasts, octeocytes and osteoclasts), both receptor types show a different expression pattern in the cortical and trabecular bones. Estrogens represent one of the most important regulators for bone metabolism, they regulate bone growth and maturation, and they also influence the differences between bone maturation and bone consolidation in men and women. These hormones have the capacity to block the osteoclastogenesis process, can interfere with the function of osteoclasts, induce them to apoptosis, and may also modify the expression of genes involved in the bone remodeling process (Slemenda et al., 1996; Kameda et al., 1997; Cummings et al., 1998)). Moreover, hormones contribute to down the expression of the Tumoral Necrosis Factor (TNF), and thereby reducing osteoclasts response to the RANK and RANKL activity (the ligand binding to the activator receptor for the kappa B factor and its ligand) (Hughes et al., 1996).

It is already known that vitamin D, through the interaction with its receptor, plays an important role in calcium homeostasis for the regulation of growth and differentiation of bone cells; that is the reason why the gene that encodes for the vitamin D receptor (VDR) is quite important in bone metabolism. Another important gene is IL6, which codifies for interleukin 6, which is a proinflammatory cytokine that has been related to several biologic processes, as bone resorption, osteoporosis and other diseases as rheumatoid arthritis, diabetes mellitus, cardiovascular diseases, cancer, etc. LRP5 gene, which encodes for protein 5 related to the low density lipoprotein receptor that participates in the development and maintenance of several tissues and represent one of the regulators for the development and proliferation of the osteoblasts (Gong et al., 2001). Other genes relevant for bone metabolism are RANK, RANK-L and OPG which encode for key proteins for bone remodeling process (Capellen et al., 2002). Other genes with higher impact on bone phenotype is the COL1A1 gene, which encodes for one of the most abundant structural proteins in bone (collagen 1A1). A great number of investigations have analyzed the association among osteoporosis and allelic and genotypic variants of these genes (Ralston et al., 2002).

There are some characteristics, for example the body mass index, that could have an impact on bone phenotype. These traits are also under genetic influence so we found genes that are related with more than one phenotype. Since several years ago it is clear that there is an important relation between bone mineral density and body mass, we already know that overweight individuals should support higher weight opposite to individuals with a lower body weight, therefore, bone mineral density is higher in overweight subjects, while thinner subjects, including the ones with alimentary disorders as anorexia or malnutrition, could present low bone quality. Some of the genes with impact on these phenotypes are ESR1, ESR2, VDR, LRP5, IL6 and OPG between others (Deng et al-. 2002; Jie et al., 2009; Frenkel et al., 2010)K. During the last years, the leptin gene and its receptor (LEP and LEPR) have been revealed as an important hormonal factors for the regulation of appetite and energetic metabolism; besides, leptin has an osteogenic effect by stimulating osteoblasts formation and plays a direct osteogenic role on bone marrow stromal cells, which allows its differentiation and maturation to osteoblasts (Esteppman et al., 2000).

Other important genes in both phenotypes are the proinsulin gene (INS), its receptor (INSR), and probably too the gene family of growth factors similar to insulin, since apparently insulin exerts a mitogenic effect on osteoblasts, which could partially explain bone mass increment that is usually noticed in obese individuals.

Table 1 despicts some of the genes related to the bone phenotype and the function that has been attributed to their products. It is evident the genetic influence on different aspects of metabolism and homeostasis of bone tissue (structure, formation, resorption and remodeling) and the number of genes involved is large and their functions are diverse. In the case of bone structure highlights the COL1A1 and COL1A2 genes which code for the type I colagen protein, which represents over 90% of the organic matrix of bone. The osteocalcin and osteopontin are also important, the first one is a calcium binding protein which is secreted by osteoblasts and is encoded by the gene OC, while the phosphoprotein known as osteopontin, encoded by the gene OPN, is essential in the mineralization process.

Hormones and their receptors		
Gene	**Chromosomal location**	**Product**
ESRα	6q25	Estrogens receptor α
ESRβ	14q22	Estrogens receptor β
AR	Xq11	Androgens receptor
VDR	12q12	D vitamin receptor
PTH	11p15	Paratohormone
PTHR1	3p22	Paratohormone receptor 1
CT	11p15	Calcitonin
CTR	7p21	Calcitonin receptor
CYP1A1	15q21	Aromatase
CASR	3q13	Receptor sensitive to calcium
ADPN	3q27	Liponectin
GR	5q31	Glucocorticoids receptor
PRL	6p22	Prolactin
LEP	7q31	Leptine
LEPR	lp31	Leptine receptor
INS	11p15	Insulin
INSR	19p13	Insulin receptor
Matrix components		
COL1A1	17p21	Collagen 1A1
COL1A2	7q22	Collagen 1A2
OC	1q25	Osteocalcin
OPN	4q21	Osteopontin
With participation in osteoblastogenic processes		
ALOX12	17p13	Araquinodate 12 lipoxigenase
ALOX15	17p13	Araquinodate 15 lipoxigenase
BMP2	20p12	Morphogenetic protein of bone 2
BMP4	14q22	Morphogenetic protein of bone 4
BMP7	20q13	Morphogenetic protein of bone 7
IGF-1	12q22	Growth factor similar to insulin
LRP5	11q13	Receptor related to lipoprotein of low density 5
LRP6	12p13	Receptor related to lipoprotein of low density 6
SOST	17q12	Sclerotin
NOG	17q22	Protein antagonist of morphogenetic proteins

With participation in osteoclastogenesis processes		
Gene	Chromosomal location	Product
P53	17p13	Tumor suppressor P53 protein
CPK	1q21	Catepsine K
OC	1q25	Osteocalcin
OPN	4q21	Osteopontin
OPG	8q24	Osteoprogeterin
RANK	18q22	Receptor activator of NF-KAPPA-B
RANK-L	13q14	Ligand of the receptor activator of NF-KAPPA-B
CLC7	16p13	Chlorine channel 7
Cytokines and their receptors		
IL1α	2q14	Interleukin 1A
IL1β	2q14	Interleukin 1B
IL6	7p21	Interleukin 6
TNF	6p21	Tumoral necrosis factor
TNFR2	1p36	Tumoral necrosis factor receptor 2
Others functions		
MTHFR	1p36	5,10-Methylenetetrahydrofolate reductase
APOE1	19q13	Apolipoprotein E
MMP-1	11q22	Metalloproteinase
MMP-2	16q13	Metalloproteinase
MMP-9	20q11	Collagenase
PON-1	7q21	Esterase
SHH	7q36	Hedgehog protein (it participates in skeleton embryogenesis)

Table 1. Genes related to bone phenotype, their chromosomal location and their products

The osteoclastogenesis and the osteoblastogenesis are fundamental processes for the homeostasis of bone tissue as the speed and intensity of bone formation and bone resorption depending on several conditions. Both mechanisms show a significant genetic influence, so the amount of genes and therefore of proteins with participation in both processes is very significant. Among them are genes that encode for the family of bone morphogenetic proteins (BMP's), the LRP5 and LRP6 genes that code for receptors for low density lipoproteins, which are involved in the osteoblastogenesis most likely to regulate the level of bone mineralization. The osteoclastogenesis is determined by the differential expression of genes of the RANK/RANK-L/OPG route. The P53 oncogene which product is very important for multiple biological processes and the cathepsin K gen (CPK) wich codes for a collagenase with preferential expression in osteoblasts, indubitably play a crucial role in bone resorption.

Different hormones involved in the bone formation and remodeling, including the sex hormones (estrogen, progesterone, androgens), growth hormone, insulin, parathyroid hormone, calcitonin, cortisol and thyroid hormones. These hormones are implicated in different ways in bone metabolism according to the different stages, including intrauterine life, in such a way that the different hormones impact on linear growth of bones, bone maturation, bone homeostasis and the size that will be achieved in adulthood. That's why there are hormonal conditions such as hypothyroidism, hyperthyroidism, postmenopause, andropause and glucocorticoid prolonged intake which are capable to impact on the quality of the bone. Finally we can not ignore that various interleukins, growth factors and their receptors have been identified and the participation in the genetic control of bone mineral density of other proteins are still under study, as in the case of ILα, ILβ, IL6, TNF, TNFR2 among others.

On the other hand, it is important to mention that during the last years some investigations have pointed out that some of the genes related with bone phenotype have been related to other disorders as cardiovascular diseases; for example, genes such as osteoprotegerin (OPG), the receptor activator for nuclear factor kappa B ligand (RANKL) and bone morphogenetic protein 2 (BMP) have been associated with osteoporosis and with cardiovascular diseases, particularly atherosclerosis, which suggest that products of these genes take part in the calcification process (Collin-Osdoby et al., 2004; Marini et al., 2010).

3. Linkage analysis as strategy in the study of osteoporosis

Linkage studies are well validated for identification of responsible genes in monogenic diseases, since the inheritance of marker alleles is related to the inheritance of a bone trait within family members. Combining the use of statistical approaches in quantitative trait loci (QTL) and genome-wide association studies (GWAS), it is possible to establish a strategy to identify chromosomal regions which contain regulating genes of some important traits in complex polygenic diseases with genetically heterogeneous traits as osteoporosis, making possible to evaluate how many of the hundreds of proposed candidate genes are really associated. Most of linkage studies in osteoporosis selected the bone mineral density as the trait of interest; however regions that regulate other relevant phenotypes, such as bone mass and skeletal geometry, have been investigated.

Former studies identified important loci linked to bone mass and geometry. A genome search study in sib pairs recruited from families with a history of osteoporosis, obtained data suggestive of linkage of 1p36, 2p23-24 and 4q32-34 with spine and hip BMD (Devoto et al., 1998; Devoto et al., 2001). Studies with healthy female sib pairs demonstrated linkage of locus 11q12-13 with BMD variation (Koller et al., 1998) and evidence suggestive of linkage of 1q21-23, 5q33-35 and 6p1-12 to femoral neck or lumbar spine BMD was obtained in a genome-wide search study performed in Caucasian and African-American healthy female sib pairs (Koller et al., 2000). Other study identified loci in 5q and 4q that showed linkage to regulation of important aspects of femoral neck geometry (Koller et al., 2001). A QTL not previously described in 22q11 showed suggestive linkage in a study with families from Belgium and France (Kaufman et al., 2008). The presence of genes controlling BMD on 1p36 was suggested too in a multivariate linkage analysis in osteoporosis pedigrees (Zhang et al., 2009). One genome-wide scan for bone loss showed that change in femoral neck BMD in Mexican-American families is significantly linked to 1q23 (Shaffer et al., 2009). Interestingly a study with pairs of brothers suggested that QTL on 7q34, 14q32 and 21q21 were male-specific (Peacock et al., 2009) and other report provides evidence of gender specific QTL on 10q21 and 18p11 (Ralston et al., 2005). Suggestive evidence of linkage of novel regions related with BMD and hip geometry on chromosomes 4, 5, 11, 16 and 20 was obtained in a sample of Caucasian Europeans (Karasik et al., 2010).

Two important large scale studies with a cohort of more than 19,000 european subjects, identified SNPs in previously proposed osteoporosis candidate genes and in regions not previously associated with femoral neck and lumbar spine BMD. SNPs from ESR1, LRP4, ITGA1, LRP5, SOST, SPP1, TNFRSF11A, TNFRSF11B AND TNFSN11 associated with either femoral neck or lumbar spine BMD in a cohort of more than 19,000 subjects. In the same study, SNPs from LRP5, SOST, SPP1 and TNFSF11A, were associated with fracture risk (Richards et al., 2009). The other study, confirmed the significant association of previously known BMD loci: ESR1, TNFRSF11B, LRP5, SP7, ZBTB40, TNFSF11 and TNFRSF11A, but interestingly they identified several loci in regions not previously associated with BMD (Rivadeneira et al., 2009). Recently, variants in CATSPERB (Koller et al., 2010), MATN3, IGF1 (Li et al., 2011), SOD2 (Deng et al., 2011) and FONG (Kou et al., 2011) genes between many others, have been involved in BMD regulation and in the pathogenesis of osteoporosis. Evidences for genes or loci association with BMD are controversial in many cases (Ralston & Uterlinden, 2010). Further large scale studies will be necessary to address the role of gene variants on BMD and osteoporosis, but the importance of this studies lies in the potential uses and clinical implications since, besides of differences in the effect of variants, the identified genes might be important for drugs design to prevention and treatment of osteoporosis.

4. Association studies

During the last years, association studies among natural variations of our genome (gene polymorphisms) and particular phenotypic characteristics such as OP, have shown that the mechanisms that condition this heritable susceptibility are defined by the presence of mutations or polymorphisms in one or several genes that influence bone phenotype. In this case, it is important clarifying that the term polymorphism refers to the presence of two or more gene variants in the same allele, in such a way that the less common variant must have a frequency equal or higher on 1% of the population, otherwise, the variation is considered as a mutation. These changes in the normal sequence may involve several bases, as in case mini-satellites or VNTR (*variable number of tandem repeat*), where the size of repeated fragments range from 15 to 70 pairs of bases in tandem. Other kind of polymorphisms are of micro-satellite also known as STR (*short tandem repeats*), which characterize for showing variations in the nucleotide number (2-6 base pairs). Recently, single nucleotide variations also known as SNPs (*single nucleotide polymorphisms*) have been analyzed; in this case, the analysis of these variations represents a very commonly used tool in studies that intend associating certain allelic variants with phenotypic characteristics, specially the ones attributed to polygenic diseases (multi-factorial and complex). Table 2 shows several single nucleotide polymorphisms studied in relation to osteoporosis and bone mineral density. It can be observed that some polymorphisms have been consistently studied with respect to particular bone traits, such as BMD in specific anatomic regions and in some cases with fracture risk.

Polymorphisms in genes as ER α and β, IL6, VDR, Aromatase (CYP19), COL IA1, RANK and RANKL are between the most studied. There are several polymorphic sites which association with BMD or with osteoporosis has been demonstrated in many different populations. The results in many cases have been controversial, for example the SNP G/A in ERα gene exon 8, have been associated with osteoporosis in Thailander (Ongphiphadhanakul et al., 2001) and in Mexican women (Gómez et al., 2007), but association was denied when it was studied in Spanish women (Riancho et al., 2006), in spite all three investigations were performed with posmenopausal women. The T/C SNP of ERα gene was associated with low BMD in Japanese women, but not in Afro-American, Caucasian or Chineese women and the A/G SNP of the same gene, was associated with low BMD only in Afro-American Women, but not in Caucasian, Chinese nor in Japanese women (Greendale et al., 2006). The differences between studies results might be due to the genetic background of studied populations, which emphasize the importance of performing studies to explore the polymorphisms in specific groups with the same characteristics to avoid the incorrect use of genetic markers. Differences between races were evident too in studies with the IL6 G572C polymorphism in which the results in Korean (Chung et al., 2003) and Japanese (Ota et al., 2001) populations were consistent associating the G allele with low BMD, meanwhile in the study performed with Caucasian US women (Ferrari et al., 2003), the G allele appears as a protective factor from bone resorption.

Discordances can certainly be seen due to the frequencies of some alleles in different populations. It is important to determine the frequency of the polymorphism in a general population study before to perform a case-control study, since some genetic sites could be not polymorphic in some populations or the variant might be present in very low frequencies and their analysis could give spurious or no association results. An example of a SNPs which could not be used as osteoporosis genetic markers in Korean population are the G174C and G/A polymorphisms in the promoter of the IL6 gene because they show a very low frequency of this polymorphisms which difficult to found associations (Chung et al., 2003). However, the same G174C SNP was analyzed in Caucasian American healthy women (Ferrari et al., 2003) and in Mexican osteoporotic and non osteoporotic women as well as in general population (Magaña, et al., 2008), obtaining that the C allele is a protective factor from bone resorption and from osteoporosis respectively. However, most of the VDR gene SNPs showed in table 2, were consistently associated with low BMD or with osteoporosis in a great variety of populations. SNPs in intron 10, exon 2 and promoter of the gene, have resulted associated in European (Bustamante et al., 2007b; Utterlinden et al., 2001) American (Kiel et al., 2007; Pérez et al., 2008; Moffet et al., 2007) and Asiatic (Mencej et al., 2009) populations and even in large scale studies with world´s population (Morrison, 2004). The colagen IA1 is one of the most studied genes involved in osteoporosis. Many SNPs have been consistently associated with BMD and osteoporosis in several populations in this gene. The G/T change has been associated with osteoporosis in almost all studied populations, for example in Mexican (Falcón-Ramírez et al., 20011) and in British (Stewart et al., 2006). Not all the polymorphisms have a functional effect on bone traits, but the presence of the polymorphism G/T in Sp1 site, alters the recognition of the Sp1 factor having effects on transcription, protein production and mechanical strength of bone.

The appropriate expression of the genes of the route of signaling RANK/RANK-L/OPG is essential in osteoclastogenesis process, and makes them some of the most investigated genes performing studies with specific allelic, genotypic and haplotypic variants in this genes searching for associations with bone mineral density. In this case, variations of a single nucleotide in the intron 1, 9, and others located in the 3´del region gene RANK have consistently shown their association with low bone mineral density in spine and hip in European populations (Paternoster et al., 2010; Styrkarsdottir et al., 2009, Xiong et al., 2006).

GEN	POLYMORPHISM	LOCATION	REFERENCES	OUTCOME
CALCR	C/T C/T	Exon 13 Intron 12	Xiong et al., 2006.	Associated with spine osteoporosis in European families
ER α	G/A	Exon 8	Ongphiphadhanakul et al., 2001. Riancho et al., 2006 Gómez et al., 2007.	Associated with osteoporosis in postmenopausal Thailander women. Not associated with BMD in postmenpausal Spanish women. Associated with spine osteoporosis in Mexican women.
	C/T	Intron 1	Ongphiphadhanakul t al., 1998. Wang et al., 2008.	Associated with high BMD of spine and radius in Thailander males. No association in Chinese of both genders.
	C/T	rs2234693	Greendale et al., 2006. Bustamante et al., 2007b	Low BMD in spine in Afro-American and Japanese women. Low BMD in femoral neck in Spanish women.
	C/G C/T	rs1884052 rs3778099	Kiel et al., 2007.	Associated with hip/spine osteoporosis, with bone mass and geometry in US families of European origin (Framingham study).
	C/T C/T	rs3020314 rs1884051	Wang et al., 2008.	Associated with hip fracture for Chinese population.
	T/C A/G	3' UTR rs728524	Greendale et al., 2006.	Low BMD in hip and/or spine in Japanese and Afro-American women, respectively.
	C/A C/G	rs726282 rs1801132	Limer et al., 2009.	Low BMD in European males.
ER β	G/C	Intron 3	Wang et al., 2008.	Associated with hip fracture in Chinese population.
	G/A	Intron 8	Massart et al., 2009.	AA and AC genotypes associated with hip fracture in Italian
	C/T C/A	Intron 2 Intron 8	Greendale et al., 2006.	Associated with low spine BMD in Caucasian and high hip BMD in Chinese women.
	T/C	Intron 3	Rivadeneira et al., 2006.	Vertebral fracture risk in carriers of haplotype 1 (CC) in Dutch population.
	C/T	Intron 8	Shearman et al., 2004.	Low hip BMD in US population (Framingham study)
	C/T T/C A/G	Intron 7 Promoter Promoter	Ichikawa et al., 2005.	Associated with spine BMD normal variations in US Caucasian men and women.
IL-6	G/C (G572C)	Promoter	Chung et al., 2003. Ota et al., 2001. Ferrari et al., 2003 Magaña et al., 2008.	C allele and increased BMD in premenopausal Korean women G allele associated with low BMD in Japanese postmenopausal women G allele as protective factor from bone resorption in healthy Caucasian US women older than 65 years.

GEN	POLYMORPHISM	LOCATION	REFERENCES	OUTCOME
IL-6	G/C (G174C)	Promoter	Chung et al., 2003.	No association with BMD of Korean premenopausal women, due to its low frequency among Korean population.
			Ferrari et al., 2003.	The C allele as a protective factor from bone resorption in healthy Caucasian US women older than 65 years.
			Magaña et al., 2008.	The C allele is associated as a protective factor in Mexican women.
	G/A	Promoter	Chung et al., 2003.	Korean premenopausal women. Not associated with BMD due to its low frequency among Korean population.
IL6R	C/T G/A A/C	Promoter Promoter Exon 9	Bustamante et al., 2007a.	C/T and G/A polymorphisms associated with femoral BMD and body mass ratio; A/C associated with lumbar spine BMD. Spanish postmenopausal women.
VDR	C/T	3' UTR	Kiel et al., 2007.	Associated with low BMD of femoral neck and spine in US population (Framingham).
			Bustamante et al., 2007b.	Associated with low BMD in Spanish postmenopausal women.
	A/C	Intron 10	Kiel et al., 2007.	Associated with low BMD femoral neck and spine in US population (Framingham).
			Morrison, 2004.	Associated with low BMD. World population.
	A/C	Intron 10	Bustamante et al., 2007b. Uitterlinden et al., 2001.	Associated with low BMD in Spanish postmenopausal women. Not associated with BMD or fracture. Meta-analysis with world population.
	A/G	Intron 10	Kiel et al., 2007.	Associated with osteoporosis and BMD of femoral neck and spine in US population (Framingham).
			Bustamante et al., 2007b. Morrison, 2004. Pérez et al., 2008.	Associated with low BMD in Spanish postmenopausal women. Associated with osteoporosis. World population. Low BMD in spine and/or femoral neck in postmenopausal-menopausal Argentinean women.
	C/T	Exon 2	Bustamante et al., 2007b. Pérez et al., 2008.	Associated with BMD; not clearly to osteoporosis in Spanish women. Low BMD in spine and/or femoral neck in postmenopausal-menopausal Argentinean women.
	A/C/G/T	Exon 2	Kiel et al., 2007.	Associated with osteoporosis and BMD of femoral neck and spine in US population (Framingham).
			Morrison, 2004. Moffett et al., 2007.	Associated with osteoporosis. World population. C/C genotype Associated with low BMD in wrist and fracture risk in Caucasian postmenopausal US women.

GEN	POLYMORPHISM	LOCATION	REFERENCES	OUTCOME
VDR	C/T	Exon 2	Uitterlinden et al., 2001.	Associated with a larger number of fractures; it does not show significant differences as risk factor for osteoporosis in Dutch women.
	A/G	Promoter	Kiel et al., 2007.	Associated with osteoporosis and BMD of femoral neck and spine in US population (Framingham).
			Morrison, 2004.	Associated with osteoporosis. World population.
			Mencej et al., 2009.	Associated with osteoporosis in Slovenia women.
	A/G	Promoter region rs2189480	Uitterlinden et al., 2001.	Associated with fractures but not with osteoporosis in Dutch women.
	A/C		Kiel et al., 2007.	Associated with low BMD of femoral neck and spine in US population (Framingham).
			Bustamante et al., 2007b.	Associated with low BMD of femoral neck and spine in postmenopausal Spanish women.
CYP19	ins/del TTC	Intron 4	Limer et al., 2009.	Low heel BMD with 1 or 2 copies of TTC in males of European countries.
	T/C	Exon 3	Riancho et al., 2005.	Low hip and spine BMD with TTC in Spanish women.
			Mendoza et al., 2006.	Low hip and spine BMD with TTC/G (rs10046) in Spanish women.
			Riancho et al., 2007.	Associated with higher vertebral fracture risk in Spanish women.
			Riancho et al., 2009.	Associated with low hip and spine BMD with TT genotype in Spanish women.
	C/T	3' UTR	Limer et al., 2009.	Low heel BMD in males of many European countries.
			Mendoza et al., 2006.	Low hip and spine BMD in Spanish women.
	C/G	5' UTR	Riancho et al., 2007.	Associated with vertebral fractures risk in Spanish women.
			Riancho et al., 2009.	Higher hip BMD with GG genotype in Spanish women.
	C/T	Exon I.6	Riancho et al., 2009.	Associated with high hip BMD with TT genotype in Spanish women.
	A/G	Between exons I.2 y I.6	Riancho et al., 2007.	Associated with vertebral fracture risk in Spanish women.
	C/G G/A	3' UTR Intron 2	Kiel et al., 2007.	Associated with osteoporosis and femoral neck BMD in US families of European origin (Framingham).
	C/T	3' UTR	Xiong et al., 2006.	Associated with hip/spine osteoporosis in US families.
	T/C C/T	Intron 8 Intron 2	Xiong et al., 2006.	Associated with hip/spine osteoporosis. US/European origin families.

GEN	POLYMORPHISM	LOCATION	REFERENCES	OUTCOME
CYP19	T/C G/A C/T	Intron 3 Intron 4 Intron 5	Hong et al., 2007.	Associated with low (T/C) and high (G/A and C/T) BMD in Chinese men.
PTHR1	A/T C/T A/G T/C	Intron 1 Intron 2 Intron 8 Intron 10	Vilariño-Güell et al., 2007.	As haplotype, they are associated with total BMD, bone mass peak, and/or loss of BMD in spine and/or hip in European families (FAMOS), in Caucasian and British women (ALSPAC).
OPG	G/A	3' UTR	Richards et al., 2008.	Associated with low BMD in spine in European population (Rotterdam study).
			Paternoster et al., 2010.	Associated with low BMD cortical. Analyzed in women of the United Kingdom (ALSPAC) and Swedish men (GOOD).
	G/C	Exon 1	García-Unzueta et al., 2008.	High BMD with CC genotype in Spanish women.
			Kim et al., 2008.	High BMD with CC genotype; dose effect of C allele in Korean women.
			Lee et al., 2010.	Low spine BMD in European and Asiatic population.
	A/G	5' proximal region	Geng et al., 2007.	BMD high con AA genotype in Chinese women.
ITGA1	C/T T/G A/C	Exon 3 Intron 5 Intron 28	Lee et al., 2007.	Associated as alleles and also as haplotypes with hip osteoporosis in Korean women.
COLIA1	G/T	Intron 1	Stewart et al., 2006.	Low BMD with haplotype -1997G/-1663 of IT/+1245T in hip and spine in British women.
			Jin et al., 2009.	Low BMD and increment of fracture risk in hip, in British men and women.
			Falcón-Ramírez et al., 2011.	Associated with spine osteoporosis in Mexican women.
	G/T	Promoter	Stewart et al., 2006.	Low BMD in hip and spine of British women. BMD increment as haplotype with other SNPs of the gene, only in spine.
	Ins/del T	Promoter	Stewart et al., 2006.	Low BMD in hip and spine in British women.
			Jin et al., 2009.	Low BMD and increment of hip fracture risk, in British men and women.
	C/A	Intron 11	Kiel et al., 2007.	Associated with the width of the femoral neck in US women.

GEN	POLYMORPHISM	LOCATION	REFERENCES	OUTCOME
RUNX2	A/T	Intron 3	Ermakov et al., 2006.	Associated with anthropometric femoral length in a study conducted in Israel.
	A/T	Intron 4		
	T/C	Intron 4		
	C/T	Promoter 2	Lee et al., 2009.	CC genotype shows a low BMD in postmenopausal Korean women in spine and hip.
	A/G	Exon 2	Vaughan et al., 2002.	The A allele was associated with an increment of BMD in Australian women.
Unknown gene	G/T	rs6696981	Styrkarsdottir et al., 2008.	Associated with hip and spine fractures in Australian, Icelandic and Danish women.
	A/G	rs7524102		
RANK		rs3018362	Paternoster et al., 2010.	Associated with low cortical BMD. Analyzed in women of the United Kingdom (ALSPAC) and Swedish men (GOOD).
			Styrkarsdottir et al., 2009.	Associated with low BMD in hip of Icelandic and European subjects.
	A/G	Intron 1	Xiong et al., 2006.	Analyzed as haplotypes, these 17 polymorphisms showed association with osteoporosis and decrease of BMD in hip and spine in European families.
	A/G	Intron 1		
	A/C	Intron 1		
	C/G	Intron 1		
	A/G	Intron 1		
	A/G	Intron 2		
	A/T	Intron 3		
	G/T	Intron 3		
	A/T	Intron 4		
	C/T	Intron 7		
	A/G	Intron 7		
	G/T	Intron 9		
	G/T	Intron 9		
	C/T	Intron 9		
	C/G	Intron 9		
	G/T	3' region		
	C/T	3' region		
	A/G	Intron 6	Koh et al., 2007.	Polymorphism associated with low BMD in ward's triangle, trocanter and femur, in Korean population.

GEN	POLYMORPHISM	LOCATION	REFERENCES	OUTCOME
RANKL	C/T	Intron 1	Xiong et al., 2006.	Associated with hip BMD decrease in European origin families.
			Mencej et al., 2006.	CC genotype Associated with a low BMD in postmenopausal Slovenia women.
			Mencej et al., 2008.	Associated with low spine BMD in osteoporotic Slovenia women.
			Mencej et al., 2009	Associated with spine BMD decrease in postmenopausal Slovenia women.
	C/T	Intron 2	Xiong et al., 2006.	Associated with hip BMD decrease in European origin families.
	C/T	Intron 1	Mencej et al., 2006.	CC genotype associated with low hip and spine BMD of postmenopausal Slovenia women.
			Mencej et al., 2008.	Association to low spine BMD of postmenopausal Slovenia women.
	C/G	Intron 1	Mencej et al., 2008.	Associated with a BMD decrease in spine in postmenopausal Slovenia women.
	C/T C/T	rs9594738 rs9594759	Styrkarsdottir et al., 2008.	Associated with low spine BMD and moderately associated with fractures, in Australian, Danish and Icelandic subjects.
HDC	C/T A/C A/C C/T	3' region 3' region 5' region 5' region	Xiong et al., 2006.	Polymorphisms associated with hip osteoporosis in European origin families.
ADCY10	G/A	Exon 7	Ichikawa et al., 2009.	Positive association to spine BMD; modest effect on the BMD peak in spine of US population (sisters study).
	C/T	Intron 14	Ichikawa et al., 2009.	US men presented association to hip BMD and trend to association to spine BMD.
TWIST1	A/G	3' region	Hwang et al., 2010.	Associated with osteoporosis in postmenopausal Korean women.

Table 2. Gene polymorphisms associated with osteoporosis and bone mineral density.

Other variations of a single nucleotide in intron 1 of the RANK-L gene have repeatedly been associated with low BMD of hip and spine in European, Asiatic and European populations (Xiong et al., 2006; Mencej et al., 2006; Mencej et al., 2008; Styrkarsdottir et al., 2008). The presence of these polymorphisms on human genome, are relatively easy to identify since birth or even in prenatal stage. These polymorphisms show a well defined inheritance pattern and their distribution may show differences not only among family groups but among populations and ethnic groups. However, in this kind of studies, we must be extremely careful and constantly consider the potentially confusing effect of some variables, such as: heterogeneity of populations, caused by genetic admixture, specially product of population's migration, the number of individuals included in studies is very important as well as the proper selection of cases and controls, and finally, the method to analyze data (Spencer et al., 2009; Duncan et al., 2002; Macarty et al., 2008). Not considering these elements in association studies would easily led us to establish spurious associations (Koller et al., 2004). Defining the genetic basis of primary osteoporosis in any population is not a simple task, we face a multi-factorial and polygenic entity present in populations that may have a great genetic heterogeneity; however the exploration of bone structure and metabolism genetic control, would allow to know the molecular basis of diseases such as osteoporosis, which represents a new window to explore therapeutic opportunities that would facilitate management of bone disorders.

5. Epigenetics and osteoporosis

During the last years attempts have been made to analyze the relation between environmental and genetic factors in the so called "complex diseases" using epigenetic studies. Epigenetics studies causal interactions among "genes" and their "products" which give place to the "phenotype", which represents the body manifestation of a specific genetic profile. Epigenetics analyzes hereditary changes in the gene expression without changes in the DNA sequence, thus representing an important nexus between genotype, environment and the presence of a disease (Dupont et al., 2009). In osteoporosis, as a polygenic entity in which environmental component plays a determinant role, several risk conditions of maternal origin as bad nutrition of the mother, particularly the lack of vitamin D, habits as smoking and exposition to chemical agents (possibly including some drugs that impact bone quality), have the capacity to induce hereditary changes on future generations, which may occur in very early stages of the embrionary development, even during the neonatal period and they can generate an "imprinting" in the pattern of gene expression; this pattern is hereditary and "semi-permanent" because epigenetic modifications are reversible (Jiang et al., 2004; Dupont et al., 2009). On the other hand, apparently there is a relationship between low weight and size at time of birth and a higher risk of osteoporotic fractures during adult stage. Then we should understand that besides genetic and environmental factors, "epigenetic" can influence genome expression, so the prevention of some maternal conditions represents a valuable opportunity to develop preventative strategies aimed to improve bone quality in future generations.

6. Conclusion

Increment in life expectancy in some populations, ageing, changes in life style, especially the ones related to nutrition quality and physical activity, plus the vertiginous technological development are characteristics of modern civilizations. This fact generates without a doubt a glaring increment in the incidence of several chronic degenerative diseases which may become crippling as occurs with osteoporosis, where the complications directly or indirectly cause great social and economic costs; thereby, they represent a social and health services challenge. Considering environment effects on the bone phenotype and the modifications in life style of populations in present time, osteoporosis could be in the future a disorder that occurs in younger population, rather than preferentially in elder people. This situation could overpass the medical services answer capacity and the governmental budget assigned to the medical care and rehabilitation of these patients; so it is important to intensify the investigations leading to elucidate the physiopathology of this disorder and the most relevant processes in bone metabolism.

Genetic association studies enable identification of new genes related to bone metabolism. Knowledge of the function of its products will allow us attaining a better understanding of some aspects of bone metabolism not entirely explored yet and will open new opportunities for therapeutic development in osteoporosis. On the other hand, clinical research from which results association studies, makes possible to identify and associate genotypic profiles (haplotypes) of risk in families and populations and even in ethnic groups. There is no doubt that progress in this scientific knowledge field, technological progress and especially the various preventative strategies at different stages of life, including prenatal stage through the integral care of maternal health, will surely contribute to achieve a better understanding of the disease, a better care and especially a better prevention.

7. References

Andrew T, Antioniades L, Scurrah KJ, Macgregor AJ & Spector TD. (2005). Risk of wrist fracture in women is heritable and is influenced by genes that are largely independent of those influencing BMD. *J Bone Miner Res*, Vol. 20, No. 1, (January 2005), pp. (67–74).

Arden NK, Baker J, Hogg C, Baan K & Spector TD. (1996). The heritability of bone mineral density, ultrasound of the calcaneus and hip axis length: a study of postmenopausal twins. *J Bone Miner Res*, Vol. 11, No. 4, (April 1996), pp. (530-534).

Asociación Mexicana de Metabolismo Óseo y Mineral. (2001). Consenso Mexicano de Osteoporosis. *Rev Invest Clin*, Vol. 5, No. 53, (September-October 2001), pp. (469-495).

Barros ER, Dias da Silva MR, Kunii IS, Hauache OM & Lazaretti-Castro M. (2007). A novel mutation in the LRP5 gene, is associated with osteoporosis-pseudoglioma syndrome. *Osteoporos Int*, Vol. 18, No. 7, (July 2007), pp. (1017-1018).

Burckardt P. (1989). The peak bone mass concept. *Clin Rehumatol*, Vol. 8, No. S2, (June 1989), pp. (16-21).

Bustamante M, Nogués X, Enjuanes A, Elosua R, García-Giralt N, Pérez-Edo L, Cáceres E, Carreras R, Mellibovsky L, Balcells S, Díez-Pérez A & Grinberg D. (2007). COL1A1, ESR1, VDR and TGFB1 polymorphisms and haplotypes in relation to BMD in Spanish postmenopausal women. *Osteoporos Int*, Vol.18, No.2, (February 2007), pp. (235-243).

Bustamante M, Nogués X, Mellibovsky L, Agueda L, Jurado S, Cáceres E, Blanch J, Carreras R, Díez-Pérez A, Grinberg D & Balcells S. (2007). Polymorphisms in the interleukin-6 receptor gene are associated with bone mineral density and body mass index in

Spanish postmenopausal women. *Eur J Endocrinol*, Vol. 157, No. 5, (November 2007), pp. (677-684).

Cappellen D, Luong-Nguyen NH, Bongiovanni S, Grenet O, Wanke C & Susa M. (2002). Transcriptional program of mouse osteoclast differentiation governed by the macrophage colony-stimulating factor and the ligand for the receptor activation of NFkappa B. *J Biol Chem*, Vol. 277, No. 24, (June 2002), pp. (21971-21982).

Chung HW, Seo JS, Hur SE, Kim HL, Kim JY, Jung JH, Kim LH, Park BL & Shin HD. (2003). Association of interleukin-6 promoter variant with bone mineral density in premenopausal women. *J Hum Genet*, Vol. 48, No. 5, (April 2003), pp.(243-248).

Clark P, Cons-Molina F, Delezé M, Ragi S, Haddock L, Zanchetta JR, Jaller JJ, Palermo L, Talavera JO, Messina DO, Morales-Torres J, Salmerón J, Navarrete A, Suárez E, Pérez CM & Cummings SR. (2009). The Prevalence of radiographic vertebral fractures in Latin American countries. The Latin American Vertebral Osteoporosis. Study (LAVOS). *Osteoporos Int*, Vol. 9, No. 20, (November 2009), pp. (275-282).

Cole ZA, Dennison EM & Cooper C. (2008). Osteoporosis epidemiology update. *Curr Rheumatol Rep*, Vol. 10, No. 2, (April 2008), pp. (92-96).

Collin-Osdoby P. (2004). Regulation of vascular calcification by osteoclast regulatory factors RANKL and osteoprotegerin. *Cir Res*, Vol. 95, No. 11, (November 2004), pp. (1046-1057).

Cummings SR, Browner WS, Bauer D, Stone K, Ensrud K, Jamal S and Ettinger B. (1998). Endogenous hormones and the risk of hip and vertebral fractures among older women. Study of Osteoporotic Fractures Research Group. *N Engl J Med*, Vol. 339, No. 11, (September 1998), pp. (733- 738).

Deng FY, Lei SF, Chen XD, Tan LJ, Zhu XZ & Deng HW. (2011). An integrative study ascertained SOD2 as a susceptibility gene for osteoporosis in Chinese. *J Bone Miner Res*, (July 2011), doi: 10.1002/jbmr.471. Epub ahead of print.

Deng HW, Chen WM, Recker S, Stegman MR, Li JL, Davies KM, ZhouY, Deng H, Heaney R & Recker RR. (2000). Genetic determination of Colles' fracture and differential bone mass in women with and without Colles' fracture. *J Bone Miner Res*, Vol. 15, No. 7, (July 2000), pp. (1243–1252).

Deng HW, Mahaney MC,Williams JT, Li J, Conway T, DaviesKM, Li JL, Deng H & Recker RR. (2002). Relevance of the genes for bone mass variation to susceptibility to osteoporotic fractures and its implications to gene search for complex human diseases. *Genet Epidemiol*, Vol. 22, No. 1, (January 2002), pp. (12–25).

Devoto M, Shimoya K, Caminis J, Ott J, Tenenhouse A, Whyte MP, Sereda L, Hall S, Considine E, Williams CJ, Tromp G, Kuivaniemi H, Ala-Kokko L, Prockop DJ & Spotila LD. (1998). First-stage autosomal genome screen in extended pedigrees suggests genes predisposing to low bone mineral density on chromosomes 1p, 2p and 4q. *Eur J Hum Genet*, Vol. 6, No. 2, (March-April 1998), pp. (151–157).

Devoto M, Specchia C, Li HH, Caminis J, Tenenhouse A, Rodriguez H & Spotila LD. (2001). Variance component linkage analysis indicates a QTL for femoral neck bone mineral density on chromosome 1p36. *Hum Mol Genet*, Vol. 10, No. 21, (October 2001), pp. (2447-52).

Duncan EL & Brown MA. (2010). Clinical review 2: Genetic determinants of bone density and fracture risk-state of the art and future directions. *J Clin Endocrinol Metab*, Vol. 95, No. 6, (June 2010), pp. (2576-2587).

Duncan EL & Brown MA. (2008). Genetic studies in osteoporosis- the end of the beginning. *Arthritis Res Ther*, Vol. 10, No. 5, (September 2008), pp. (214-225).

Duncan EL & Brown MA. (2010). Mapping genes for osteoporosis-Old dogs and new tricks. *Bone*, Vol. 46, No. 5, (May 2005), pp. (1219-1225).

Dupont C, Armant DR & Brenner CA. (2009). Epigenetics: Definition, Mechanisms and Clinical Perspective. *Semin Reprod Med*, Vol. 27, No. 5, (September 2009), pp. (351-357).

Elliot-Gibson V, Bogoch ER, Jamal SA & Beaton DE. (2004). Practice patterns in the diagnosis and treatment of osteoporosis after a fragility fracture: a systematic review. *Osteoporos Int*, Vol. 15, No. 10, (July 2004), pp. (767-778).

Ermakov S, Malkin I, Kobyliansky E & Livshits G. (2006). Variation in femoral length is associated with polymorphisms in RUNX2 gene. *Bone*, Vol.38, No. 2, (February 2006), pp. (199-205).

Falcón-Ramírez E, Casas-Avila L, Miranda A, Diez P, Castro C, Rubio J, Gómez R & Valdés-Flores M. (2011). Sp1 polymorphism in collagen I alpha1 gene is associated with osteoporosis in lumbar spine of Mexican women. *Mol Biol Rep*, Vol. 38, No. 5, (June 2011), pp. (2987-2992).

Ferrari SL, Ahn-Luong L, Garnero P, Humphries SE & Greenspan SL. (2003). Two promoter polymorphisms regulating interleukin-6 gene expression are associated with circulating levels of C-reactive protein and markers of bone resorption in postmenopausal women. *J Clin Endocrinol Metab*, Vol. 88, No. 1, (January 2003), pp. (255-259).

Fox KM, Cummings SR, Powell-Threets K & Stone K. (1998). Family history and risk of osteoporotic fracture. Study of Osteoporotic Fractures Research Group. *Osteoporos Int*, Vol. 8, No. 6, (November 1998), pp. (557-562).

Frenkel B, Hong A, Baniwal SK, Coetzee GA, Ohisson C, Khalid O & Gabet Y. (2010). Regulation of adult bone turnover by sex steroids. *J Cell Physiol*, Vol. 224, No. 2, (August 2010), pp. (305-310).

García-Unzueta MT, Riancho JA, Zarrabeitia MT, Sañudo C, Berja A, Valero C, Pesquera C, Paule B, González-Macías J & Amado JA. (2008). Association of the 163A/G and 1181G/C osteoprotegerin polymorphism with bone mineral density. *Horm Metab Res*, Vol. 40, No. 3, (March 2008), pp. (219-224).

Geng L, Yao ZW, Luo JY, Han LL & Lu Q. (2007). Association between Val80 polymorphism of the CYP19 gene, A163G polymorphism of the OPG gene and bone mineral density in post-menopausal Chinese women. *Yi Chuan*, Vol. 29, No. 11, (November 2007), pp. (1345-1350).

Gómez R, Magaña JJ, Cisneros B, Pérez-Salazar E, Faugeron S, Véliz D, Castro C, Rubio J, Casas L & Valdés-Flores M. (2007). Association of the estrogen receptor alpha gene polymorphisms with osteoporosis in the Mexican population. *Clin Genet*, Vol. 72, No. 6, (December 2007), pp. (574-581).

Gong Y, Slee RB, Fukai N, Rawadi G, Roman-Roman S, Reginato AM, Wang H, Cundy T, Glorieux FH, Lev D, Zacharin M, Oexle K, Marcelino J, Suwairi W, Heeger S, Sabatakos G, Apte S, Adkins WN, Allgrove J, Arslan-Kirchner M, Batch JA, Beighton P, Black GC, Boles RG, Boon LM, Borrone C, Brunner HG, Carle GF, Dallapiccola B, De Paepe A, Floege B, Halfhide ML, Hall B, Hennekam RC, Hirose T, Jans A, Jüppner H, Kim CA, Keppler-Noreuil K, Kohlschuetter A, LaCombe D,

Lambert M, Lemyre E, Letteboer T, Peltonen L, Ramesar RS, Romanengo M, Somer H, Steichen-Gersdorf E, Steinmann B, Sullivan B, Superti-Furga A, Swoboda W, van den Boogaard MJ, Van Hull W, Vikkula M, Votruba M, Zabel B, Garcia T, Baron R, Olsen BR & Warman ML. (2001). LDL receptor-related protein 5 (LRP5) affects bone accrual and eye development. *Cell*, Vol. 107, No. 4, (November 2001), pp. (513-523).

Greendale GA, Chu J, Ferrell R, Randolph JF Jr, Johnston JM & Sowers MR. (2006). The association of bone mineral density with estrogen receptor gene polymorphisms. *Am J Med*, Vol. 119, Suppl 1, (September 2006), pp. (S79-S86).

Greespan SL, Maitland LA, Krasnow MB & Kido TH. (1994). Femoral bone loss progresses with age: a longitudinal study in women over age 65. *J Bone Miner Res*, Vol. 9, No. 12, (December 1994), pp. (1959-1965).

Gu JM, Xiao WJ, He JW, Zhang H, Hu WW, Hu YQ, Li M, Liu YJ, Fu WZ, Yu JB, Gao G, Yue H, Ke YH & Zhang ZL. (2009). Association between VDR and ESR1 gene polymorphisms with bone and obesity phenotypes in Chinese male nuclear families. *Acta Pharmacol Sin*, Vol. 30, No. 12, (Dicember 2009), pp. (1634-1642).

Guéguen R, Jouanny P, Guillemin F, Kuntz C, Pourel J & Siest G. (1995). Segregation analysis of bone mineral density in healty families. *J Bone Miner Res*, Vol. 10, No. 12, (December 1995), pp. (2017-2022).

Hong X, Hsu YH, Terwedow H, Arguelles LM, Tang G, Liu X, Zhang S, Xu X & Xu X. (2007). CYP19A1 polymorphisms are associated with bone mineral density in Chinese men. *Hum Genet*, Vol. 121, No. 3-4, (May 2007), pp. (491-500).

Hughes DE, Dai A, Tiffee JC, Li HH, Mundy GR & Boyce BF. (1996). Estrogen promotes apoptosis of murine osteoclasts mediated by TGF-beta. *Nat Med*, Vol. 2, No. 10, (October 1996), pp. (1132-1136).

Hwang JY, Kim SY, Lee SH, Kim GS, Go MJ, Kim SE, Kim HC, Shin HD, Park BL, Kim TH, Hong JM, Park EK, Kim HL, Lee JY & Koh JM. (2010). Association of TWIST1 gene polymorphisms with bone mineral density in postmenopausal women *Osteoporos Int*, Vol. 21, No. 5, (May 2010), pp. (757-764).

Ichikawa S, Koller DL, Peacock M, Johnson ML, Lai D, Hui SL, Johnston CC, Foroud TM & Econs MJ. (2005). Polymorphisms in the estrogen receptor beta (ESR2) gene are associated with bone mineral density in Caucasian men and women. *J Clin Endocrinol Metab*, Vol. 90, No. 11, (November 2005), pp. (5921-5927).

Ichikawa S, Koller DL, Curry LR, Lai D, Xuei X, Edenberg HJ, Hui SL, Peacock M, Foroud T & Econs MJ. (2009). Association of adenylate cyclase 10 (ADCY10) polymorphisms and bone mineral density in healthy adults. *Calcif Tissue Int*, Vol. 84, No. 2, February 2009), pp. (97-102).

Ismail AA, Cooper C, Felsenberg D, Varlow J, Kanis JA, Silman AJ & O'Neill TW. (1999). Number and type of vertebral deformities: epidemiological characteristics and relation to bake pain and height loss. European Vertebral Osteoporosis Study Group. *Osteoporos Int*, Vol. 9, No. 3, (March 1999), pp. (206-213).

Jiang YH, Bressler J & Beaudet AL. (2004). Epigenetics and human disease. *Annu Rev Genomics Hum Genet*, Vol. 5, (September 2004), pp. (479-510).

Jin H, Stewart TL, Hof RV, Reid DM, Aspden RM & Ralston S. (2009). A rare haplotype in the upstream regulatory region of COL1A1 is associated with reduced bone quality and hip fracture. *J Bone Miner Res*, Vol. 24, No. 3, (March 2009), pp. (448-454).

Kameda T, Mano H, Yuasa T, Mori Y, Miyasawa K, Shiokawa M, Yukiya Nakamaru, Emi Hirol, Kenji Hiura, Akira Kameda, Na N. Yang, Yoshiyuji Hakeds & Masayushi Kumegaea. (1997). Estrogen inhibits bone resorption by directly inducing apoptosis of the bone-resorbing osteoclasts. *J Exp Med*, Vol. 186, No. 4, (August 1997), pp. (489-95).

Kanis JA, Melton LJ 3rd, Christiansen C, Johnston CC & Khaltaev N. (1994). The diagnosis of osteoporosis. *J Bone Miner Res*, Vol. 9, No. 8, (August 1994), pp. (1137–1141).

Kannus P, Palvanen M, Kaprio J, Parkkari J & Koskenvuo M. (1999). Genetic factors and osteoporotic fractures in elderly people: prospective 25 year follow up of a nationwide cohort of elderly Finnish twins. *BMJ*, Vol. 319, No. 7221, (November 1999), pp. (1334–1337).

Karasik D, Dupuis J, Cho K, Cupples LA, Zhou Y, Kiel DP & Demissie S. (2010). Refined QTLs of osteoporosis-related traits by linkage analysis with genome-wide SNPs: Framingham SHARe. *Bone*, Vol. 46, No. 4, (April 2010), pp. (1114-1121).

Kaufman JM, Ostertag A, Saint-Pierre A, Cohen-Solal M, Boland A, Van Pottelbergh I, Toye K, de Vernejoul MC & Martinez M. (2008). Genome-wide linkage screen of bone mineral density (BMD) in European pedigrees ascertained through a male relative with low BMD values: evidence for quantitative trait loci on 17q21-23, 11q12-13, 13q12-14, and 22q11. *J Clin Endocrinol Metab*, Vol. 93, No. 10, (October 2008), pp. (3755-3762).

Kiel DP, Demissie S, Duppuis J, Lunetta KL, Murabito JM & D Karasik. (2007). Genome-wide association with bone mass and geometry in the Famingham Heart Study. *BMC Medical Genetics*, Vol. 8, Suppl 1, (September 2007), pp.(S14–S27).

Kim JG, Kim JH, Lee DO, Kim H, Kim JY, Suh CS, Kim SH & Choi YM. (2008). Changes in the serum levels of osteoprotegerin and soluble receptor activator for nuclear factor kappaB ligand after estrogen-progestogen therapy and their relationships with changes in bone mass in postmenopausal women. *Menopause*, Vol. 15, No. 2, (March-April 2008), pp. (357-362).

Koh JM, Park BL, Kim DJ, Kim GS, Cheong HS, Kim TH, Hong JM, Shin HI, Park EK, Kim SY & Shin HD.(2007). Identification of novel RANK polymorphisms and their putative association with low BMD among postmenopausal women. *Osteoporos Int*, Vol. 18, No. 3, (March 2007), pp. (323-331).

Koller DL, Econs MJ, Morin PA, Christian JC, Hui SL, Parry P, Curran ME, Rodriguez LA, Conneally PM, Joslyn G, Peacock M, Johnston CC & Foroud T. (2000). Genome screen for QTLs contributing to normal variation in bone mineral density and osteoporosis. *J Clin Endocrinol Metab*, Vol. 85, No. 9, (September 2000), pp. (3116-3120).

Koller DL, Ichikawa S, Lai D, Padgett LR, Doheny KF, Pugh E, Paschall J, Hui SL, Edenberg HJ, Xuei X, Peacock M, Econs MJ & Foroud T. (2010). Genome-wide association study of bone mineral density in premenopausal European-American women and replication in African-American women. *J Clin Endocrinol Metab*, Vol. 95, No. 4, (April 2010), pp. (1802-1809).

Koller DL, Liu G, Econs MJ, Hui SL, Morin PA, Joslyn G, Rodriguez LA, Conneally PM, Christian JC, Johnston CC Jr, Foroud T & Peacock M. (2001). Genome screen for quantitative trait loci underlying normal variation in femoral structure. *J Bone Miner Res*, Vol. 16, No. 6, (June 2001), pp. (985-991).

Koller DL, Peacock M, Lai D, Foroud T & Econs MJ. (2004). False Positive Rates in Association Studies as a Function of Degree of Stratification. *J Bone Miner Res*, Vol. 19, No. 8, (August 2004), pp. (1291-1295).

Koller DL, Rodriguez LA, Christian JC, Slemenda CW, Econs MJ, Hui SL, Morin P, Conneally PM, Joslyn G, Curran ME, Peacock M, Johnston CC & Foroud T. (1998). Linkage of a QTL contributing to normal variation in bone mineral density to chromosome 11q12-13. *J Bone Miner Res*, Vol. 13, No. 12, (December 1998), pp. (1903-1908).

Kou I, Takahashi A, Urano T, Fukui N, Ito H, Ozaki K, Tanaka T, Hosoi T, Shiraki M, Inoue S, Nakamura Y, Kamatani N, Kubo M, Mori S & Ikegawa S. (2011). Common variants in a novel gene, FONG on chromosome 2q33.1 confer risk of osteoporosis in Japanese. *PLoS One*, Vol. 6, No. 5, (May 2011), pp. (e19641).

Krall EA & Dawson-Hughes B. (1993). Heritable and life-style determinants of bone mineral density. *J Bone Miner Res*, Vol. 8, No. 1, (January 1993), pp. (1-9).

Lee HJ, Kim SY, Koh JM, Bok J, Kim KJ, Kim KS, Park MH, Shin HD, Park BL, Kim TH, Hong JM, Park EK, Kim DJ, Oh B, Kimm K, Kim GS & Lee JY. (2007). Polymorphisms and haplotypes of integrinalpha1 (ITGA1) are associated with bone mineral density and fracture risk in postmenopausal Koreans. *Bone*, Vol. 41, No. 6, (December 2007), pp. (979-986).

Lee HJ, Koh JM, Hwang JY, Choi KY, Lee SH, Park EK, Kim TH, Han BG, Kim GS, Kim SY & Lee JY. (2009). Association of a RUNX2 promoter polymorphism with bone mineral density in postmenopausal Korean women. *Calcif Tissue Int*, Vol. 84, No. 6, (June 2009), pp. (439-445).

Lee YH, Woo JH, Choi SJ, Ji JD & Song GG. (2010). Associations between osteoprotegerin polymorphisms and bone mineral density: a meta-analysis. *Mol Biol Rep*, Vol. 37, No. 1, (January 2010), pp. (227-234).

Li GH, Deng HW, Kung AW & Huang QY. (2011). Identification of genes for bone mineral density variation by computational disease gene identification strategy. *J Bone Miner Metab*, (June 2011), doi: 10.1007/s00774-011-0271-y. Epub ahead of print.

Limer KL, Pye SR, Thomson W, Boonen S, Borghs H, Vanderschueren D, Huhtaniemi IT, Adams JE, Ward KA, Platt H, Payne D, John SL, Bartfai G, Casanueva F, Finn JD, Forti G, Giwercman A, Han TS, Kula K, Lean ME, Pendleton N, Punab M, Silman AJ, Wu FC & O'Neill TW. (2009). EMAS Study Group. Genetic variation in sex hormone genes influences heel ultrasound parameters in middle-aged and elderly men: results from the European Male Aging Study (EMAS). *J Bone Miner Res*, Vol. 24, No. 2, (February 2009), pp. (314-323).

MacGregor A, Snieder H & Spector TD. (2000). Genetic factors and osteoporotic fractures in elderly people. Twin data support genetic contribution to risk of fracture. *BMJ*, Vol. 320, No. 7225, (June 2000), pp. (1669-1670).

Magaña JJ, Gómez R, Cisneros B, Casas L & Valdés-Flores M. (2008). Association of interleukin-6 gene polymorphisms with bone mineral density in Mexican women. *Arch Med Res*, Vol. 39, No. 6, (August 2008), pp. (618-624).

Marini F & Brandi ML. (2010). Genetic Determinants of osteoporosis: common bases to cardiovascular diseases?. *Int J of Hypertens*, (March 2010), doi: 10.4061/2010/394579. Epub ahead of print.

Massart F, Marini F, Bianchi G, Minisola S, Luisetto G, Pirazzoli A, Salvi S, Micheli D, Masi L & Brandi ML. (2009). Age-specific effects of estrogen receptors' polymorphisms on the bone traits in healthy fertile women: the BONTURNO study. *Reprod Biol Endocrinol*, Vol. 7, No. 1, (April 2009), pp. (32-40).

McCarthy MI & Hirschhorn JN. (2008). Genome-wide association studies; potential next steps on a genetic journey. *Hum Mol Genet*, Vol. 17, No. 2, (October 2008), pp. (R156-R165).

Mencej S, Albagha OM, Prezelj J, Kocjan T & Marc J. (2008). Tumour necrosis factor superfamily member 11 gene promoter polymorphisms modulate promoter activity and influence bone mineral density in postmenopausal women with osteoporosis. *J Mol Endocrinol*, Vol. 40, No. 6, (June 2008), pp. (273-279).

Mencej S, Prezelj J, Kocijancic A, Ostanek B & Marc J. (2006). Association of TNFSF11 gene promoter polymorphisms with bone mineral density in postmenopausal women. *Maturitas*, Vol. 55, No. 3, (October 2006), pp. (219-226).

Mencej S, Prezelj J, Kocjan T, Teskac K, Ostanek B, Smelcer M & Marc J. (2009). The combinations of polymorphisms in vitamin D receptor, osteoprotegerin and tumour necrosis factor superfamily member 11 genes are associated with bone mineral density. *J Mol Endocrinology*, Vol. 42, No. 3, (March 2009), pp. (239-247).

Mendoza N, Morón FJ, Vázquez F, Quereda F, Sáez ME, Martínez-Astorquiza T, González-Pérez A, Sánchez-Borrego R & Ruiz A. (2006). Weighting the effect of CYP19A gene in bone mineral density of postmenopausal women. *Bone*, Vol. 38, No. 6, (June 2006), pp. (951-953).

Michaelsson K, Melhus H, Ferm H, Ahlbom A & Pedersen NL. (2005). Genetic liability to fractures in the elderly. *Arch Intern Med*, Vol. 165, No. 16, (September 2005), pp. (1825–1830).

Moffett SP, Zmuda JM, Cauley JA, Ensrud KE, Hillier TA, Hochberg MC, Li J, Cayabyab S, Lee JM, Peltz G & Cummings SR. (2007). Association of the VDR translation star site polymorphism and fracture risk in older women. *J Bone Mineral Res*, Vol. 22, No. 5, (May 2007), pp. (730-736).

Morrison N. (2004). Commentary: vitamin D receptor polymorphism and bone mineral density: effect size in Caucasians means detection is uncertain in small studies. *Int J Epidemiol*, Vol. 33, No. 5, (October 2004), pp. (989-994).

NIH Consensus Development Panel On osteoporosis Prevention, Diagnosis and Therapy. (2001). *JAMA*, Vol. 285, No. 6, (February 2001), pp. (785-795).

Ongphiphadhanakul B, Chanprasertyothin S, Payattikul P, Saetung S, Piaseu N, Chailurkit L & Rajatanavin R. (2001). Association of a G2014A transition in exon 8 of the estrogen receptor-alpha gene with postmenopausal osteoporosis. *Osteoporos Int*, Vol. 12, No. 12, (December 2001), pp. (1015-1019).

Ongphiphadhanakul B, Rajatanavin R, Chanprasertyothin S, Piaseu N & Chailurkit L. (1998). Serum oestradiol and oestrogen-receptor gene polymorphism are associated with bone mineral density independently of serum testosterone in normal males. *Clin Endocrinol* (Oxf), Vol. 49, No. 6, (December 1998), pp. (803-809).

Ota N, Nakajima T, Nakazawa I, Suzuki T, Hosoi T, Orimo H, Inoue S, Shirai Y & Emi M. (2001). A nucleotide variant in the promoter region of the interleukin-6 gene associated with decreased bone mineral density. *J Hum Genet*, Vol. 46, No. 5, (February 2001), pp. (267-272).

Paternoster L, Ohlsson C, Sayers A, Vandenput L, Lorentzon M, Evans DM & Tobias JH. (2010). OPG and RANK polymorphisms are both associated with cortical bone mineral density: findings from a metaanalysis of the Avon longitudinal study of parents and children and gothenburg osteoporosis and obesity determinants cohorts. *J Clin Endocrinol Metab*, Vol. 95, No. 8, (August 2010), pp. (3940-3948).

Peacock M, Koller DL, Lai D, Hui S, Foroud T & Econs MJ. (2009). Bone mineral density variation in men is influenced by sex-specific and non sex-specific quantitative trait loci. *Bone*, Vol. 45, No. 3, (September 2009), pp. (443-448).

Pérez A, Ulla M, García B, Lavezzo M, Elías E, Binci M, Rivoira M, Centeno V, Alisio A & Tolosa de Talamoni N. (2008). Genotypes and clinical aspects associated with bone mineral density in Argentine postmenopausal women. *J Bone Miner Metab*, Vol. 26, No. 4, (July 2008), pp. (358-365).

Ralston SH. (2002). Genetic control of susceptibility to osteoporosis. *J Clin Endocrinol Metab*, Vol. 87, No. 6, (June 2002), pp. (2460–2466).

Ralston SH, Galwey N, MacKay I, Albagha OM, Cardon L, Compston JE, Cooper C, Duncan E, Keen R, Langdahl B, McLellan A, O'Riordan J, Pols HA, Reid DM, Uitterlinden AG, Wass J & Bennett ST. (2005). Loci for regulation of bone mineral density in men and women identified by genome wide linkage scan: the FAMOS study. *Hum Mol Genet*, Vol. 14, No. 7, (April 2005), pp. (943-951).

Ralston SH & de Crombrugghe B. (2006). Genetic regulation of bone mass and susceptibility to osteoporosis. *Genes Dev*, Vol. 20, No. 18, (September 2006), pp. (2492-2506).

Ralston SH & Uitterlinden AG. (2010). Genetics of osteoporosis. *Endocr Rev*, Vol. 31, No. 5, (October 2010), pp. (629-662).

Raspe A, Matthis C, Scheidt-Nave C & Raspe H. (1998). European study of vertebral osteoporosis (EVOS): design and implementation in 8 German study centers. *Med Klin (Munich)*, Vol. 93, No. 2, (March 1998), pp. (12-18).

Riancho JA, Sañudo C, Valero C, Pipaón C, Olmos JM, Mijares V, Fernández-Luna JL & Zarrabeitia MT. (2009) Association of the aromatase gene alleles with BMD: epidemiological and functional evidence. *J Bone Miner Res*, Vol. 24, No. 10, (October 2009), pp. (1709-1718).

Riancho JA, Valero C, Naranjo A, Morales DJ, Sañudo C & Zarrabeitia MT. (2007). Identification of an aromatase haplotype that is associated with gene expression and postmenopausal osteoporosis. *J Clin Endocrinol Metab*, Vol. 92, No. 2, (February 2007), pp. (660-665).

Riancho JA, Zarrabeitia MT, Valero C, Sañudo C, Hernández JL, Amado JA, Zarrabeitia A & González-Macías J. (2005). Aromatase gene and osteoporosis: relationship of ten polymorphic loci with bone mineral density. *Bone*, Vol. 36, No. 5, (May 2005), pp. (917-925).

Riancho JA, Zarrabeitia MT, Valero C, Sañudo C, Mijares V & González-Macías J. A. (2006). Gene-to-gene interaction between aromatase and estrogen receptors influences bone mineral density. *Eur J Endocrinol*, Vol. 155, No. 1, (July 2006), pp. (53-59).

Richards JB, Rivadeneira F, Inouye M, Pastinen TM, Soranzo N, Wilson SG, Andrew T, Falchi M, Gwilliam R, Ahmadi KR, Valdes AM, Arp P, Whittaker P, Verlaan DJ, Jhamai M, Kumanduri V, Moorhouse M, van Meurs JB, Hofman A, Pols HA, Hart D, Zhai G, Kato BS, Mullin BH, Zhang F, Deloukas P, Uitterlinden AG & Spector TD. (2008). Bone mineral density, osteoporosis, and osteoporotic fractures: a genome-wide association study. *Lancet*, Vol. 371, No. 9623, (May 2008), pp. (1505–1512).

Richards JB, Kavvoura FK, Rivadeneira F, Styrkársdóttir U, Estrada K, Halldórsson BV, Hsu YH, Zillikens MC, Wilson SG, Mullin BH, Amin N, Aulchenko YS, Cupples LA, Deloukas P, Demissie S, Hofman A, Kong A, Karasik D, van Meurs JB, Oostra BA, Pols HA, Sigurdsson G, Thorsteinsdottir U, Soranzo N, Williams FM, Zhou Y, Ralston SH, Thorleifsson G, van Duijn CM, Kiel DP, Stefansson K, Uitterlinden AG, Ioannidis JP & Spector TD. (2009). Genetic Factors for Osteoporosis Consortium. Collaborative meta-analysis: associations of 150 candidate genes with osteoporosis and osteoporotic fracture. *Ann Intern Med,* Vol. 151, No. 8, (October 2009), pp. (528-537).

Riggs BL & Melton LJ. (1986). Involutional osteoporosis. *N Engl J Med,* Vol. 314, No. 26, (June 1986), pp. (1676-1686).

Rivadeneira F, Styrkársdottir U, Estrada K, Halldórsson BV, Hsu YH, Richards JB, Zillikens MC, Kavvoura FK, Amin N, Aulchenko YS, Cupples LA, Deloukas P, Demissie S, Grundberg E, Hofman A, Kong A, Karasik D, van Meurs JB, Oostra B, Pastinen T, Pols HA, Sigurdsson G, Soranzo N, Thorleifsson G, Thorsteinsdottir U, Williams FM, Wilson SG, Zhou Y, Ralston SH, van Duijn CM, Spector T, Kiel DP, Stefansson K, Ioannidis JP & Uitterlinden AG. (2009). Genetic Factors for Osteoporosis (GEFOS) Consortium. Twenty bone-mineral-density loci identified by large-scale meta-analysis of genome-wide association studies. *Nat Genet,* Vol. 41, No. 11, (November 2009), pp. (1199-1206).

Rivadeneira F, van Meurs JB, Kant J, Zillikens MC, Stolk L, Beck TJ, Arp P, Schuit SC, Hofman A, Houwing-Duistermaat JJ, van Duijn CM, van Leeuwen JP, Pols HA & Uitterlinden AG. (2006). Estrogen receptor beta (ESR2) polymorphisms in interaction with estrogen receptor alpha (ESR1) and insulin-like growth factor I (IGF1) variants influence the risk of fracture in postmenopausal women. *J Bone Miner Res,* Vol. 21, No. 9, (September 2006), pp. (1443-1456).

Shaffer JR, Kammerer CM, Bruder JM, Cole SA, Dyer TD, Almasy L, Maccluer JW, Blangero J, Bauer RL & Mitchell BD. (2009). Quantitative trait locus on chromosome 1q influences bone loss in young Mexican American adults. *Calcif Tissue Int,* Vol. 84, No. 2, (February 2009), pp. (75-84).

Shearman AM, Karasik D, Gruenthal KM, Demissie S, Cupples LA, Housman DE, Kiel DP. (2004). Estrogen receptor beta polymorphisms are associated with bone mass in women and men: the Framingham Study. *J Bone Miner Res,* Vol. 19, No. 5, (2004 May), pp. (773-781).

Slemenda C, Longcope C, Peacock M, Hui S & Johnston CC. (1996). Sex steroids, bone mass and bone loss. *J Clin Invest,* Vol. 97, No. 1, (January 1996), pp. (14-21).

Slemenda CW, Turner CH, Peacock M, Christian JC, Sorbel J, Hui SL & Johnston CC. (1996). The genetics of proximal femur geometry, distribution of bone mass and bone mineral density. *Osteoporos Int,* Vol. 6, No. 2, (March 1996), pp. (178-182).

Spencer CC, Su Z, Donnelly P & Marchini J. (2009). Designing Genome-Wide Association Studies: Sample Size, Power, Imputation, and the Choice of Genotyping Chip. *PLoS Genetics,* Vol. 5, No. 5, (May 2009), doi: 10.1371/journal.pgen.1000477. Epub ahead of print.

Steppan CM, Crawford DT, Chidsey-Frink KL, Ke HZ & Swick AG. (2000). Leptin is a potent stimulator of growth in ob/ob mice. *Regul Pept,* Vol. 92, No. 1-3, (August 2000), pp. (73-78).

Stewart TL, Jin H, McGuigan FE, Albagha OM, Garcia-Giralt N, Bassiti A, Grinberg D, Balcells S, Reid DM & Ralston SH. (2006). Haplotypes defined by promoter and intron 1 polymorphisms of the COLIA1 gene regulate bone mineral density in women. *J Clin Endocrinol Metab*, Vol. 91, No. 9, (September 2006), pp. (3575-3583).

Styrkarsdottir U, Halldorsson BV, Gretarsdottir S, Gudbjartsson DF, Walters GB, Ingvarsson T, Jonsdottir T, Saemundsdottir J, Center JR, Nguyen TV, Bagger Y, Gulcher JR, Eisman JA, Christiansen C, Sigurdsson G, Kong A, Thorsteinsdottir U & Stefansson K. (2008). Multiple genetic loci for bone mineral density and fractures. *N Engl J Med*, Vol. 358, No. 22, (May 2008), pp. (2355-2365).

Styrkarsdottir U, Halldorsson BV, Gretarsdottir S, Gudbjartsson DF, Walters GB, Ingvarsson T, Jonsdottir T, Saemundsdottir J, Snorradottir S, Center JR, Nguyen TV, Alexandersen P, Gulcher JR, Eisman JA, Christiansen C, Sigurdsson G, Kong A, Thorsteinsdottir U & Stefansson K. (2009). New sequence variants associated with bone mineral density. *Nat Genet*, Vol. 41, No. 1, (January 2009), pp. (15-17).

Thomas DC & Witte JS. Point: Population Stratification: A Problem for Case-Control Studies of Candidate-Gene Associations?. (2002). *Cancer Epidemiol Biomarkers Prev*, Vol. 11, No. 6, (June 2002), pp. (505-512).

Uitterlinden AG, Weel AE, Burger H, Fang Y, van Duijn CM, Hofman A, van Leeuwen JP & Pols HA. (2001). Interaction between the vitamin D receptor gene and collagen type Ialpha1 gene in susceptibility for fracture. *J Bone Miner Res*, Vol. 16, No. 2, (February 2001), pp. (379-385).

Vaughan T, Pasco JA, Kotowicz MA, Nicholson GC & Morrison NA. (2002). Alleles of RUNX2/CBFA1 gene are associated with differences in bone mineral density and risk of fracture. *J Bone Miner Res*, Vol. 17, No. 8, (August 2002), pp. (1527-1534).

Vilariño-Güell C, Miles LJ, Duncan EL, Ralston SH, Compston JE, Cooper C, Langdahl BL, Maclelland A, Pols HA, Reid DM, Uitterlinden AG, Steer CD, Tobias JH, Wass JA & Brown MA. (2007). PTHR1 polymorphisms influence BMD variation through effects on the growing skeleton. *Calcif Tissue Int*, Vol. 81, No. 4, (October 2007), pp. (270-278).

Wang JT, Guo Y, Yang TL, Xu XH, Dong SS, Li M, Li TQ, Chen Y & Deng HW. (2008). Polymorphisms in the estrogen receptor genes are associated with hip fractures in Chinese. *Bone*, Vol. 43, No. 5,(November 2008), pp.(910-914).

Williams FM & Spector TD. (2006). Recent advances in the genetics of osteoporosis. *J Musculoskelet Neuronal Interact*, Vol. 6, No. 1, (January-March 2006), pp. (27-35).

World Health Organization. (1994). Assessment of fracture risk and its aplication to screening for postmenopausal osteoporosis. *Technical Report series*, 843 Genova: World Health Organization.

Xiong DH, Shen H, Zhao LJ, Xiao P, Yang TL, Guo Y, Wang W, Guo YF, Liu YJ, Recker RR & Deng HW. (2006). Robust and comprehensive analysis of 20 osteoporosis candidate genes by very high-density single-nucleotide polymorphism screen among 405 white nuclear families identified significant association and gene-gene interaction. *J Bone Miner Res*, Vol. 21, No. 11, (November 2006), pp. (1678-1695).

Zhang H, Sol-Church K, Rydbeck H, Stabley D, Spotila LD & Devoto M. (2009). High resolution linkage and linkage disequilibrium analyses of chromosome 1p36 SNPs identify new positional candidate genes for low bone mineral density. *Osteoporos Int*, Vol. 20, No. 2, (February 2009), pp. (341-346).

Biomechanics of Osteoporosis: The Importance of Bone Resorption and Remodeling Processes

Gholamreza Rouhi
[1]Faculty of Biomedical Engineering,
Amirkabir University of Technology, Tehran,
[2]Department of Mechanical Engineering & School of Human Kinetics,
University of Ottawa, Ontario,
[1]Iran
[2]Canada

1. Introduction

Bone is a vital, dynamic connective tissue that gives form to the body, supporting its weight, protecting vital organs, and facilitating locomotion by providing attachments for muscles to act as levers. It also acts as a reservoir for ions, especially for calcium and phosphate, the homeostasis of which is essential to life. These functions place serious requirements on the mechanical properties of bone, which should be stiff enough to support the body's weight and tough enough to prevent easy fracturing, as well as it should be able to be resorbed and/or formed depending on the mechanical and biological requirements of the body. Under normal physiological conditions, the structure/function relationships observed in bone, coupled with its role in maintaining mineral homeostasis, strongly suggest that it is an organ of optimum structural design. To fulfill these structure/function relationships adequately, bone is constantly being broken down and rebuilt in a process called remodeling. Bone has the potential to adapt its architecture, shape, and mechanical properties via a continuous process termed adaptation in response to altered loading conditions (Burr et al., 2002; Forwood & Turner, 1995; Hsieh & Turner, 2001). Under normal states of bone homeostasis, the remodeling activities in bone serve to remove bone mass where the mechanical demands of the skeleton are low, and form bone at those sites where mechanical loads are transmitted sufficiently and repeatedly. An early hypothesis about the dependence of the structure and form of bones, and the mechanical loads they carry, was proposed by Galileo in 1638 (Ascenzi, 1993), and was first described in a semiquantitative manner by Wolff (Wolff, 1892). The adaptive response of bone has been a subject of research for more than a century and many researchers have attempted to develop mathematical models for functional adaptation of bone.

In this chapter, a brief explanation about the bone structure and mechanics will be provided first. Then, the bone remodeling process and its relation with osteoporosis will be discussed. The important issue of bone quality makes another section of this chapter.

Two mixture models of bone resorption, a bi- and a tri-phasic model of bone resorption will be reviewed, followed by a 2D model investigating the effects of osteocytes number and mechanosensitivity on bone loss. Discussion and conclusions make the last section of this chapter.

2. Bone structure and mechanics

Bone is the main constituent of the skeletal system and differs from the connective tissues in rigidity and hardness. The rigidity and hardness of bone enable the skeleton to maintain the shape of the body; to protect the vital organs; to supply the framework for the bone marrow; and also to transmit the force of muscular contraction from one part to another during movement. It is made basically of the fibrous protein collagen, impregnated with a mineral closely resembling calcium phosphate (Currey, 2002). The mineral content of bone acts as a reservoir for ions, particularly calcium (almost 99% of the calcium of our body is stored in bone), and it also contributes to the regulation of extracellular fluid composition. It also contains water, which is very important mechanically, some not well understood proteins and polysaccharides, living cells and blood vessels. The organic matrix of bone consists of 90% collagen, the most abundant protein in the body, and about 10% of various noncollagenous proteins (Behari, 1991). The protein part, mainly collagen type I, forms a model for the subsequent deposition of hydroxyapatite, the mineral phase of bone which provides rigidity to the structure. From mechanical point of view, bone is a nonhomogeneous and anisotropic material. Spongy and cortical bones can be considered as orthotropic and transversely isotropic materials, respectively. In the physiological range of loading, bone can be assumed as a linear elastic material, with negligible viscoelastic effects (Rouhi, 2006a). Bone is stronger in compression than in tension, and much greater young's moduli of elasticity than shear modulus (Bartel et al., 2006).

Outstanding mechanical properties of bone can be achieved by a very complex hierarchical structure of bone tissue, which has been explained in a number of reviews (Weiner and Wagner, 1998; Fratzl et al., 2004; Fratzl and Weinkamer, 2007). The mechanical performance of bone tissue depends on all levels of hierarchy. The term composite is usually employed for those materials in which two or more distinct phases are separated on a scale larger than the atomic, and in which their material properties such as stiffness and strength are altered compared with those of a homogeneous material. On the basis of the definition of a composite and also by considering bone structure, it is clear that bone is a composite material. Bone, as a biocomposite, shows hierarchical structures at different scales (Lakes, 1993). For example, in cortical bone, on the microstructural level, there are osteons or Haversian systems, which are large hollow fibers (200 to 250 μm outer diameter) composed of concentric lamellae and of pores. The lamellae are made up of fibers, and the fibers contain fibrils.

At the molecular level, the sophisticated structural interaction between the organic and inorganic phases is one of the fundamental determinants of the astonishing mechanical properties of bone. The underlying assumption is that a strong bonding between mineral and collagen allows the former to stiffen the collagen matrix through shear stress transfer. There are some important questions related to the composite nature of bone, which need to be addressed in order to make one able to understand the mechanics of bone as a composite at different hierarchical levels, such as: What are the properties of organic and mineral phases of bone?; How do the organic and the inorganic phases of bone interact to offer the superior mechanical properties?; How do the cross-links within and between collagen fibrils contribute to the mechanical properties of the collagen?; and How is load and stress distributed between the collagen and mineral?. It is known that improperly mineralized tissues are often resulted when there is flaw in organic phase of bone for mineral deposition (Lucchinetti, 2001). At the nanoscale, bone is a composite of a collagen-rich organic matrix and mineral nanoparticles made from carbonated hydroxyapatite. The basic building block of the bone material is a mineralized collagen fibril of between 50 and 200 nm diameter. The collagen fibrils are filled and coated by mineral crystallites (Rubin et al., 2004); the latter are mainly flat plates that are mostly distributed parallel to each other in a fibril, and parallel to the long axis of the collagen fibrils (Landis, 1996). These well organized structural features have been associated with various unique structural properties of bone. For instance, the stiffness of bone is related to the composite structure of mineral micro-crystals and collagen fibers (Lakes & Saha, 1979); and the cement lines as weak interfaces convey a degree of toughness to bone (Piekarski, 1970).

Bone is a porous structure with different values of porosity depending on its macrostructure. At the macroscopic level, there are basically two types of bone structures: cortical (compact or Haversian) and cancellous (spongy, or trabecular) bone. Cortical bone is a dense, solid mass with only microscopic channels, and with a maximal density of about 1.8 gr/cm3. Approximately 80% of the skeletal mass in the adult human is cortical bone, which forms the outer wall of all bones and is largely responsible for the supportive and protective function of the skeleton. The main structural unit of the cortical bone is called osteon, or a Haversian system (Rouhi, 2006a). A typical osteon is a hollow cylinder with the outer and inner diameters of about 200 (or 250) and 50 μm, respectively. An osteon is made up of 20 to 30 concentric lamellae, and surrounding the outer border of each osteon there is a cement line, a 1-2 μm thick layer of mineralized matrix deficient in collagen fibers, which it is believed they act as crack stoppers when cracks are present. On the other hand, cancellous (spongy or trabecular) bone is a lattice of narrow rods and plates (70 to 200 μm in thickness) of calcified bone tissue called trabeculae, with an average thickness of 100-150 μm (Van der Meulen & Prendergast, 2000). The trabeculae are surrounded by bone marrow that is vascular and provides nutrients and waste disposal for the bone cells. The symmetry of structure in cancellous bone depends upon the direction of applied loads. If the stress pattern in spongy bone is complex, then the structure of the network of trabeculae is also complex and highly asymmetric. Comparison of micrograph structures with the density maps show that low density, open cell, rod like structure develops in regions of low stress while greater density, closed cell, plate like structures appear in regions of higher density in cancellous bone (Gibson, 1985). There are no blood vessels within the trabeculae, but there are vessels immediately adjacent to the tissue. Trabecualr bone is less mineralized than cortical bone, and experimental evidence and data suggest that spongy bone is much more active in remodeling than that of cortical bone (Guo & Goldstein, 1997). With ageing there are changes in the microarchitecture of bone. There is thinning of the cortex and of trabeculae, and a loss of connectivity, in particular of the horizontal trabeculae. The major cellular elements of bone include osteoclasts (bone resorbing cells), osteoblasts (bone making cells), osteocytes (bone sensor cells) and bone lining cells (inactive cells on the resting surfaces of bone) (Burger & Klein-Nulend, 1999). While osteoblasts and osteoclasts have opposite functions and have different developmental origins, they exhibit several parallel features, particularly with respect to their life cycles. Osteoblasts and osteoclasts are both temporary cells with relatively short life spans (Parfitt, 1995).

3. Bone remodeling process and osteoporosis

During growth, bone is formed in the necessary places and resorbed as needed to attain the final shape, in a process called modeling. Modeling involves resorption drifts and formation drifts that remove or add bone over wide regions of bone surfaces. Thus, in modeling, bone resorbing and making cells act independently and at different spots. Modeling controls the growth, shape, size, strength, and anatomy of bones and joints. Collectively, modeling leads to increasing the outside cortex and marrow cavity diameters, shaping the ends of long bones. Modeling allows not only the development of normal architecture during growth, but also the modulation of this architecture and mass when the mechanical condition changes. When bone strains exceed a modeling threshold window, the minimum effective strain, modeling in the formation mode is turned on to increase bone mass and strength, and lower its strains toward the bottom of the window. When strains remain below the modeling threshold, mechanically controlled formation drifts stay inactive. As the forces on bone increases 20 times in size between birth and maturity, modeling in the formation mode keeps making bones strong enough to keep their strains from exceeding the modeling threshold, and therefore from reaching the microdamage threshold (Jee, 2001). In the adult age, the localized and independent activities of cells in modeling, are replaced by a distributed and coordinated work of the cells, resulting in a dynamic state called remodeling process. The actual remodeling occurs in two steps: the osteoclasts attach to the bone surface, dissolve the mineral, and later the organic phase of the bone, opening a hole that is subsequently filled by a number of osteoblasts, which produce the collagen matrix and secrete a protein which stimulates the calcium phosphate deposition. In the bone remdoeling process, resorption of extra-cellular matrices by osteoclasts (Teitelbaum & Ross 2003) is followed by osteoblastic invasion of the cavity, and subsequent secretion of extra-cellular matrix that is then mineralized (Ducy et al. 2000). These two processes, which together are called bone remodeling, occur continuously from birth to death and are in balance in a healthy bone (Riggs et al. 2002). This state can be shifted in favour of bone formation or resorption by mechanical stimulation, hormonal effects, nutrition, or diseases among other factors (Rouhi, 2006). Optimal remodeling is responsible for bone health and strength throughout life. An imbalance in bone remodeling may cause diseases such as osteoporosis. Bone remodeling occurs throughout life in thousands of sites within the human skeleton. The cellular link between bone resorbing cells or osteoclasts, and bone forming cells or osteoblasts, is known as coupling. How bone resorption and bone formation are linked is not entirely understood, but the consequences of accentuating one or the other preferentially leads to disease.

It was postulated that bone remodeling occurs to repair microdamage in bone (Frost, 1985; Mori & Burr, 1993). It was suggested that disruption of the canlicular connections occur when microcracks cut across them and can provide the stimulus to launch remodeling. It is well accepted that an unharmed gap junction intercellular communication or osteocyte-canalicular system inhibits the activation of osteoclast resorption and that interruption of the connection, for instance osteocyte apoptosis or microdamage, prevent the inhibition signals to osteoclasts and so bone resorption starts (Martin, 2000). Gradual and diffusive osteocyte death has been reported with aging that can lead to enhanced bone remodeling and bone loss. Moreover, osteocyte death can make bones more brittle and vulnerable to fatigue damage, and bone remodeling bone loss (Jee, 2001). There are several reasons for the necessity of remodeling process, for examples: immature bone formed at the metaphyses is structurally inferior to mature bone; or the quality of adult bone deteriorates with time; or microcracks produced in bone by daily activity should be removed to attain a desired strength in bone; and/or ions concentration (e.g. calcium) should be adjusted to lie in an acceptable range; and, most likely, other factors that will be known in the future (Rouhi, 2006a). Assuming normal rates of adult bone remodeling, cortical bone has a mean age of 20 years and cancellous bone 1 to 4 years (Parfitt, 1983). Numerous theories related to the bone remodeling process have been proposed so far (see for instance, (Cowin & Hegedus, 1976; Hegedus & Cowin, 1976; Beaupre et al., 1990; Mullender et al., 1994; Jacobs et al., 1997; Rouhi et al., 2004 & 2006b))

Many diseases are related to global shift in the bone remodeling balance, for example: Osteoporosis, which is caused by increased osteoclast activity; Osteopetrosis, which is an abnormal increase in bone density by reduced osteoclast activity, Osteopenia, which is the bone loss by decreased osteoblast activity. The balance between bone resorption and bone formation is maintained through a complex regulatory system of systemic local factors acting on bone cells, such as calcium regulating factors, sex hormones, growth factors, and cytokine. The signal responsible for termination of bone resorption and initiation of bone formation are not well understood; however, evidence suggests that liberation of matrix embedded insulin- like growth factor system components may induce the shift. During bone turnover, surplus products synthesized by the osteoblasts during bone formation or fragments released during bone resorption are found in blood and urine. Too much bone resorption at the expense of formation results in osteoporosis, a loss of bone strength and integrity, resulting in fractures after minimal trauma. This leads to a disturbance in the bone's microarchitecture, which increases the probability of fractures. Osteoporosis is often called a "silent disease" because there are no symptoms until a bone breaks. Osteoporosis is a condition characterized by low bone mineral density and microstructural deterioration of bone tissue, leading to enhanced bone fragility and structural failure of the skeleton under low loads. Osteoporosis is a disease of enormous socioeconomic impact that is characterized by increase bone fragility (Seeman and Delmas, 2006). Such fragility is generally associated with an abnormal loss in bone volume, deterioration in the quality of the bone microarchitecture, an increased bone turnover rate, and also a shift of bone mineral density towards a lower mineralization density. Bone fragility can be defined from the pathophysiological point of view as "...the consequence of a stochastic process, that is, multiple genetic, physical, hormonal and nutritional factors acting alone or in concert to diminish skeletal integrity (Marcus, 1996)". The treatment of the bone diseases is based on drugs that intend to restore the remodeling equilibrium. Most of the work on osteoporosis, probably the most important of these diseases, seems to be currently in the osteoclast inhibition side (Rodan & Martin, 2000; Teitelbaum, 2000; Rouhi et al., 2007).

Peak bone mass (PBM) corresponds to the amount of bony tissue present at the end of skeletal maturation. It is a major determinant of the risk of fracture later in life, because there is an inverse relationship between fracture risk and areal bone mineral density, in women, as well as in men. Interaction between genetic and non-genetic factors on bone mineral mass and structure changes during puberty. Genetic factors are either acting directly on bone or indirectly by modulating the sensitivity to environmental factors. Similarly, environmental factors are acting either directly on bone or indirectly by modulating the genetic potential. Human bone mass increases during growth, levels off in young adult life, and after about 30 years it starts to decrease. The most common sites of bone fracture are spine, hip, and wrist. The main cause of osteoporosis is the continuous loss of bone during life, which is intensified in female after menopause and male with andropause. At age 70 years, 70% of the young adult mass can remain (Wanich, 1999). It is known that with ageing, bone is lost from all parts of the skeleton, but not in equal amounts. Another factor is a lesser bone production during maturation, which cause a reduction in peak bone mass. Both cortical and cancellous bones are primarily thinned by the removal of bone at the endosteal surfaces adjacent to bone marrow. Cortical bone loss occurs mostly at the cortical endosteal surface and to a small degree from the increase in the radius of the Haversian canals. A small net gain of bone partly offsets this lost at the periosteal surface (Martin and Burr, 1989; Frost, 1999a). Age-related cancellous bone loss is because of the imbalance in bone remodeling with excessive bone resorption relative to bone formation. The sequence of Activation-Resorption-Formation is often uncoupled because of reducing the available trabecular rods/plates surfaces for bone formation. In elderly people, the most common cause of increased bone resorption is calcium and vitamin D deficiency, which will result in secondary hyperparathyroidism. Muscle mass and strength increases during growth and plateaus in young adults and then declines. Interesting to know that muscles apply the largest loads on bone, and bones normally adapt their mass and strength to the largest load. Thus, age-related reduction in muscle mass and strength can be deemed as a major factor for the age-related reduction in bone apparent density and strength (Bucwalter, et al., 1993; Frost, 1999 a&b; Burr, 1997). Needless to emphasize that loss of muscle mass and strength will increase the tendency to fall, and thus will increase the fracture risk.

4. Factors determining bone quality

The quality of bone tissue relates to its composition and microstructure, whereas its quality as an organ depends also on its macrostructure. The strength of a bone and its ability to perform these physical functions depend on its structure and the intrinsic properties of the materials of which it is composed. The amount of bone, its spatial arrangement, its composition, and its turnover are all determinants of its ability to perform mechanical functions and to resist fracture. Bone quality is determined by at least four factors as follows: Properties of the organic and mineral phases of bone, also the collagen-HAp composite structure; Microdamage accumulation; Architecture and geometry of cancellous and cortical bone; and finally Rate of bone turnover and remodeling. Organic and mineral phases, i.e. collagen and hydroxyapatite, and architecture changes with age, bone diseases, such as osteoporosis, and therapeutic treatment. The risk of fracture in a 75-year-old woman can be 4-7 times that of a 45-yr-old woman with identical bone mass, demonstrating a bone quality component of fragility that is independent of bone mass.

The fracture resistance of bone results from the ability of its microstructure to dissipate deformation energy, without the propagation of large cracks leading to eventual material failure (Currey, 1999; Currey, 2003; Taylor et al., 2007). One striking feature of the fracture properties in compact bone is the anisotropy of the fracture toughness, which differs by almost two orders of magnitude between a crack that propagates parallel or perpendicular to the fibril direction. This dependence of fracture properties on collagen orientation underlines the general importance of the organic matrix and its organization for bone toughness (Seeman & Delmas, 2006). Mechanical properties of bone are determined by a number of structural features, including: the mineral concentration inside the organic matrix; the size and mechanical properties of mineral particles; the quality of the collagen, in term of its amino-acid sequence, crosslinks and hydration; the quality and composition of the extrafibrillar organic matrix between the collagen fibrils; and the orientation distribution of the mineralized collagen fibrils. The mineral concentration inside the organic bone matrix is a major determinant of bone stiffness and strength (Seeman & Delmas, 2006; Currey, 2001; Currey, 2002). However, the mineral content within both the trabecular and the cortical bone is far from homogeneous. At least two processes that occur in bones over the whole lifetime of an adult individual are responsible for this situation: bone remodeling and kinetics of matrix mineralization. The newly formed bone matrix is initially unmineralized (osteoid), but after an initial maturation time of about 2 weeks, the bone goes through a stage of rapid mineralization, where 70% of the full matrix mineral content is achieved in a few days (primary mineralization). Then, the mineral content increases very slowly to reach full mineralization within years (secondary mineralization) (Boivin & Meunier, 2003).

Fracture risk increases with age, partly as a function of changes in bone mineral density. Aging is associated with a reduction in collagen content. In osteoporosis, there is an increase in both synthesis and degradation of collagen, and an increase in the number of immature cross-links. Osteoporotic bone may be more fragile due to fewer collagen fibers and weaker cross-linking. Questions such as: How do therapeutic treatments for osteoporosis alter collagen quality (contents, cross linking, turnover rate)?; and How does increased bone turnover affect collagen quality?, are still open and need to be addressed in the future. Although changes in bone mineral content are widely recognized to occur in aging and osteoporosis, the physicochemical properties of the mineral crystal may also be changed. Mineral crystallinity increases with age, and this in itself may make the tissue more brittle. Anti-resorptive therapies increase tissue mineralization by increasing the mean tissue age. Whether this is beneficial or deleterious is not clear yet. However, the increase in mineralization never achieves the level of mineral in normal non-osteoporotic age-matched controls, so it is likely to be a positive change. However, anti-resorptive therapies also have a tendency to make the tissue mineralization more uniform, from a fracture mechanics point of view, and this would make it more likely for cracks that are introduced into the matrix to grow. There are still many questions in regard to the mineral phase of bone, such as: How is bone crystallinity affected by long-term antiresorptive therapies?; What role do osteocytes play in matrix mineralization?; What is the relationship between mineral crystallinity and brittleness?; What is the mechanical effect of reduced variability in bone mineral distribution (i.e. increasing homogeneity of tissue properties)?, which need to be addressed in the future. Structural changes, some of which are independent of bone mass, also occur in osteoporosis. In osteoporosis, there is a tendency to convert to a more rod-like and more anisotropic structure, whereas bisphosphonate treatments tend to make the bone more plate-like and more isotropic.

Complete trabecular perforations increase as the remodeling rate increase. These may weaken the structure more than expected based on the loss of bone mass alone. Regarding the effects of bone architecture on its quality and mechanical properties, there are some questions such as: Does maintenance of anisotropy reduce bone fracture risk?; To what extent do resorption bays in trabeculae waken bone?; and What is the relative role of trabecular and cortical bone in vertebral and hip fracture risk?, which need to be answered.

A reduction in fracture toughness of bone with age was reported in the literature, which was caused either because of an increase in mineralization (Currey et al., 1996; Zioupos et al., 1998) or alterations in the collagen matrix (Zioupos et al., 1999). In an animal model of disuse osteoporosis, a reduction in collagen cross-links can be seen (Yamauchi et al., 1988). Other experimental evidence supports the idea that the concentration of collagen cross-links is considerably lower in osteoporotic individuals compared to age-matched controls (Oxlund et al., 1996). It should be noted that the initial cross-links between collagen molecules are unstable, but as bone matures, the cross-links also mature into more stable nonreducible forms. So, there is an increase in collagen matrix's density, stiffness, and strength during maturation (Bailey & Paul, 1999). It should also be noted that the content of mature cross-links is lower in cancellous bone as compared to cortical bone, due to the greater rate of the cancellous bone remodeling (Eyre et al., 1988). The bone collagen cross-links are usually modified in the mineralization process.

5. A bi-phasic mixture model of bone resorption process

Osteoporosis, regardless of etiology, always represents enhanced bone resorption relative to formation. Thus, insights into the pathogenesis of this disease, and progress in its prevention and/or cure, depend on understanding the mechanisms by which bone is degraded. The osteoclast is the principal resorptive cell of bone, and the most successful treatments of osteoporosis, to date, target osteoclastic bone resorption. The osteoclast is a multinucleated cell whose capacity to degrade hard tissues, among other factors, depends on cell/matrix contact. All forms of adult osteoporosis reflect enhanced bone resorption relative to formation, and should be viewed in the context of the remodeling cycle. The reason for using this way of treatment is the lack of information about all various factors affecting osteoclasts' activity. Biological tissues, including bones, are all composed of multiphase constituents, and there are chemical reactions and/or diffusions between different components of them. Cells, as live organs in the biological tissues, can dictate rate of growth and adaptation, and their activities are affected by different, including mechanical, chemical, and biological factors.

Here a brief explanation about a recently proposed biphasic mixture model of bone resorption is presented (Rouhi et al., 2007). This model aims at shedding some light on the bone resorption process using a multi-constituents continuum mechanics model. In this model, bone is treated as a biphasic mixture of matrix and fluid, and bone resorption is considered as an exchange of mass between the solid and fluid phases. This exchange is caused by the secretion of H+ and Cl− from osteoclasts, which creates an acidic environment in a sealed microenvironment between the osteoclasts and the bone matrix (Blair 1998; Rousselle and Heymann 2002). The governing equations for bone resorption can be derived using the conservation laws, entropy inequality, and the appropriate constitutive equations.

In the conservation of mass equations, the rate of mass transferred to different constituents is assumed to be given by an empirical relation arising from the dissolution kinetics of the solid phase. In the constitutive equations, it is assumed that dependent variables, such as free energy, are a function of temperature, deformation gradient, rate of deformation gradient, and the extent of chemical reactions (Rouhi et al., 2007).

It should be noted that bone mineral (hydroxyapatite) and organic (collagen I) matrix are degraded independently. Thus, a bone resorption model needs two separate expressions, one because of the each phase. Because of the lack of information about the dissolution of the organic phase, we only considered the mineral phase dissolution and assumed that it is equivalent to the dissolution of the bone matrix. Microscopic observations suggest that degradation of collagen closely follows mineral degradation (Chambers et al. 1984), so our assumption may be justified. Dissolution of minerals occurs at the bone surface. A major source of uncertainty is the surface reactivity, which depends on chemical composition, atomic structure, and surface topography. The free energy of surface sites changes as a function of the aforementioned factors. Thus, no universal expression for the dissolution kinetics exists and experimental studies are needed to derive a dissolution kinetics relation for each case. The dissolution kinetics of hydroxyapatite has been the subject of numerous studies so far (Christoffersen et al. 1996; Dorozhkin 1997a; 1997b; 1997c; Thomann et al. 1989; 1990; 1991; Margolis and Moreno 1992; Hankermeyer et al. 2002; Fulmer et al. 2002; Chow et al. 2003). Because of the small dimensions of the resorption microenvironment between the osteoclasts and the bone matrix assuming that dissolution is governed by the reaction kinetics seems logical and acceptable.

In order to develop a general framework for the description of bio-chemo-mechanically driven bone resorption, some basic assumptions should be made as follows: Bone is a biphasic mixture of a solid phase and a fluid phase; The transfer of mass, energy and entropy between the solid and the fluid phases are a result of biochemical reactions that occur between the osteoclasts and the matrix; The characteristic time of chemical reactions is several orders of magnitude greater than the characteristic time associated with a complete perfusion of the blood plasma in bone, so the resorption process can be considered isothermal; The bone matrix is isotropic and linearly elastic; Mechanical, chemical, and biological factors affect the rate of bone resorption, thus they all appear in the bio-chemo-mechanical affinity as the driving forces of the chemical reactions; and finally Dissolution of the matrix is the same as resorption of the mineral phase. Furthermore, it is assumed that the degree of saturation is a function of the bio-chemo-mechanical affinity, but not just of the Gibbs free energy.

Bone resorption can be simplified to (see (Blair 1998; Dorozhkin 1997a; 1997b; 1997c)):

$$Ca_{10}(PO_4)_6(OH)_2 + 2H^+ \longrightarrow 10Ca^{2+} + 6PO_4^{-3} + 2H_2O \tag{1}$$

The chemical driving force for bone resorption, i.e., the chemical reaction shown in Equation (1), can be expressed by the Gibbs free energy variation per mole. In 1992, Margolis and Moreno (Margolis & Moreno, 1992) performed dissolution experiments with hydroxyapatite crystals, in which they measured pH, calcium and phosphate concentrations at a constant temperature. They proposed the following equation for the rate of dissolution of the mineral phase of the bone matrix:

$$J = k(1 - DS)^m [H^+]^n \tag{2}$$

where J is the mineral flux across the real surface of the mineral phase, DS is the degree of saturation, $[H^+]$ is the concentration of hydrogen ion, and k, m, and n are empirical constants. As stated earlier, it is assumed that the mineral flux, J, is almost the same as the dissolution rate of the solid phase, i.e. hydroxyapatite + collagen fibers.

The degree of saturation (DS) is expressed as:

$$DS = \{([Ca^{2+}]^5 [PO_4^{-3}]^3 [OH^-])/Kso\}^{1/9} \tag{3}$$

where $[X]$ is the concentration of ion X, and Kso is the solubility product of hydroxyapatite (Margolis and Moreno 1992).

Since biological, chemical, and mechanical factors have a definite effect on the rate of dissolution, it is hypothesized that a bio-chemo-mechanical driving force should be considered in the dissolution relation, instead of just a chemical driving force (i.e. just changes in the Gibbs free energy). Dissipation law can be used to find the bio-chemo-mechanical affinity, and it is defined as the difference between the external work rate and the rate of change in free energy. According to the Second Law of Thermodynamics, this quantity should be nonnegative. Using the dissipation law and after some manipulations, the driving force for the dissolution process of bone can take the following form:

$$A = \psi_{mech.} + P + C_s (\mu_s - \mu_{ext}) \tag{4}$$

where $\psi_{mech.}$ is the mechanical part of the free energy, P is the hydrostatic pressure, C_s is defined as ρ/M, where ρ and M are the density and the molar mass of the matrix, respectively, and μ_s & μ_{ext} are the chemical potential of the solid phase in the unstressed condition and the external potential energy, respectively.

Our bi-phasci mixture model of bone resorption shows that the activity of osteoclasts and, thus, the rate of bone resorption are not only dictated by biological factors (e.g., hormone levels), but also by engineering quantities, i.e. hydrostatic pressure, strain energy density, and concentration of different ions before and after the resorption process. Interesting to note that the exact stimulus for the initiation of the remodeling process of bone is not known yet and is a place of debate (Rouhi, 2006a). In 1990, Brown and co-workers have shown experimentally that strain energy density can be a likely stimulus for bone remodeling (Brown et al. 1990), and it was used extensively in many theoretical modeling of bone adaptation; for instance (Jacobs et al. 1997; Huiskes et al. 2000; Doblar'e and Garc'ia 2001; Garcia et al. 2002; Ruimerman et al. 2005). As can be seen in Eq. 4, in this bi-phasic model, strain energy density is appeared as an effective mechanical stimulus for the bone resorption. Moreover, using our bi-phasic model, hydrostatic pressure was introduced as another mechanical stimulus for the bone resorption process (see Eq. (4)). Using this model, it was also shown that increasing either strain energy density or hydrostatic pressure will increase rate of bone resorption. The former point can be used as a theoretical justification for many experimental observations (e.g., (Burr et al. 1985; Burr and Martin 1993; Mori and Burr 1993; Schaffler and Jepsen 2000; Li et al. 2001; Martin 2003; Van Der Vis et al. 1998; Skripitz and Aspenberg 2000; Astrand et al. 2003). This model also shows that an increase in the concentration of H^+, or a decrease in the concentrations of PO_4^{-3} and Ca^{2+} can cause a reduction in the rate of bone resorption. Experimental data can be found in support of this model's predictions of the effect of Ca^{2+} concentration on the rate of bone resorption (Lorget et al. 2000). Using the Second Law of

Thermodynamics, it was also shown that the maximum rate of bone resorption in cortical bone is greater than that of cancellous bone. This behaviour of cortical and trabecular bone, which is well accepted experimentally (Martin & Burr, 1989), can also be predicted using the axiom of mass balance in this bi-phasic model.

For more detailed information about the basic assumptions, also governing equations of the bi-phasic model of bone resorption, interested readers are encouraged to consult the following reference (Rouhi et al., 2007).

6. A tri-phasic mixture model of bone resorption process

Recently, a tri-phasic model of bone resorption using mixture theory with chemical reactions was proposed (Rouhi, 2011). In this model, three different constituents (matrix, fluid, and cells) have been considered. Bone resorption is considered as a chemical reaction caused by the secretion of H^+ and Cl^- from osteoclasts which creates an acidic environment in a sealed zone between osteoclasts and bone matrix. It is assumed that the solid phase obeys small deformation theory and is isotropic and linearly elastic. The velocity of the matrix and cells is assumed to be zero. The fluid phase is assumed to be viscous, and inertial effects are neglected because of the slow velocities that are at play. A non-rotational fluid is assumed for deriving the final form of the entropy inequality for the mixture as a whole. In the constitutive equations, similar to our bi-phasic model (Rouhi et al., 2007), it is assumed that the free energy, enthalpy, specific entropy, heat flux, and stress tensor are functions of temperature, deformation gradient, and the extent of chemical reactions. Bone resorption was considered as an isothermal and a quasi-static process. For the sake of simplicity, presence of ostocytes in the bone matrix was discarded in this model, despite the fact that fluid flow in the bone matrix (e.g. in the lacuno-canalicular network) has a definite effect on the osteocytes, and, most likely, on the osteoclasts and thus on the rate of bone resorption. Using these assumptions, the governing equations for bone resorption were derived using the conservation laws (mass, momentum, and energy), as well as entropy inequality and the appropriate constitutive equations.

By using mixture theory with chemical reactions, first, contribution of different phases present in the mixture can be observed. Secondly, using consistency requirement for energy balance, it was found that rate of bone resorption is a function of different factors including apparent density of bone matrix and bone fluid; fluid velocity; momentum supply to the fluid or solid phase; and internal energy densities of different constituents. Thirdly, using the relation between momentum supply to the solid and fluid phase, one can conclude that rate of bone resorption is inversely proportional to the bone fluid velocity. Also, it was found that in spongy bone, by increasing the porosity, rate of resorption will decrease and vice versa. Based on our results, it is speculated that bone resorption in cortical and cancellous bones might be affected by a control system which is resulted from the relation between the specific surface of bone and its apparent density and volume fraction. As it is known, one reason of osteoporosis is the lack of calcium ions in our body, so in the case of need of calcium, where is better than a rich reservoir, i.e. bones, to take away calcium ions via bone resorption process and giving back in the bone formation process. It seems necessary and feasible, as a future task, to investigate the relation between calcium concentration in the bone fluid and the rate of bone resotrpiton using mixture theory.

For more detailed information about the basic assumptions, also governing equations of the tri-phasic model of bone resorption, interested readers are encouraged to consult the following reference (Rouhi, 2011).

7. The effects of osteocytes number and mechanosensitivity on bone loss

Based on the experimental data and evidence, it is known that osteocyte density (the number of osteocytes per unit surface of bone) changes with aging and also in osteoporotic bones (Gong et al., 2008; Mullender et al., 1996). Moreover, they interestingly found that the osteocyte density increased in osteoporotic patients compared to that of healthy adults, although excessive bone loss and reduced spongy bone wall thickness have been described as characteristic for osteoporotic bones. Experimental evidence for altered mechanosensitivity of osteocytes derived from osteoporotic patients has also been reported (Sterck et al., 1998). According to the semi-mechanistic bone remodeling theory (Huiskes et al., 2000; Ruimerman et al., 2005), and based on the fact that the number of osteocytes per unit surface of bone decreases with aging, we hypothesized that bone loss with the age is correlated with the reduction of either the number of osteocytes, or the strength of the recruitment signal sent by osteocytes to osteoblasts (Li, 2011; Li & Rouhi, 2011).

In the semimechanistic model of Huiskes and co-workers, bone remodeling is considered as a coupling process of bone resorption and bone formation on the bone free surfaces. Osteoclasts are assumed to resorb bone stochastically. Osteocytes are suggested to act as strain energy density (SED) rate sensing cells, and to play a role in the regulation of bone remodeling. It is assumed that osteocytes locally sense the SED rate perturbation generated by either the external load or by cavities made by osteoclasts (bone resorbing cells), and then recruit osteoblasts to form bone tissue to fill the resorption cavities. Osteoclasts are assumed to resorb a constant amount of bone per day. The probability of osteoclast activities may be regulated by the presence of either micro-cracks or in the case of disuse. Since the changes in bone structure because of osteoporosis are similar to changes resulting from disuse (Frost, 1988; Rodan, 1991), it was assumed that one of the causes for bone loss in osteoporotic bones can be the reduction in osteocyte mechanosensitivity.

In our study, we developed a two dimensional finite element model of spongy bone using a semi-mechanistic bone remodeling theory (Huiskes et al., 2000) to simulate spongy bone remodeling and investigate the validity of our hypotheses (Li, 2011; Li & Rouhi, 2011). Results of our study showed that the osteocyte density has a significant role in the final geometry of spongy bone in the bone remodeling process. It was also shown that by decreasing the osteocyte density (knowing that the osteocyte density decrease as a healthy adult ages), bone loss will occur and there will be a decrease in bone apparent density. Moreover, it was shown that when osteocyte mechanosensitivity is less than a certain level, osteoporotic patients lose more spongy bone than healthy old adults even though osteoporotic patients have greater osteocyte number than in healthy old adults. Figure 1 shows the final simulation results of spongy bone with different mechanosensitivities of osteocytes, but the same osteocytes' number and the same form of osteocyte distribution. As can be seen, by decreasing the mechanosensitivity of osteocytes, there will be a reduction in spongy bone apparent density. Results of this study were in favour of our hypothesis stating that "by decreasing the osteocyte mechanosensitivity, as is the case in an osteoporotic bone, bone apparent density will also decrease even by increasing the number of osteocytes".

Some of the possible explanations for the abnormal bone loss in an osteoporotic bone suggested by different researchers are as follows: (1) a higher percentage of the bone forming cells is embedded in bone matrix as osteocytes (Mullender et al., 1996), so a reduction in the number of bone forming cells can be seen; (2) the bone forming activity of osteoblasts is reduced (Mullender et al., 1996; Ruimerman et al., 200?), thus less bone apposition will occur; (3) the average life-span of osteoblasts is reduced (Mullender et al., 1996; Eriksen and Kassem, 1992); (4) a reduction in bone sensor cells mechanosensitivity (Sterck et al., 1998), thus they cannot make a true picture of the mechanical environment of the bone and so there will be a reduction in the smartness of bone structure. It seems reasonable to assume that bone loss in the case of osteoporosis is the result of a combination of all the above mentioned, and likely some other, factors.

For more detailed information about this work, interested readers are encouraged to consult the following references (Li & Rouhi, 2011; Li, 2011).

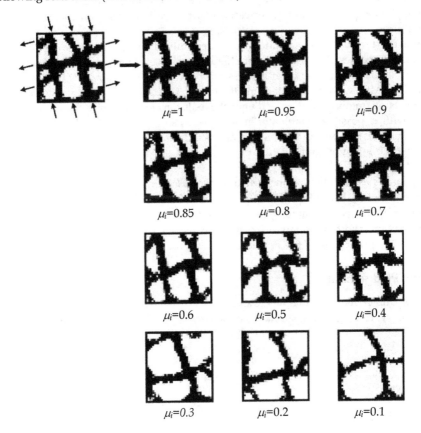

Fig. 1. Results of simulation of the spongy bone remodeling for different levels of osteocyte mechanosensitivity (μi), representing the level of activity of bone sensor cells (Li, 2011).

8. Discussion and conclusions

Unlike Engineering materials and structures, biological materials including bone, are sensitive to the mechanical stimuli placed on them. Moreover, their mechanical properties are changing continuously as a function of time, mechanical load, and biological factors (e.g. various hormones levels and nutrition). Osteoporosis is caused when there is an imbalance in the bone remodeling process. So, in order to be able to find a solid cure for this disease, a clear and comprehensive understanding of the bone remodeling process at different level of considerations, i.e. molecular; cellular; and tissue level, is needed. A wealth of evidence has been accumulated during the past few years supporting the concept that the study of bone micro- and nano-structures will not only improve our understanding of the mechanisms that underlie bone fragility, but also help to discover the effects of treatments. For instance, nanomedicine and its application to bone research can undoubtedly broaden our knowledge of patho-physiology and improve the diagnostic, prevention and treatment of bone diseases including osteoporosis. Considering the complexity and multifactorial aspect of the remodeling process, the best way to tackle this problem seems to be working in a multidisciplinary group including researchers from various disciplines of medicine and bioengineering.

Based on the fact that skeletal integrity is determined by the outstanding and variant mechanical properties of bone at different hierarchical levels of its structure, it becomes clear that a simple diagnostic parameter such as hip bone mineral density (BMD) does not have enough diagnostic strength to determine the complex patho-physiological mechanisms that determine bone fragility. Thus, new diagnostic tools developed by bioengineering scientists, coupled with a possible combinatorial approach using different methods to define the material qualities of bone at different hierarchical levels of bone's structure, are needed in identifying the initiation and also the progression of the silent and dangerous disease, so-called osteoporosis.

The responsiveness to either an increase or a decrease in mechanical stimulus is very likely greater in growing than adult bones. So, the concept of public health programs aimed at increasing physical activity among healthy children and adolescents in order to maximize peak bone mass, and thus to minimize the probability of bone fracture due t low strength, seems reasonable and should be considered seriously.

9. Acknowledgement

Amirkabir University of Technology, Iran & University of Ottawa, Canada, as well as Dr. M. Esptein, Dr. W. Herzog, Dr. L. Sudak from the University of Calgary, and Mr. X. Li.

10. References

Ascenzi, A. (1993). Biomechanics and Galileo Galilei, *Journal of Biomechanics*, Vol. 26, pp. 95–100.

Astrand, J.; Skripitz, R., Skoglund, B. & Aspenberg, P. (2003). A rat model for testing pharmacologic treatments of pressure-related bone loss, *Clinical Orthopaedics and Related Research*, Vol. 409, pp. 296–305.

Bailey, A.J. & Paul, R.G. (1999). The mechanisms and consequences of the maturation and ageing of collagen, *Journal of Chemical Sciences*, Vol. 111, Number 1, pp. 57-69.

Bartel, L.B.; Dwight T.D. & Keaveny T.M. (2006). Orthopaedic Biomechanics Mechanics and Design in Musculoskeletal Systems, Chap. 3, Pearson Prentice Hall.

Beaupre, G.S.; Orr, T.E. & Carter, D.R. (1990). An approach for time-dependent bone modeling and remodeling—theoretical development, *Journal of Orthopaedic Research*, Vol. 8, Issue 5, pp 651–661.

Behari, J. (1991). Solid state bone behaviour, *Progress in Biophysics & Molecular Biology*, Vol. 56, pp. 1-41.

Blair, H.C. (1998). How the osteoclast degrades bone, *BioEssays*, Vol. 20, Issue 10, pp. 837–846.

Boivin, G. & Meunier, P.J. (2003). The mineralization of bone tissue: a forgotten dimension in osteoporosis research, *Osteoporosis International*, Vol. 14, Suppl. 3, S19-S24.

Brown, T.D.; Pedersen, D.R.; Gray, M.L.; Brand, R.A. & Rubin, C.T. (1990). Toward an identification of mechanical parameters initiating periosteal remodeling: a combined experimental and analytic approach, *Journal of Biomechanics,* Vol. 23, Issue 9, pp. 893–897.

Bucwalter, J.A.; Woo, S.LY.; Goldberg, V.M.; Hadley, E.C.; Booth, R.; Oregema, T.R. & Eyre, D.R. (1993). Soft tissue aging and musculoskeletal function, *Journal of Bone and Joint Surgery*, Vol. 75A, Issue 10, pp. 1533-1548.

Burger, E.H. & Klein-Nulend, J. (1999). Mechanotransduction in bone-role of the lacunocanalicular network, *FASEB Journal.* Vol. 13, pp. S101-S112.

Burr, D.B. (1997). Muscle strength, bone mass and age related bone loss, *Journal of Bone and Mineral Research*, Vol. 12, Issue 10, pp. 1547-1551.

Burr, D.B.; Martin, R. B.; Schaffler, M.B. & Radin, E.L. (1985). Bone remodeling in response to in vivo fatigue microdamage, *Journal of Biomechanics*, Volume 18, Issue 3, pp. 189–200.

Burr, D.B. & Martin, R.B. (1993). Calculating the probability that microcracks initiate resorption spaces, *Journal of Biomechanics*, Vol. 26, Issue 4-5, pp. 613–616.

Burr, D.B.; Robling, A.G.& Turner, C.H. (2002). Effects of biomechanical stress on bones in animals, *Bone*, Vol. 30, Issue 5, pp. 781–786.

Chambers, T.J.; Revell, P.A.; Fuller, K. & Athanasou, N.A. (1984). Resorption of bone by isolated rabbit osteoclasts, *Journal of Cell Science*, Vol. 66, Issue 1, pp. 383–399.

Chow, L.C.; Markovic, M. & Takagi, S. (2003). A dual constant-composition titration system as in vitro resorption model for comparing dissolution rates of calcium phosphates biomaterials, *Journal of Biomedical Material Research*, Vol. 65B, Issue 2, pp. 245–251.

Christoffersen, J.; Christoffersen, M.R. & Johansen, T. (1996). Kinetics of growth and dissolution of fluorapatite, *Journal of Crystal Growth*, Vol. 163, Issue 3, pp. 295–303.

Cowin, C.S. & Hegedus, D.H. (1967). Bone remodeling I: a theory of adaptive elasticity, *Journal of Elasticity*, Vol. 6, Issue 3, pp. 313-326.

Currey, J.D. (2001). Bone strength: what are we trying to measure?, *Calcified Tissue International*, Vol. 68, Number 4, pp. 205-210.

Currey, J.D. (2002). Bone- Struture and Mechanics, Princeton University Press, Princeton.

Currey, J.D. (1999). The design of mineralised hard tissues for their mechanical functions, *The Journal of Experimental Biology*, Vol. 202, pp. 3285-3294.

Currey, J.D. (2003). How well are bones designed to resist fracture?, *Journal of Bone and Mineral Research*, Vol. 18, Issue 4, pp. 591-598.

Currey, J.D.; Brear, K. & Zioupos, P. (1996). The effects of ageing and changes in mineral content in degrading the toughness of human femora, *Journal of Biomechanics*, Vol. 29, Issue 2, pp. 257-260.

Doblaré, M. & García, J.M. (2001). Application of an anisotropic bone-remodeling model based on a damage-repair theory to the analysis of the proximal femur before and after total hip replacement, *Journal of Biomechanics*, Vol. 34, Issue 9, pp. 1157-1170.

Dorozhkin, S. V. (1997a). Acidic dissolution mechanism of natural fluorapatite,I: milli- and microlevels of investigations, *Journal of Crystal Growth*, Vol. 182, Issue 1-2, pp. 125-132.

Dorozhkin, S. V. (1997b). Acidic dissolution mechanism of natural fluorapatite,II: nanolevel of investigations, *Journal of Crystal Growth*, Vol. 182, Issue 1-2, pp. 133-140.

Dorozhkin, S. V. (1997c). Surface reactions of apatite dissolution, *Journal of Colloid and Interface Science*, Vol. 191, Issue 2, pp. 489-497.

Ducy, P.; Schinke, T. & Karsenty, G. (2000). The osteoblast: a sophisticated fibroblast under central surveillance, *Science*, Vol. 289, Number 5484, pp. 1501-1504.

Eriksen, E.F. & Kassem, M. (1992). The cellular basis of bone remodeling, Triangle, Sandoz *Journal of Medical Science*, Vol. 31, Issue 2/3, pp. 45-57.

Eyre, D.R.; Dickson, I.R. & Van Ness, K. (1988). Collagen cross-linking in human bone and articular cartilage. Age-related changes in the content of mature hydroxypyridinium residues. *Biochemical Journal*, Vol. 252, Issue 2, pp. 495-500.

Forwood, M.R.& Turner, C.H. (1995). Skeletal adaptations to mechanical usage: results from tibial loading studies in rats. *Bone*, Vol. 17, Issue 4, pp. 197S-205S.

Fratzl, P.; Gupta, H.S.; Paschalis, E.P. & Roschger, P. (2004). Structure and mechanical quality of the collagen-mineral nano-composite in bone, *Journal of Materials Chemistry*, Vol. 14, pp. 2115-2123.

Fratzl, P. & Weinkamer, R. (2007). Nature's hierarchical materials, *Progress in Materials Science*, Vol. 52, pp. 1263-1334.

Frost, H.M. (1985). Bone microdamage: factors that impair its repair, in Current Concepts in Bone Fragility, Uhthoff, H.K, Ed., Springer, Berlin.

Frost, H.M. (1988). Vital biomechanics: proposed general concepts for skeletal adaptations to mechanical usage, *Calcified Tissue International*, Vol. 42, Issue 3, pp. 145-156.

Frost, H.M. (1999a). Perspective, why do bone strength and "mass" in aging adults become nonresponsive to vigorous exercise? Insights of the Utah paradigm, *Journal of Bone and Mineral Metabolism*, Vol. 17, Number 2, pp. 90-97.

Frost, H.M. (1999b). On the estrogen-bone relationship and postmenopausal bone loss: a new model, *Journal of Bone and Mineral Research*, Vol. 14, Number 9, pp. 1473-1477.

Fulmer, M. T.,; Ison, I.C.; Hankermayer, C.R.; Constantz, B.R. & Ross, J. (2002). Measurements of the solubilities and dissolution rates of several hydroxyapatites, *Biomaterials*, Vol. 23, Issue 3, pp. 751-755.

Garcia, J. M.; Doblare, M. & Cegonino, J. (2002). Bone remodeling simulation: a tool for implant design, *Computational Materials Science*, Vol. 25, Issue 1-2, pp. 100-114.

Gibson, L.J. (1985). The mechanical behaviour of cancellous bone, *Journal of Biomechanics*, Vol. 18, pp. 317-328.

Gong, H.; Fan, Y. & Zhang, M. (2008). Numerical simulation on the adaptation of forms in trabecular bone to mechanical disuse and basic multi-cellular unit activation threshold at menopause, *Acta Mechanica Sinica*, Vol. 24, pp. 207-214.

Guo, X.E. & Goldstein, S.A. (1997). Is trabecular bone tissue different from cortical bone?, *Forma*, Vol. 12, pp. 3-4.

Hankermeyer, C.R.; Ohashi, K.L.; Delaney, D.C.; Ross, J. & Constantz, B.R. (2002). Dissolution rates of carbonated hydroxyapatite in hydrochloric acid, *Biomaterials*, Vol. 23, Issue 3, pp. 743-750.

Hegedus, D.H. & Cowin, C.S. (1976). Bone remodeling II: small strain adaptive elasticity, *Journal of Elasticity*, Vol. 6, Issue 4, pp. 337-352.

Hsieh, Y.F. & Turner, C.H. (2001). Effects of loading frequency on mechanically induced bone formation, *Journal of Bone and Mineral Research*, Vol. 16, Issue 5, pp. 918–924.

Huiskes, R.; Ruimerman, R.; Van Lenthe, G.H. & Janssen, J.D. (2000). Effects of mechanical forces on maintenance and adaptation of form in trabecular bone, *Nature*, Vol. 405, pp. 704–706.

Jacobs, C.R.; Simo, J.C.; Beaupré, G.S. & Carter, D.R. (1997). Adaptive bone remodeling incorporating simultaneous density and anisotropy considerations, *Journal of Biomechanics*, Vol. 30, Issue 6, pp. 603–613.

Lakes, R.S. & Saha, S. (1979). Cement line motion in bone, *Science*, Vol. 204, pp. 501-503.

Lakes, R. (1993). Materials with structural hierarchy, *Nature*, Vol. 361, pp. 511-515.

Landis, W.J. (1996). Mineral characterization in calcifying tissues: atomic, molecular and macromolecular perspectives, *Connective Tissue Research*, Vol. 35, pp. 1-8.

Li, J.; Mashiba, T. & Burr, D.B. (2001). Bisphosphonate treatment suppresses not only stochastic remodeling but also the targeted repair of microdamage, *Calcified Tissue International*, Vol. 69, Issue 5, pp. 281–286.

Li, X. (2011). Investigation into spongy bone remodeling through a semi-mechanistic bone remodeling theory using finite element analysis, MASc Thesis, University of Ottawa, ON, Canada.

Li, X. & Rouhi G. (2011). An investigation into the effects of osteocyte density and mechanosensitivity on the spongy bone loss in aging and osteoporotic individuals, (Accepted subject to revision).

Lucchinetti, E. (2001). Dense bone tissue as a molecular composite, in *Bone Mechanics Handbook* (Ed. Cowin, S.C.), Chap.13.

Lorget, F.; Kamel, S.; Mentaverri, R.; Wattel, A.; Naassila, M.; Maamer M. & Brazier, M. (2000). High extracellular calcium concentrations directly stimulate osteoclast apoptosis, *Biochemical and Biophysical Research Communications*, Vol. 268, Issue 3, pp. 899–903.

Marcus, R. (1996). The nature of osteoporosis, *The Journal of Clinical Endocrinology and Metabolism*, Vol. 81, Issue 1, pp. 1-5.

Margolis, H.C. & Moreno, E.C. (1992). Kinetics of hydroxyapatite dissolution in acetic, lactic, and phosphoric-acid solutions, *Calcified Tissue International*, Vol. 50, Issue 2, pp. 137–143.

Martin, R.B. & Burr, D.B. (1989). Mechanical adaptation, in Structures, Functions and Adaptation of Compact Bone, Raven Press, New York.

Martin, R.B. (2000). Toward a unifying theory of bone remodeling, *Bone*, Vol. 26, Issue 1, pp. 1-6.

Martin, R. B. (2003). Fatigue microdamage as an essential element of bone mechanics and biology, *Calcified Tissue International*, Vol. 73, Issue 2, pp. 101–107.

Mori, S. & Burr, D.B. (1993). Increased intracortical remodleing following fatigue damage, *Bone*, Vol. 14, Issue 2, pp. 103-109.

Mullender, M.G., Huiskes, R. & Weinans, H. (1994). A physiological approach to the simulation of bone remodeling as a self-organizational control process, *Journal of Biomechanics*, Vol. 27, Issue 611, pp. 1389–1394.

Mullender, M.G.; van Der Meer, D.D.; Huiskes, R. & Lips, P. (1996). Osteocyte density changes in aging and osteoporosis, *Bone*, Vol. 18, Issue 2, pp. 109-113.

Oxlund, H.; Mosekilde, L. & Ortoft, G. (1996). Reduced concentration of collagen reducible cross links in human trabecular bone with respect to age and osteoporosis, *Bone*, Vol. 19, Issue 5, pp. 479-484.

Parfitt, A.M. (1995). Problems in the application of *in vitro* systems to the study of human bone remodeling, *Calcified Tissue International*, Vol. 56 (Suppl. 1), pp. S5-S7.

Piekarski, K.J. (1970). Fracture of bone, *Journal of Applied Physics*, Vol. 41, pp. 215-223.

Riggs, B.L.; Khosla, S. & Melton, L.J. (2002). Sex steroids and the construction and conservation of the adult skeleton, *Endocrine Reviews*, Vol. 23, Number 3, pp. 279–302.

Rodan, G.A. (1991). Mechanical loading, estrogen deficiency, and the coupling of bone formation to bone resorption, *Journal of Bone and Mineral Research*, Vol. 6, Issue 6, pp. 527-530.

Rouhi, G.; Herzog, W.; Sudak, L.; Firoozbakhsh, K. & Epstein, M. (2004). Free surface density instead of volume fraction in the bone remodeling equation: theoretical considerations, *Forma*, Vol. 19, Issue 3, pp. 165-182.

Rouhi, G. (2006a). Theoretical aspects of bone remodeling and resorption processes, *PhD Dissertation*, University of Calgary, AB, Canada.

Rouhi, G.; Epstein, M.; Herzog, W. & Sudak, L. (2006b). Free surface density and microdamage in the bone remodeling equation: theoretical considerations, *International Journal of Engineering Sciences*, Vol. 44, Issue 7, pp. 456–469.

Rouhi, G.; Epstein M.; Sudak, L. & Herzog W. (2007). Modeling bone resorption using mixture theory with chemical reactions, *Journal of Mechanics of Materials and Structures*, Vol. 2, Number 6, pp. 1141-1156.

Rouhi G. (2011). A tri-phasic mixture model of bone resorption: Theoretical investigations, *Journal of the Mechanical Behavior of Biomedical Materials*, Vol. 4, Issue 8, pp. 1947-1954.

Rousselle, A.V. & Heymann, D. (2002). Osteoclastic acidification pathways during bone resorption, *Bone*, Vol. 30, Issue 4, pp. 533–540.

Rubin, M.A.; Rubin, J. & Jasiuk, W. (2004). SEM and TEM study of the hierarchical structure of C57BL/6J and C3H/HeJ mice trabecular bone, *Bone*, Vol. 35, Issue 1, pp. 11-20.

Ruimerman, R.; Huiskes, R.; van Lenthe, G.H & Janssen, J.D. (2001). A computer-simulation model relating bone-cell metabolism to mechanical adaptation of trabecular bone, *Computer Methods in Biomechanics and Biomedical Engineering*, Vol. 4, Issue 5, pp. 433-448.

Ruimerman, R.; Hilbers, P.; van Rietbergen, B. & Huiskes, R. (2005). A theoretical framework for strain related trabecular bone maintenance and adaptation, *Journal of Biomechanics*, Vol. 38, Issue 4, pp. 931–941.

Teitelbaum, S.L. & Ross, F.P. (2003). Genetic regulation of osteoclast development and function, *Nature Reviews Genetics*, Vol. 4, Issue 8, pp. 638–649.

Thomann, J. M.; Voegel, J.C.; Gumper, M. & Gramain, P. (1989). Dissolution kinetics of human enamel powder, II: a model based on the formation of a self-inhibiting surface layer, *Journal of Colloid and Interface Science*, Vol. 132, Issue 2, pp. 403–412.

Thomann, J. C.; Voegel, J.C. & Gramain, P. (1990). Kinetics of dissolution of calcium hydroxyapatite powder, III: PH and sample conditioning effects, *Calcified Tissue International*, Vol. 46, Issue 2, pp. 121–129.

Thomann, J.M.; Voegel, J.C. & Gramain, P. (1991). Kinetics of dissolution of calcium hydroxyapatite powder, IV: interfacial calcium diffusion controlled process, *Colloids and Surfaces*, Vol. 54, Issue 1-2, pp. 145–159.

Schaffler, M.B. & Jepsen, K.J. (2000). Fatigue and repair in bone, *International Journal of Fatigue* , Vol. 22, Issue 10, pp. 839–846.

Seeman, E. & Delmas, P.D. (2006). Bone quality – the material and structural basis of bone strength and fragility, *The New England Journal of Medicine*, Vol. 354, Number 21, pp. 2250-2261.

Skripitz, R. & Aspenberg, P. (2000). Pressure-induced periprosthetic osteolysis: a rat model, *Journal of Orthopaedic Research*, Vol. 18, Issue 3, pp. 481–484.

Sterck, J.G.H.; Klein-Nulend, J.; Lips, P. & Burger, E.H. (1998). Response of normal and osteoporotic human bone cells to mechanical stress in vitro, *American Journal of Physiology- Endocrinology and Metabolism*, Vol. 274, Issue 6, pp. 11113-1120.

Taylor, D.; Hazenberg, J.G. & Lee T.C. (2007). Living with cracks: damage and repair in human bone, *Nature Materials*, Vol. 6, pp. 263-268.

Van der Meulen, M.C.H. & Prendergast, P.J. (2000). Mechanics in skeletal development, adaptation and disease, *Philosophical Transactions for the Royal Society of London A*, Vol. 358, pp. 565-578.

Van Der Vis, H. M.; Aspenberg, P.; Marti, R. K.; Tigchelaar, W. & Van Noorden, C. J. (1998). Fluid pressure causes bone resorption in a rabbit model of prosthetic loosening, *Clinical Orthopaedics and Related Research*, Vol. 350, pp. 201–208.

Wanich, R.D. (1999). Epideminology of osteoporosis, in Primer on the Metabolic Bone Diseases and Disorders of Mineral Metabolism, 4th ed., Favus, M.J. Ed., Lippincott/Williams & Wilkines, chap. 46.

Weiner, S. & Wagner, H.D. (1998). The material bone: structure-mechanical function relations, *Annual reviews of Materials Science*, Vol. 28, pp. 271-298.

Wolff, J. (1892). *The Law of Bone Remodeling* (original publication 1892 translated in 1986 by P. Maquet and R. Furlong), Springer, Berlin.

Yamauchi, M.; Young, D.R.; Chandler, G.S. & Mechanic, G.L. (1988). Cross linking and new bone collagen synthesis in immobilized and recovering primate osteoporosis, *Bone*, Vol. 9, Issue 6, pp. 415-418.

Zioupos, P. & Currey, J.D. (1998). Changes in the stiffness, strength, and toughness of human cortical bone with age, *Bone*, Vol. 22, Issue 1, pp. 57-66.

Zioupos, P.; Currey, J.D. & Hamer, A.J. (1999). The role of collagen in the declining mechanical properties of ageing human cortical bone, *Journal of Biomedical Material Research*, Vol. 45, Issue 2, pp. 108-116.

3

Bone Mineral Quality

Delphine Farlay[1,2] and Georges Boivin[1,2]
[1]INSERM, UMR 1033, F-69372 Lyon,
[2]Université de Lyon, F-69008 Lyon,
France

1. Introduction

The main function of bone is to promote locomotion and protection of vital organs. Bone is also an important mineral ions reservoir, essential to maintain phosphocalcic homeostasis. Bone mineral is a calcium phosphate named "apatite", which form naturally in the Earth's crust (Wopenka & Pasteris 2005). Compared to others minerals, apatite is more "tolerant" and is very accommodating to chemical substitutions. This ability to easily absorb ions confers to bone a detoxification property, with some ions normally absent of bone and which are captured by bone mineral. But the substitutions in bone mineral change the structure of apatite, conferring to bone several properties such as solubility, morphology, hardness, strain etc.

Thanks to those remarkable properties, bone has the ability to continually adapt to changes to its mechanical environment (Bouxsein 2005). Bone is an anisotropic composite material tissue, and highly hierarchical viscoelastic (Bouxsein 2005). When a load is applied to bone, this produces energy, and as this energy can not be destroy, the bone has to absorbed it (Seeman & Delmas 2006). The elastic properties of bone allow to absorb this energy by deforming reversibly. But if the load exceeds the ability of the bone to carry this load, it can deform permanently by plastic deformation (Fig.1). This produces microcracks allowing

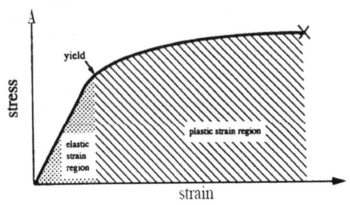

Fig. 1. Stress-strain curve divided into the elastic and plastic regions. The fracture occurs at the end of the curve (marked with **X**). Reprinted from Turner & Burr, 1993, with permission from Elsevier.

energy release. If the microcracks remain small, this has no impact on bone. However, if the microcracks become numerous and/or too long, the bone fractures. Thus, to resist to a fracture, the bone need to find the best compromise between *stiffness* and *flexibility* (to resist deformation) (Seeman & Delmas 2006). A high mineral content increases *stiffness* reducing *flexibility*, and if the bone is too flexible, it will deform beyond its peak strain and crack. Several studies showed that mineral part is involved in the elastic properties of bone, whereas organic part is rather involved in the plastic deformation (Bala et al., 2011b; Bouxsein 2005; Currey 2003; Follet et al., 2004).

2. Determinants of bone quality

Bone is constituted by three major components which are the organic matrix (≈30%, mainly type I collagen), mineral (≈60%, carbonated apatite) and water (≈10%). Organic matrix is essentially constituted by ~ 90% of a network of type I collagen fibrils, and ~10% of non-collagenous proteins. Type I collagen molecules are formed by three polypeptides α chains [2 α1(I) and 1 α2(I)] forming a tight triple helix structure with a repetition of Gly-X-Y triplets (Myllyharju & Kivirikko 2004). To provide the stability of type I collagen fibrils, several mechanisms of maturation and ageing of bone collagen occurs, including enzymatic collagen cross-linking and non-enzymatic modifications (Saito & Marumo 2010; Viguet-Carrin et al., 2006). In parallel, the organic matrix mineralizes, and the organization of type I collagen network determines the specific arrangement of mineral crystals (Höhling et al., 1990; Riggs et al., 1993). The crystals first grow in length, typically plate-like (Landis, 1995; Roschger et al., 1998), then they become thicker but stay relatively thin (Roschger et al., 1998). Concomitantly, the crystals number increases up to physiologic limits of mineralization (Bala et al., 2010; Boivin et al., 2008; Boivin & Meunier 2002).

The quantity of bone mineral (assimilated to the quantity of total bone) is usually measured by bone mineral density (BMD), using dual X-ray absorptiometry (DXA). However, about one-half of fractures occur in women having a T-Score above the World Health Organization (WHO) diagnosis threshold of osteoporosis (≤-2.5) (Siris et al., 2004; Sornay-Rendu et al., 2005) suggesting that other factors than bone quantity are involved in the apparition of fractures. These factors, involved in bone quality, are called intrinsic determinants. Both extrinsic determinants (including bone mass, macro/microarchitecture) and intrinsic determinants are involved in bone strength, and are directly dependent of bone remodeling activity (Fig.2).

DXA measurement gives information on bone mineral mass but not on its mineral quality. For example, when fluoride salts was used to treat post menopausal osteoporosis, an increase in bone mineral density was measured by DXA, but the bones of patients treated with fluoride salts were much more brittle than untreated patients. In fact, fluoride ions in bone mineral impaired the bone mineral quality increasing the size of bone (large crystals), and thus reducing the contact area with collagen matrix, despite a higher amount of bone mineral density.

The determinants of bone quality, called "intrinsic determinants", are thus essential in bone strength. Those determinants include mineral quality, collagen quality, and presence of microcracks. A good collagen quality is required to an optimal bone strength. For example, osteogenesis imperfecta, which is an heritable brittle-bone disease, is characterized by a type-I collagen mutation, leading to collagen fibrils abnormally thin, and to an excessive bone fragility (Rauch & Glorieux 2004). Among these determinants, microcracks are normally present in bone, and permit to dissipate energy when bone is submitted to a load. However, the presence of too long microcracks is not good for bone. Thus, all together those extrinsic and intrinsic determinants are involved in bone strength.

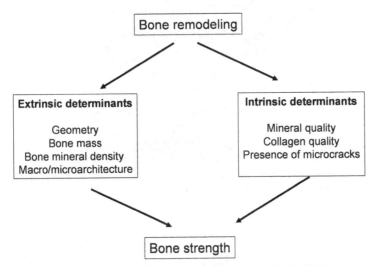

Fig. 2. Description of determinants of bone strength (INSERM UMR 1033)

Bone mineral properties are important determinants of bone strength. Those properties include material (degree of mineralization, hardness…) and crystalline (crystallinity, mineral maturity, ionic substitutions…) characteristics. The importance of the components of bone quality is thus evident and the relationships between the determinants of bone quality are essential to maintain an overall mechanical competent bone. Indeed, bone mineral is complex and knowledge of its composition is important to better understand the mechanisms of bone fragility.

The main purpose of this present chapter is to bring a best approach of bone mineral quality, mineralization process, mineral crystals and mineral composition.

3. Mineralization process: A dynamic process

As bone is submitted to a constant remodeling during all the adult life, old Bone Structural Units (BSUs, named the osteons in cortical bone and the trabecular packets in cancellous bone) will be resorbed by osteoclasts, and replaced by new formed bone. Thus, the recently formed BSUs will be less mineralized than the older BSUs present in interstitial bone and not already resorbed. This heterogeneity of mineralization in the different BSUs can be easily visualized on a X rays microradiograph (Fig. 3). This mineralization process related to bone remodeling can be decomposed into two steps: a primary mineralization which corresponds to a very rapid deposition of first crystals, and a secondary mineralization which is much longer, with a slow and gradual increase in size, perfection and number of crystals.

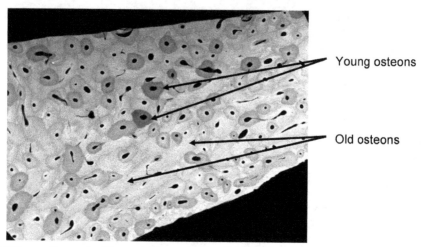

Fig. 3. Microradiograph of human femur illustrating the heterogeneity of the mineralization (cortical bone of a man, 48 year-old) (INSERM UMR 1033)

3.1 Primary and secondary mineralization processes

The process of primary mineralization is a very rapid process, starting in the unmineralized bone matrix (osteoid) deposited by the osteoblasts; in humans, the new matrix begins to mineralize after 5 to 10 days after the deposition of osteoid. The primary mineralization can be measured using double tetracycline labeling (Frost 1969) (Fig. 4). The double labeling involves the administration of two short courses of tetracycline which is deposited along the calcification front as two distinct lines visualized on bone sections under ultraviolet (UV) light. This allows the measurement of the mineral apposition rate (MAR). Usually, a labeling procedure is 10 mg/kg/day demethylchlortetracycline or tetracycline hydrochloride orally for 2 days, 12 days off, 4 days on. The bone biopsy is then taken 4-6 days later (Frost 1969).

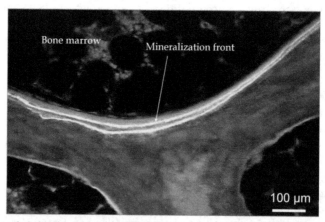

Fig. 4. Histological slide of bone tissue observed under UV light and illustrating a double tetracycline labelling (yellow lines) in trabecular bone and showing the front of mineralization (INSERM UMR 1033).

In adult, MAR varies from 0.60 to 0.80 µm/day whatever the age and the sex (Vedi et al., 1983). MAR is slightly increased in young children, reaching 1 µm/day (Glorieux et al., 2000). During the process of primary mineralization, the first depositions of mineral correspond to about 50 to 60 % of the maximal mineral charge in bone tissue (Meunier & Boivin 1997). This process is extremely rapid, and the first depositions of mineral are used as nucleator for the secondary mineralization. The secondary mineralization corresponds to a slow and gradual increase in both crystal size and number. This process increases until a physiological limit: once the maximum number of crystals attained in a given volume, it is not possible to exceed this limit. Thus in bone remodeling, there is no process of "hypermineralization", because a given BSU can not contain more crystals than its physiological capacity.

The duration of the secondary mineralization is unknown in humans. This duration has been reported in rabbits (Fuchs et al., 2008) and more recently in an animal model (ewes) having a remodeling activity close to the Humans (Bala et al., 2010). The chronology of secondary mineralization has been identify by injection of different fluorescent labels every six months, in order to date the "age" of the BSUs (Bala et al., 2010). In this study, it has been shown that the secondary mineralization lasts approximatively for 24 to 30 months, suggesting that after this time, no increase in degree of mineralization occurs (Fig. 5).

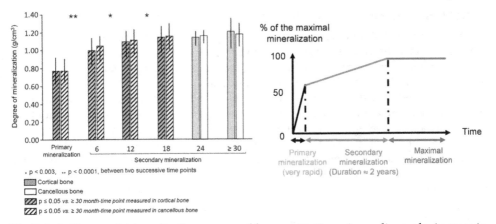

Fig. 5. Left: Degree of mineralization measured by quantitative microradiography in ewes in cortical and cancellous bone, every 6 months (on 512 BSUs; Reprinted from Bala et al., 2010, with permission from Elsevier). Right: Schematic representation of the duration of primary and secondary mineralizations.

This duration of mineralization should be taking into account into anti-resorptive treatment of post menopausal osteoporosis, because once that all the BSUs have attained their maximal mineralization, no gain in term of DMB will occurs.

3.2 Methods to measure degree of mineralization

Several methods are used to measure the degree of mineralization of bone. The technique used in the laboratory is the quantitative microradiography, which is a computerized microdensitometric method based on the X-rays absorption (Boivin & Meunier 2002). Others methods are used to measure the degree of mineralization, as the quantitative backscattering electron or synchrotron infrared microspectroscopy.

3.2.1 Quantitative microradiography

3.2.1.1 Specimen preparation

Undecalcified iliac bone samples were generally used in humans, fixed in 70% alcohol for ten days or more (depending on the size of the samples), and then specimens are placed two days in absolute alcohol to complete dehydration. Alcohol baths are changed every day and specimens are substituted in methylcyclohexane again for two days, before embedding in methyl methacrylate (MMA). The latter is a transparent and hard plastic having a very low X-ray absorption power. Samples are kept for two days in MMA monomer alone, at 4°C, two days in MMA with 1% of catalyst (anhydrous dibenzoyl peroxide) and 2 days in MMA with 2% of catalyst. Then the specimens are placed in an oven (30°C) for final polymerization to obtain hard blocks. After polymerization, thick sections are cut from the embedded bone samples with a precision diamond wire saw, progressively ground to a thickness of 100μm and polished with an alumina suspension. The thickness of the section was measured with an accuracy of 1 μm using a precision micrometer. After ultrasonic cleaning in demineralised water, the bone sections were microradiographed. If orientation of the blocks is possible before sectioning, the cutting plane perpendicular to the haversian canals of cortical bone is preferred.

3.2.1.2 Measurement of degree of mineralization (DMB) (Boivin & Meunier 2002)

Soft X-rays are produced in a X-ray generator (Philips compact PW1830/40 X-ray diffraction generator, Limeil Brévannes, France), equipped with a diffraction tube PW 2273/20. A monochromatic X-ray beam is employed, i.e., nickel-filtered copper Kα radiation with a wavelength of 1.54 Å for which the ratio of the mass- absorption coefficients of aluminium to apatite is 0.561. The distance between the X-ray source and the specimen is about 25-30 cm. In a dark room, the 100 μm-thick bone sections are placed on a photographic emulsion covered by a thin polyester (mylar) film transparent to X-rays, and placed in a specimen holder. An aluminium step-wedge is also exposed on each microradiography. Aluminium was chosen because it is convenient material having an atomic number not far from the effective atomic number of hydroxyapatite. The section is firmly pressed flat by tightening the specimen holder cap and evacuating the air situated between the mylar and the emulsion by means of a vacuum pump, thus bringing the section in direct contact with the emulsion. The specimen holder is placed in a camera perpendicular to the X-ray beam and locked into position during X-ray exposure, during 20 min at 25 kV and 25 mA.

After X-ray exposure, the film (VRP-M green sensitive emulsion from Geola, Slavich International Wholesale Office, Vilnius, Lithuania) is developed for 5 min in Kodak D19 at 20°C, rinsed and then fixed for 5 min in Ilford Hypam. The film is washed and dried, then mounted between two slides. The DMB is quantified using an automatic program for analyzing grayness levels (MorphoExpert and Mineralization, ExploraNova, La Rochelle, France). A digital camera (resolution: 1600 x 1200 pixels or 800 x 600 after binning), captures the microscopic image of the microradiograph. After calibration with the aluminium reference system, the measured regions of bone tissue are automatically selected, and the gray levels are segmented after bone thresholding. The values of the gray levels are then obtained at pixel level (for a magnification x2.5, the size of the pixel is 2.82 μm). Finally, gray-level are converted into DMB measurements with the construction of a calibration curve based on the measurements obtained on the aluminium step-wedge. DMB is finally expressed in gram of mineral over cm^3 of bone (g/cm^3) and measured separately in cortical and cancellous bone. The main parameters, extracted from the DMB measurements, are the mean DMB, the mean highest and most frequent DMB (DMB Freq. Max) and the mean index of heterogeneity of the distribution of DMB expressed as the mean of the widths at half-maximum measured on the individual DMB curves.

3.2.2 Quantitative backscattering electron imaging (qBEI)

The mineral content of bone samples has also been evaluated (Roschger et al., 1995, 1998, 2003; Ruffoni et al. 2007) by quantitative Backscattered Electron Imaging (qBEI). This method, based on the detection of electrons backscattered (BSE) on the surface of the bone specimen, is generally used on the same type of bone biopsy fixed in alcohol and embedded in MMA. As the intensity of the BSE signal is strongly related to the atomic number (Z) of the specimen, BSE images provide information about the distribution of different elements in the sample. A calibration of the BE signal with carbon and aluminium as references was performed. Osteoid and hydroxyapatite were also employed as references to convert gray level values into calcium weight % values. In bone, the main signal is related to Ca (Z=20) and P (Z=15) which are the main mineral elements (Roschger et al., 1998). These authors have correlated BE gray levels of bone with calcium content (in weight percent Ca) based on the Ca $K\alpha$-line intensities detected from identical bone areas (Roschger et al., 1995). The intensity of the backscattered electron signal from the sample is directly proportional to the bone calcium concentration and can therefore be used for the generation of bone mineralization density distribution (BMDD). BMDDs display the frequency of certain calcium concentrations and are analyzed for the weighted mean calcium concentration (Ca mean), the most frequent calcium concentration (Ca peak) and the homogeneity of mineralization (Ca width). The BMDD of trabecular bone from healthy, adult individuals was shown to be nearly constant over several biological factors (gender, age, ethnicity, skeletal site). Technical and biological variations showed that it is a method sensitive for subtle changes in mineralization.

3.2.3 Synchrotron radiation microtomography (SRµCT)

Aside from the difficulty of access to synchrotron radiation facilities, a main advantage of this technique is the use of a mono-energetic synchrotron beam, thus avoiding beam-hardening effects. Indeed, the reconstructed gray levels of tomographic images correspond directly to a map of a linear attenuation coefficient within the sample. The SRµCT method has been tested on human bone tissue (Borah et al., 2005, 2006; Nuzzo et al., 2002) but it is still an equipment with difficulty accessible. The availability of a three-dimensional (3D) measuring technique coupled to specific image processing method opens new possibilities. SRµCT may provide 3D images with spatial resolution as high as one micrometer. The acquisition of 3D bone samples images at high spatial resolution using SRµCT has proved to be very accurate for quantifying human bone micro-architecture. Moreover SRµCT is a non destructive, fast, and very precise procedure to determine the DMB in 3D, simultaneously to the micro-architecture. The calibration procedure used homogeneous phantoms of water solutions at different concentrations of K_2HPO_4 (Nuzzo et al., 2002). This method was compared with the quantitative microradiography technique on the same bone samples, and showed that the values of the DMB are both in the range 0.5-1.6 g/cm^3 of bone, both in cortical and cancellous bone, with a mean difference around 4.7%, slightly higher in trabecular region (Nuzzo et al., 2002).

3.3 Bone microhardness at the tissue level

Another important characteristic of bone mineral is its hardness (Currey 2003; Nalla et al., 2003). Thanks to indentation techniques, it has been shown that microhardness of bone osteon was strongly related to its mineral content (Amprino 1958; Bala et al., 2010; Boivin et al., 2008; Carlstrom 1954; Weaver 1966). From a mechanical point of view, microhardness parameter is related to both elastic and plastic deformations, and an indentation technique has been developed to measure directly both elastic modulus (E) and contact hardness (Hc) on small area of bone tissue (Oliver & Pharr 1992). However, this technique has been developed for isotropic materials. While it is known that the bone tissue is complex with an anisotropic structure, the measurements of E is usually performed with a defined Poisson's ratio ($v=0.3$). It has been shown that contact hardness was linearly interdependent with elastic modulus (Oyen 2006). Therefore, contact hardness can give an evaluation of bone stiffness which is directly related to its brittleness. Contact hardness can be evaluated at the microstructural (BSU) or nanostructural (lamellar) levels. At the microstructural level in bone, the pyramidal square-based Vickers indenter is often used (Fig. 6) (Boivin et al., 2008), and nanoindentation is rather used at the lamellar level using Berckovich indenter (Ammann & Rizzoli 2003). Very recently, it has been shown, by instrumented nanoindentation, that contact hardness was correlated both to DMB and collagen maturity (Bala et al., 2011b). Mineralization is a major determinant of microhardness, with about two-thirds of the variance, and one-third being explained by the organic matrix (Boivin et al., 2008). In human control bone, the microhardness does not vary with age and sex, in cortical and cancellous bone, as for the degree of mineralization. In 19 human control bones, the hardness in cortical bone is about 49.30 ± 2.16 kg/mm² and in cancellous bone about 48.92 ± 1.57 kg/mm².

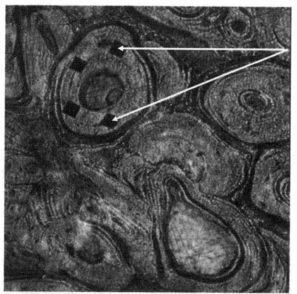

Vickers indents

Fig. 6. Iliac bone from ewe showing a Bone Structural Units (BSU) with 4 Vickers indents (INSERM UMR 1033).

4. Characteristics of bone mineral crystals

Human bone mineral is a non-stoichiometric and poorly crystallized apatite. Bone apatite structure is hexagonal with space group $P6_{3/m}$, with lattice parameters a=9.42Å and c=6.88Å. It is a calcium (Ca)-deficient apatite analog, contains major elements like calcium, [Ca^{2+} (40 wt %)], phosphate [PO_4^{3-}(18 wt %)], carbonates [CO_3^{2-} (6-7 wt %)], minor elements such as magnesium (Mg^{2+}) or sodium (Na^{2+}), and trace elements (LeGeros & LeGeros 1983; LeGeros et al., 1968). Bone mineral also contains ions normally absent from body fluids (lead, fluoride, aluminium etc). Indeed, the apatite lattice is very tolerant to substitutions and vacancies. Compared to dental enamel, the bone mineral contains much more vacancies. In fact, apatite is able to incorporate itself, in its atomic structure, the half of the elements in the periodic chart (Wopenka & Pasteris 2005). Apatite lattice contains about 40 ions, and the unit cell is the smallest basic unit which is a sample of the entire lattice array (Glimcher 1998). In the apatite unit cell, four different types of crystallographic positions (or "sites") have been identified (Fig.7): (1) tetrahedral sites for six P^{5+}-ions, each in 4-fold coordination with oxygen, (2) Ca[1] sites for four of the Ca^{2+} ions, (3) Ca[II] sites for the six other Ca^{2+} ions, and (4) the channel site, occupied by two monovalent anions (OH-, F- and/or Cl-) (Posner 1969; Wopenka & Pasteris 2005). The small ions (Cd^{2+}, Zn^{2+}, Mg^{2+}) are preferentially incorporated into Ca[I], whereas bigger ions (Sr^{2+}, Ba^{2+}, Pb^{2+}) are incorporated into Ca[II] (Fig. 7). The reason why apatite is the mineral component of vertebral skeleton is not known, but it was shown that apatite is the only calcium-phosphate mineral phase that is stable at both a neutral and basic pH (Glimcher 2006; Omelon et al., 2009). Another explanation is coming from the presence of denses granules containing polyphosphates near the mineralizing cartilage and resorbing bone (Omelon et al., 2009). Indeed, when the mineral apatite is dissolved after acidification and resorption by osteoclasts, there is no reprecipitation within the resorption pits, even the return to a neutral pH. The hypothesis of the authors was that polyphosphates formation provides a mechanism for accumulating phosphate, controlling the apatite at locations sites previously mentioned. Enzymatic action can thus control apatite supersaturation at neutral pH, directly by controlling orthophosphate ion activity (Omelon et al., 2009).

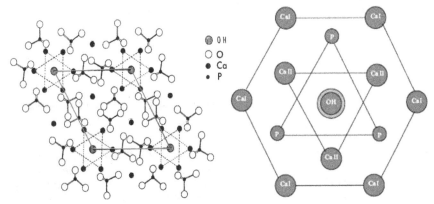

Fig. 7. (Left) Hexagonal system of apatite lattice, showing the disposition of atoms. (Right) The Ca ions occupy two crystallographic non-equivalent sites (Ca I and Ca II). From (Reprinted from Li et al., 2007, with permission from Elsevier). Small ions (Cd^{2+}, Zn^{2+} and Mg^{2+}) are preferentially incorporated into Ca[I], whereas bigger ions (Sr^{2+}, Ba^{2+} and Pb^{2+}) are incorporated into Ca[II].

4.1 Bone crystal size and shape

The crystal structure and morphology of bone minerals have often been controversial, mainly due to the different techniques used to characterize bone mineral. Today, with the use of more accurate method (atomic force microscopy, high resolution transmission electron microscopy), it is clear that the bone mineral crystals are very small and platelet-shaped (length $\approx$ 200-600 Å, width $\approx$ 100-200 Å, thickness $\approx$ 20-50 Å, Figs. 8 and 9). Compared to bone crystals, enamel crystals are needle-shape and much bigger. This small bone crystal size has several advantages. First, it permits an extended surface area (100-200 m^2/g). Two factors are involved in the surface activity: the surface area expressed in m^2/g and the physical and chemical properties of the surface. These properties determine the type of reactions, while the surface area determines the number of reactions. The combination of both factors makes the bone mineral substance metabolically very active; consequently, crystals have a very large interface with extracellular fluids. For example, the crystals contain in a small lumbar vertebra (L1 or L2) having a dry wet of 30 g, have a specific surface comparable to that of the playing field of soccer. Bone mineral is metabolically active, various and numerous interactions between ions from the extracellular fluid and ions constituting apatite crystals, are thus possible. Second, another interest of the small crystal sizes is mechanic. Indeed, the highly ordered location and orientation of very small crystals within the collagen fibrils permits an acceptable range of flexibility without fracture or disruption of the bone substance (Glimcher 1998; Landis 1995).

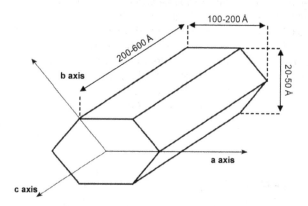

Fig. 8. Schematic representation and crystal size of bone apatite with the 3 axis (INSERM UMR 1033)

4.2 Relationships between water, organic matrix and mineral

In bone, the process of crystal nucleation in bone matrix is heterogenous, and is formed within the "hole" band of type I collagen (670 Å) (Glimcher et al., 1957). During the process of mineralization, the apatite crystals replaced some of the molecules of water so their content is inversely proportional to that of water (Elliott & Robinson 1957; Robinson 1975). Once deposited, the mineral phase induces compaction of the collagen fibril structure. Neutron and X-ray diffraction have shown that the Bragg-spacing of collagen strongly decreases with increasing mineral content (Lees 1987). Computer modeling and SAXS confirmed the process of closer packing of the collagen molecules when clusters of mineral crystals replaced the water within the fibrils (Fratzl et al., 1993). The expansion of mineral crystals compressed the collagen molecule packing, thus decreasing the molecular spacing. This indicated the close relationship between water and the mineral deposition process. Modification of the collagen packing probably influences secondary structure of organic matrix. More recently, in intact bovine bone, the effects of dehydration have been studied using solid-state NMR spectroscopy (Zhu et al., 2009). Interestingly, well-resolved peaks broadened with dehydration, suggesting a conformational disorder and structural changes of bone matrix. This is in agreement with other studies showing a collagen conformational change with dehydration (Naito et al, 1994 ; Saito et al, 1984, 1992).

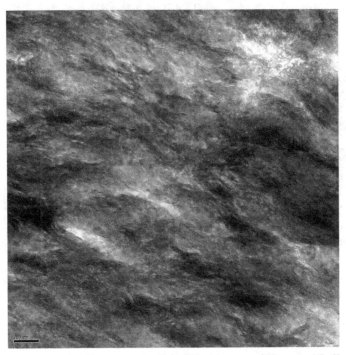

Fig. 9. Electron micrograph of human cancellous bone (woman, 80 year-old) illustrating the bone crystals within the type I collagen (INSERM UMR 1033).

It was suggested that water could play a role in the mechanical behavior of cortical bone (Nyman et al., 2006) and the removal of water alter crystallographic structure of synthetic apatites (LeGeros et al., 1978). As the water content decreases in bone with age (Jonsson et al., 1985; Mueller et al., 1966), it was suggested that water could be involved in bone fragility. Three main types of water exist in bone: the freely mobile water located into vascular lacunar canalicular spaces, the water bound to the collagen network, and the water bound to the mineral. More precisely, there is two type of water bound to the mineral: (a) the water bound to the surface of bone crystals, and (b) the water located within the apatite lattice. Water bound to the collagen fibrils provides post-yield toughness to bone and when water was removed, the strength and stiffness was increased whereas the toughness was decreased (Nyman et al., 2006). The role of the loss of water bound to the mineral on bone strength was not clear in this study, while it was suggested that the loss of water located in apatite lattice could change the size of the bone mineral crystals (Nyman et al., 2006), since it was already observed in dehydrated enamel or precipitated apatites (LeGeros et al., 1978). Consequently, the decrease in bone strength and toughness related to age could be due to a change in water distribution.

4.3 Chemical composition of bone mineral

The composition of bone mineral was for a long time assimilated to hydroxyapatite, but it is not. Several studies showed the lack of OH-, by inelastic neutron scattering, Raman of infrared spectroscopies (Loong et al., 2000; Pasteris et al., 2004; Rey et al., 1995b). Solid state-NMR shows that the percentage of OH- does not exceed 20% of the amount expected in stoichiometric apatite in human cortical bone (Cho et al., 2003). In fact, the small crystal size could be one of the reasons for the absence of OH- ions in the bone apatite. Indeed, Wopenka and Pasteris have suggested that the small crystal size and the great the atomic disorder within the unit cells of the crystal was not energetically favourable for apatite for incorporate OH- into its channel (Pasteris et al., 2004). Another reason for the lack of OH- ions in bone apatite could be due to the type–B substitution of PO4 by CO3, creating a vacancy in the channel site to maintain electrostatic equilibrium.

Nature of apatite	Chemical formula
Hydroxyapatite	$Ca_{10} (PO_4)_6 (OH)_2$
Bone mineral	$Ca_{8.3} \square_{1.7} (PO_4)_{4.3} (HPO_4) (CO_3)_{1.7} (OH)_{0.3} \square_{1.7}$
Dental enamel	$Ca_{9.4} \square_{0.6} (PO_4)_{5.4} (HPO_4) (CO_3)_{0.6} (OH)_{1.4} \square_{0.6}$

Table 1. Chemical formula of different apatites ($\square$: vacancy) (adapted from Cazalbou et al., 2004a)

When an ion with the same electric charge is substituted within the bone apatite, no effect is produced on the structure lattice. If ions have a different electric charge (CO_3^{2-} substituted for PO_4^{3-}), a vacancy is created to maintained electrostatic equilibrium. Some ions can be replaced by other ions of almost identical radius. These ions induce only minor changes in shape at crystal level and do not affect the structure of the crystal. Such substitutions occur during formation of the crystal or through ionic exchanges with the existing crystals. In vitro, some interactions between mineral substance and the solution lead to the diffusion of ions within the hydrated shell, the exchanges at the crystal surface and the exchanges inside the crystal. Similar mechanisms are likely to occur in vivo during remodeling of bone tissue (Blumenthal 1990; LeGeros 1981; Posner 1985). Some cations of similar size and charge as the Ca^{2+} (Sr^{2+}, Na^+), as well as others that cannot substitute for the Ca^{2+} in the apatite structure (Ba^{2+}, Ra^{2+}, Mg^{2+}, K^+), are easily exchangeable from the solution to the surface Ca^{2+} ions. Such substitutions lead to modifications in the a and c parameters of the apatite unit cell. Substitutions with Mg^{2+} are only partial. In biomimetic apatite nanocrystal, the incorporation of Mg has been recently studied to analyze the effect of substitution with Ca^{2+} on particule morphology (Bertinetti et al., 2009). Incorporation of Mg^{2+} does not affect apatitic nature, nonetheless, a lower degree of crystallinity was observed by XRD (Bertinetti et al., 2009). Moreover, it was shown that apatites enriched with Mg^{2+} retain more water at their surface than Mg^{2+}-free apatites (Bertinetti et al., 2009). Calcium can be easily substituted by significantly larger ions, but less frequently by smaller ions (Blumenthal 1990). An ion can only be substituted to another if its ionic radius is less than 10% higher than the radius of the ion replaced. The exchange of anions (PO_4^{3-}, F^-) around the crystal surface is also well known. The substitution of F^- with OH^- ions can not be reversed because it leads to the formation of a more stable compound: F^- ions are more similar to Ca^{2+} ions than OH^- ions and the electrostatic links between Ca^{2+} and F^- are stronger than the ones between Ca^{2+} and OH^-. The more insoluble apatite is the fluoroapatite [chemical formula: $Ca_{10}(PO_4)_6F_2$]. To be resorbed by osteoclasts, the bone mineral have to be more soluble than hydroxyapatite, and the vacancies present in bone mineral enable this dissolution. Carbonates can be found in apatite crystals as CO_3^{2-} ions, which can substituted for either PO_4^{3-} or OH^- ions. When the volume of CO_3^{2-} ions increases, the a parameter of the crystal unit cell decreases, while the c parameter increases.

Some foreign ions can increase or decrease the bone crystal size. In the case of Mg^{2+}, *in vitro* studies have shown that Mg^{2+} bound to the hydroxyapatite crystals retarded nucleation and growth of the crystal. In vivo studies show a decrease in crystal size in Mg-deficient rats, thus Mg interferes with the mineralization process (Bigi et al., 1992; Blumenthal et al., 1977; Boskey et al., 1992).

Others ions, as Fe^{3+} ions, have a direct effect on hydroxyapatite, inhibiting the growth and changing the quality of crystals (decrease in crystallinity and increase in carbonate substitution) (Guggenbuhl et al., 2008). Aluminium also affects bone mineralization, and osteomalacia renal osteodystrophy has been associated, in patients on long-term hemodialysis, with Al^{3+} accumulation in bone (Blumenthal & Posner 1984). A recent study on rats showed that a long-term Al^{3+} exposure reduces the levels of mineral and trace elements in bone (Zn, Fe, Cu, Mn, Se, B, and Sr) (Li et al., 2010b). This is accompagnied by a decrease in BMD especially in cancellous bone. An high amount of ions which are normally present in small proportion in bone mineral can cause alteration of bone substance. As previously mentioned, fluoride ions at high doses cause osteomalacia and defects of mineralization (Balena et al., 1998). On the other hand, small doses of some ions can have positive effect on bone strength. For example, Sr^{2+} (Strontium ranelate is an osteoporosis treatment) reduces both the vertebral and non vertebral fractures (Meunier et al., 2004; Reginster et al., 2005). Besides the effect of Sr^{2+} on bone cells (stimulating bone formation and decreasing bone resorption) (Grynpas & Marie 1990; Marie et al., 1993), the presence of Sr^{2+} is shown in the bone mineral formed during treatment, in osteoporotic women treated with strontium ranelate for 3-5 years (Boivin et al., 2010; Doublier et al, 2011a, b). The concentration of Sr^{2+} is very low, and do not exceed in human a maximum of 0.5 ions Sr^{2+} for 10 Ca^{2+} (Li et al., 2010a). Moreover, the thickness and length of the plate-shaped bone mineral crystals were not affected by the strontium ranelate treatment (Li et al., 2010a). Presence of Sr^{2+} causes no osteomalacia, no modification in the mineralization process or crystal size. However, the Sr^{2+} increases the bone strength, thus the presence of Sr^{2+} in bone mineral has certainly positive effects, but this mechanism is to date unknown.

4.4 Bone apatite: A particular structure, with a hydrated layer around an apatitic core
The surface of bone crystals, formed in the water of extracellular fluid, exhibits a "hydrated layer" (Fig. 10). Ions in this layer are very labile and reactive, and constitute the non-apatitic domain, surrounding the relatively inert and more stable apatite domain of the bone crystal (Cazalbou et al., 2004; Termine et al., 1973). Newly deposited bone mineral contains many labile non-apatitic domains [HPO_4, PO_4, and CO_3], located in the

well-developed hydrated layer involved in the high surface reactivity of mineral (Cazalbou et al., 2004). Labile PO_4 and CO_3 groups are easily and reversibly exchangeable with other ions in the hydrated layer. During maturation, the decrease in labile non-apatitic environments is associated with an increase in stable apatitic environments (Cazalbou et al., 2004). A particularity of the bone mineral is its non-stoichiometry, leading to the presence of numerous vacancies in the apatite crystal. Consequently, bone crystal is mainly maintained by electrostatic cohesion, thus bone crystals are easily soluble relative to stoichiometric apatite (Barry et al., 2002) . As bone becomes more mature, both the size and number of crystals increase.

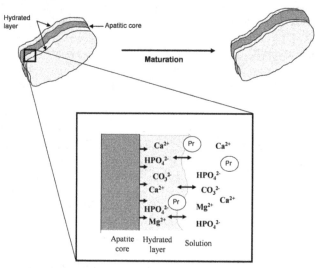

Fig. 10. Evolution of the hydrated layer and apatite core from bone crystal. During the maturation and growth of the crystal, the hydrated layer, involved in a high surface reactivity, progressively decreases and led to a stable apatitic domain. The structure of the hydrated layer constitutes a pool of loosely bound ions which can be incorporated in the growing apatite domains and can be exchanged by foreign ions in the solution and charged groups of proteins (Pr) (Adapted from Rey et al., 2009).

During mineral maturation, the hydrated layer decreases while the stable apatite domain grow, corresponding to the evolution of non-apatitic environments into apatitic environments detected by Fourier Transform InfraRed spectroscopy (FTIR). This hydrated layer, different from a hydration layer (Stern double layer), corresponds to the mode of formation of apatite crystals in physiologic conditions. The existence of these two domains (hydrated layer and apatite core) in biomimetic nanocrystals, has been recently confirmed by solid-state NMR (Jager et al., 2006). The hydrated surface layer contains loosely bound ions, which are easily exchangeable, and determine the surface properties of the nanocrystalline apatites (Cazalbou et al., 2004; Termine et al., 1973). In bone, those loosely bound ions can be also exchanged with charged groups of proteins present in collagen and non-collagenous proteins. The role of charged proteins on mineralization is well known (Boskey et al, 1989, 1998; Boskey 1989; Georges & Veis 2008; Landis et al., 1993; Malaval et al., 2008; Traub et al., 1992).

4.5 Measurement of mineral crystallinity

Crystallinity is defined as the degree of structural order in a crystal. The atoms in the crystal are arranged in a regular and periodic manner. The referent method to measure *absolute crystallinity* is the X-rays diffraction, and is based on the elastic scattering of the X-rays. This technique can be used to determine the crystal structure (Le Bail & Loüer 1978; Rietveld 1969) or chemical composition of a sample through the power diffraction bank data file (Powder diffraction file). The WAXS (wide angle X-rays scattering) is based on scattering angles 2θ larger than $5°$, and SAXS (small X-ray scattering) gives informations on angles 2θ close to $0°$. This method gives informations on the size, strain and orientation of crystals. A peak broadening can be due the small crystal size or microstrains. The crystal size can be determined by the *Scherrer* equation.

Vibrational spectroscopy techniques, such as Fourier Transform InfraRed Spectroscopy (FTIRS), Synchrotron InfraRed or Raman Spectroscopy, have been extensively used to study calcified tissues (Ager et al., 2005; Akkus et al., 2003; Boskey et al., 2005; Cazalbou et al., 2004; Farlay et al., 2010b; LeGeros 1981; Miller et al., 2001; Paschalis et al., 1996; Pleshko et al., 1991; Rey et al., 1990, 1991). Spectroscopic techniques allow assessment of physicochemical modifications of mineral induced by mechanical tests (Ager et al., 2005; Akkus et al., 2003; Carden et al., 2003; Morris & Mandair 2011; Tarnowski et al., 2004), age-related modifications (Ager et al., 2005; Akkus et al., 2003; Miller et al., 2007), and pathologic or treatment-related changes (Boskey et al., 2005; Carden & Morris 2000; Fratzl 2004; Huang et al., 2003; Siris et al., 2004). The application of Fourier Transform InfraRed Microspectroscopy and Imaging (FTIRM, FTIRI) for bone allows in situ analysis of embedded bone samples at the BSU level. These techniques are based on the vibrations of the atoms of a molecule and give complementary informations. The functional groups present in the sample absorb infrared light (or scatter light for Raman) at different wavelengths. In bone, infrared and Raman spectroscopies were used to obtain information on bone mineral and organic matrix, the two major components of bone. The main advantage of these techniques is that they can be used on embedded bone biopsies, on thin sections (2μm-thick MMA sections), keeping the integrity of the bone microarchitecture. By infrared spectroscopy, different vibrations can be analyzed in bone mineral: the phosphate mode vibrations with the $v_1v_3PO_4$ corresponding to an antisymmetric stretch, the v_4PO_4 (bending stretch), the carbonate vibrations v_2CO_3 and v_3CO3. Organic matrix can be analyzed through the Amides I, II and III vibrations. Different parameters can be deduced from these vibrations, as the mineral maturity, crystallinity, carbonate substitution, mineral to matrix ratio, providing informations on bone mineral quality (Boskey et al., 1998, 2005; Miller et al., 2007; Paschalis et al., 1996, 1997a; 1997b; Paschalis & Mendelsohn 2000, Pleshko et al., 1991, Rey et al., 1989, 1995a). By Raman spectroscopy, crystallinity, carbonate type B substitution, and mineral to matrix ratio can be determined (Akkus et al., 2003; Morris & Mandair 2011).

Others techniques as vibrational methods have been extensively used to obtain informations on the structural and compound identification, especially on the relative crystallinity (also called crystallinity index).

4.6 Maturity and crystallinity of bone crystals

As mentioned previously, with maturation, stable apatitic domains grow, whereas hydrated layer decreases. Thus, when bone crystals mature, their crystallinity also increases. These two variables can be assessed separately in infrared spectroscopy (Fig.11). Mineral maturity and mineral crystallinity are two parameters temporally linked and often well correlated in synthetic apatite. The ratio 1030/1020 cm⁻¹ (apatitic phosphate over non apatitic phosphate, v_3PO_4 vibration) was well correlated in synthetic apatites to the crystallinity measured by XRD, and it was established that the ratio 1030/1020 cm⁻¹ was an index of mineral maturity/crystallinity. From that, mineral maturity and crystallinity were associated in a lot of studies (Boskey et al., 2005; Paschalis et al., 1996, 1997a, 1997b). We have defined a new ratio to assess mineral maturity, the 1030/1110 cm⁻¹, (apatitic phosphate over non apatitic phosphate, v_3PO_4 vibration) equivalent to the 1030/1020 cm⁻¹ but more sensitive (Farlay et al., 2010b). We agree with the fact that the 1020/1030 cm⁻¹ ratio, which is an index of mineral maturity, evolves simultaneously with crystallinity in synthetic samples or normal bone. However, by definition, those two parameters are different, as mineral maturity corresponds to a stage of maturation, and crystallinity corresponds to the organization of the apatite lattice. We have defined a new mineral crystallinity index, measured by FTIRM on the peak 604 cm⁻¹ (bending vibration of phosphates) (Farlay et al., 2010b). This vibration is often inaccessible for microscopic infrared imaging, due to the cut-off of the detector. A wide band detector allows the access to this vibration and we have shown that the value of the full width at half maximum of the 604 cm⁻¹ peak, was inversely correlated to the crystallinity (Farlay et al., 2010b). This crystallinity index is well correlated, on the same samples, with another crystallinity index measured on the same vibration, the Shemesh ratio (Shemesh 1990) which is itself derived from the splitting factor of Termine & Posner, 1966. In human bone, it has been shown that those two parameters could evolve separately, and thus can independently affect the mineral characteristics. Indeed, mineral maturity can be affected by modification of bone remodeling (and by formative or antiresorptive treatments), whereas crystallinity can be influenced by ionic substitutions. This was verified in bone samples from patients with skeletal fluorosis (Farlay et al., 2010b). Skeletal fluorosis is a pathology caused by an excessive consumption of fluoride, and characterized by ionic substitution of hydroxyl ions by fluoride ions in bone mineral. In these samples, mineral maturity was decreased, due to a stimulation of osteoblasts on bone formation by fluoride, but crystallinity was increased due to the substitution of OH⁻ by F⁻.

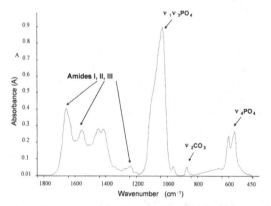

Fig. 11. Infrared spectra of human cortical bone (iliac bone) showing the mineral ($v_1v_3PO_4$, v_4PO_4,v_2CO_3) and the organic (amides) vibrations (INSERM UMR 1033).

In the study previously mentioned for determining the chronology of secondary mineralization on ewes (Bala et al., 2010), it has been shown that kinetic of mineral maturity was very close to the kinetic of the degree of mineralization, whereas the crystallinity index was biphasic, showing a rapid increase for the six first months, then stabilizing until 18 months, and showing another increase toward highest values after 24 months (Fig.12). In another study performed in women long term-treated by bisphosphonates, an increase in mineral maturity was observed, associated with a decrease in crystallinity, reinforcing the statement that mineral maturity and crystallinity have to be cautiously separately analyzed (Bala et al., 2011).

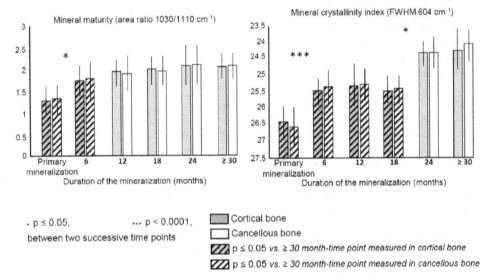

Fig. 12. Histograms showing (left) the rapid increase of mineral maturity during the 6 first months of mineralization, followed by a slowdown and stabilization; (right) the biphasic evolution of mineral crystallinity index, with an increase the 6 first months, a stabilization, and then a resumption at 18 months (Reprinted from Bala et al., 2010, with permission from Elsevier).

Finally, in a study on 53 human vertebrae, it was shown that with age of donor, crystallinity was increased and mineral maturity unchanged (Farlay et al., 2010a). This increase in crystallinity was previously shown in osteoporotic bone (Boskey, 2003), suggesting that with aging, an increase in crystal size/perfection occurs, independently of the bone remodeling (Farlay et al., 2010a).

4.7 Carbonates in bone mineral

In bone mineral, carbonates ions represent about 6-7% of the total mineral ions, thus a non negligible proportion. CO_3^{2-} can be incorporated into bone mineral by substitution in the apatite lattice either to PO_4^{3-} (major site, type-B carbonate) or to OH^- (minor site, type-A carbonate). A third site of CO_3^{2-} ions corresponds to labile carbonates which decrease with the maturation of the apatite crystal (Rey et al., 1989, 1991). The carbonates decrease the regularity of the atomic arrangement in hydroxyapatite (Blumenthal et al., 1975), thus altering the crystallinity. CO_3^{2-} determine physical properties of materials, or biological behavior of cells in scaffold or ceramics. The CO_3^{2-} A/B ratio is very constant among different species, suggesting that CO_3^{2-} incorporation in bone is a highly regulated process. Carbonates are also important for mineral dissolution (LeGeros 1981). It is well-established in literature that, in synthetic apatites, CO_3^{2-} content increases with time of maturation (Cazalbou et al., 2004b; LeGeros & LeGeros 1983; LeGeros et al., 1968; Rey et al., 1989, 1995a). However, in bone, there is a controversy with some studies showing an increase of CO_3/PO_4 with mineral maturation (Petra et al., 2005) or a decrease (Farlay et al., 2006; Ou-Yang et al., 2001; Paschalis et al., 1996). In very young bone, labile carbonates and HPO_4 are high, and progressively decreased with time of maturation, this being associated with an increase in mineral crystallinity (Magne et al., 2001). The amount of carbonate ions can be measured by different methods (chemical dosage, thermogravimetric analysis, vibrational spectroscopies…). In infrared spectroscopy, carbonate content is generally determined using the v_2CO_3 line (out-of-plane bending vibration) which is free of contribution of amide vibrations, and was generally calculated as CO_3/PO_4 area ratio. The role of carbonate in bone mineral is not entirely elucidated. The hypothesis of Wopenka and Pasteris is that carbonate could control bone crystal size, and that high concentration of carbonate could play an important role in constraining bone crystals to the nanometer scale (Wopenka & Pasteris 2005). Indeed, dentin, in which the amount of carbonate concentration is the same than in bone, has also a crystal size similar to bone. However, enamel crystals, which are very much larger size, have only about half the carbonate concentration as bone does.

5. Modifications of bone mineral characteristics with age or in post-menopausal osteoporosis

Bone loss occurs in all individuals after middle life. This bone loss can be moderated (osteopenia), or can become more important (osteoporosis). Osteoporosis is a metabolic bone disease, leading to a decrease in the amount of mineralized bone and an increase in the risk of fracture. In post menopausal osteoporosis, the oestrogen deficiency lead to an acceleration of bone remodeling, the balance between resorption and formation is disturbed in favour of resorption. This lead to a decrease in the more mineralized bone, which is only partially replaced by young less mineralized bone, reducing material stiffness.

5.1 Modifications of bone mineral at tissue level

Several studies performed in bone from osteoporotic women have shown not only that bone mass is decreased but that the bone mineral content was decreased, due to the fact the newly formed BSUs have not the time to achieve their mineralization before to be resorbed. Thus the mean age of matrix is decreased, leading to a decrease to the mean degree of mineralization.

5.1.1 Degree of mineralization (DMB) in control humans (Boivin et al., 2008)

Bone samples from persons of both sexes (sudden died and without known pathology) were studied. This control group was composed of iliac bone samples taken at necropsy form 30 women (aged 48.4 ± 3.7 years; range 20-93 years) and 13 men (aged 66.0 ± 4.4 years; range 43-86 years). The mean DMB expressed in g mineral/cm^3 (mean $\pm$ SEM) was 1.082 ± 0.017 in cortical bone and 1.099 ± 0.018 in cancellous bone (Figure 13).

In iliac crests, no significant influence of sex or age on the mean DMB was observed (Boivin et al., 2008). In cancellous bone, another study by qBEI showed the absence of influence of sex, age, ethnicity or skeletal sites in BMDD measurements (≈22% in w% Ca) (Roschger et al., 2003). A recent study on vertebral bone of 53 donors (age range: 54-95 year-old, 21 men, 27 women) showed no influence of sex and age on the DMB (Follet et al., 2010).

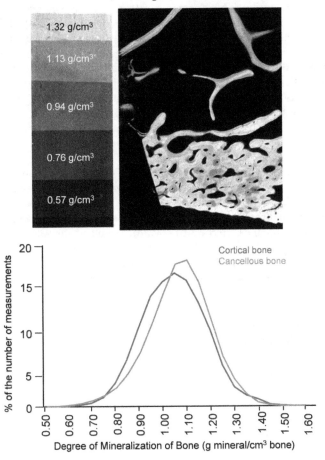

Fig. 13. Quantitative microradiography: (top) aluminium step wedge and microradiograph of bone tissue. (bottom) Distribution of the degrees of mineralization in human iliac bone (INSERM UMR 1033).

5.1.2 Bone mineralization at tissue level in bone of post-menopausal women treated with anti-osteoporotic treatments

In adult bone, the DMB, i.e., the bone mineral density at the tissue level depends on the rate of remodeling. Thus, agents (parathyroid hormone) or events (menopause, ovariectomy) which provoke an augmentation in the « birthrate » or activation frequency of Basic Multicellular Units (BMUs), induce a decrease of the « lifespan » of BSUs, in other words on the time available for the secondary mineralization. This leads to the fact that new BSUs are resorbed before they have fully completed their secondary mineralization, as proven by the presence of a large amount of uncompletely mineralized BSUs and a low mean DMB (Arlot et al., 2005; Boivin & Meunier 2003; Misof et al., 2003). In a study on men and women with idiopathic osteoporosis, a decrease in DMB was observed compared to controls (-7%) (Boivin et al., 2008). However, a decrease in heterogeneity index of mineralization was observed in this study, indicating a homogeneization of the mineralization. This decrease is also accompanied, in men only, by a decrease in microhardness (-10%) (Boivin et al., 2008). However, it is important to mention that, both in control or osteoporotic bone, no variation in DMB or microhardness was correlated with age. Conversely, antiresorptive agents (bisphosphonates, calcitonin, estrogen, SERMs) which cause a marked reduction in the « birthrate » of BMUs, prolong the « lifespan » of the BSUs, allowing a more complete secondary mineralization and an increase of DMB (Bala et al., 2011a, 2011b; Boivin et al., 2000, 2003; Borah et al., 2005, 2006). A dissociating agent (Strontium Ranelate), acting both on resorption and formation, is now used in the treatment of post-menopausal osteoporosis (Meunier et al., 2004; Reginster et al., 2005). After short- and long-term treatment, the DMB was not significantly different from the physiological range (Boivin et al., 2010; Doublier et al., 2011a). Recently, also with a microradiographic method, it has been shown, in hip-fracture patients, an increase in DMB heterogeneity in both interstitial and osteons compared to controls (Bousson et al., 2011). Thus, some differences exist, considering osteoporotic or hip-fractures cases, in term of heterogeneity of mineralization.

The mineralization index measured by FTIRM, calculated as the ratio of $v_1v_3PO_4$/amide I vibration (Paschalis et al., 1996) is a relative index which has been correlated to ash content (Faibish et al., 2005) and DMB (Farlay et al., unpublished data). The mineralization index (or mineral to matrix ratio) has been shown to be higher in bone of post menopausal woman treated with alendronate (Boskey et al., 2009).

5.2 Modifications of bone crystal characteristics

Concerning crystal characteristics, it has been shown, by XRD technique that, with age, there was an increase in crystal size. In 117 iliac bone samples (range of age: 0-90 years), there was an increase, between 0-30 years, in crystallinity in c-axis, corresponding to the crystal length, and a decrease in the a axis (Hanschin & Stern 1995). After 30 years, modifications were less evident, only a slight increase in crystallinity within the basal plane was observed.

Modifications of bone crystal size impaired mechanical characteristic of bone. Indeed, it was observed that the bones of older animals or that osteoporotic bone, two cases in which bone fractures easily, contained more large crystals than normal (Boskey 2003). Conversely, young animals, which have mechanically strong bones, have a mixture of small and large crystals. In a recent study performed by Raman microspectroscopy in human femurs (age range: 52-85 years old), an overall reduction in heterogeneity of mineralization, crystallinity, and type-B carbonation was observed (Yerramshetty et al., 2006). In this study, bone became more mineralized and more highly type-B carbonated with age, whereas crystallinity was unchanged. In a study performed by FTIRM on 53 human vertebrae (range of age: 54-93 years), a significant increase in crystallinity was observed (Farlay et al., 2010a). This means that, in vertebrae, either crystal size or crystal perfection is increased. In those vertebrae, the bone volume was also significantly decreased. The reason of the increase in crystallinity is unclear, but it is possible that it corresponds to a mechanism of adaptation of bone, in order to compensate the bone loss due to age. In the same study, a decrease in CO_3/PO_4 ratio was observed suggesting an alteration of the physico-chemical composition of bone mineral with age. Thus, comparing the results obtained in human femora and vertebrae in term of physico-chemical composition, some differences appears. However, the techniques were different (FTIR and Raman microspectroscopies), and the bones were not extracted from the same donors.

6. Perspectives and conclusion

Different factors increase the risk of fracture, independent of bone mineral density. Among these factors, bone mineral features are important in determining some mechanical behavior, especially elastic properties. Besides the decrease in bone mineral volume occurring with age, the alteration of mineral quality plays also a major role in bone fragility. The study of bone mineral quality is a instrumental challenge, due to [1] the dimension and the nature itself of crystal apatite (nanocrystalline), [2] the fact that bone is a composite material (organic matrix intimately linked to bone mineral), and [3] because bone is a complex tissue with different levels of organization (organ, BSU, crystal).

Thus, the using of different complementary techniques (spectroscopic, diffraction, electron microscopy techniques) has been very useful in the comprehension of bone mineral structure the last 50 years. Despite very important findings, there are still lacks in the understanding of the role of certain ions (minor or trace elements) in the biological or biomechanical properties (such as carbonates, strontium ions etc.).

Bone is a fascinating tissue governed by the remodeling activity and the plasma composition. It underlies several characteristics which are interdependent. For example, carbonate ions substitutions into apatite promote the platelet-shape in bone crystals rather than needle-shape found in enamel. But the presence of carbonates, moreover, as mentioned previously, inhibits the incorporation of OH^- in bone apatite. Thus, the study of correlations between different variables is still indispensable to understand the relationship between physicochemical and mechanical properties.

From the previous studies performed on bone mineral, it seems that a small crystal size associated with a heterogeneity of crystal size (nanometer size-scale) is important to an optimal mechanical strength. Indeed, the presence of too large crystal is not good for bone strength. Fluoride, as mentioned previously, induces the formation of large crystals, and the formation of a "brittle" bone, despite a high BMD. Moreover, concerning mineralization and its heterogeneity at the tissue level, values comprised between 0.8 and 1.30 g/cm^3 of bone could be a great deal to maintain stiffness of the bone. The preservation of mineralization heterogeneity is necessary for bone mechanical strength, allowing, for example, the stopping of microcracks propagation. No modification in degree of mineralization is observed with age or sex, but some differences exist in hip- fracture or osteoporotic cases. Thus a modification in the calcium absorption or an increase in the bone remodeling can lead to a decrease to the degree of mineralization. Differences also exist in studies in degree of mineralization due to the fact that either weight or non-weight-bearing bones are analyzed. We have an ongoing study on these different types of bone (weight or non-weight-bearing bones) in a same donor, in order to analyze the structural and mechanical bone mineral properties.

In conclusion, despite a lot of studies have permitted to understand the characteristics of bone mineral, further studies are needed to clarify the mechanisms of bone fragility at the different levels of investigation.

7. Acknowledgments

The authors gratefully acknowledge Christian Rey, Yohann Bala, Gérard Panczer, Baptiste Depalle, Audrey Doublier, Hélène Follet, Pascale Chavassieux and Pierre Jean Meunier for their collaboration to the major studies referenced in the present chapter.

8. References

Ager, J. W.; Nalla, R. K.; Breeden, K. L. & Ritchie, R. O. (2005). Deep-ultraviolet Raman spectroscopy study of the effect of aging on human cortical bone. *J Biomed Opt*, Vol.10, No.3, pp. 034012.

Akkus, O.; Polyakova-Akkus, A.; Adar, F. & Schaffler, M. B. (2003). Aging of microstructural compartments in human compact bone. *J Bone Miner Res*, Vol.18, No.6, pp. 1012-1019.

Ammann, P. & Rizzoli, R. (2003). Bone strength and its determinants. *Osteoporos Int*, Vol.14 Suppl 3, pp. S13-18.

Amprino, R. (1958). Investigations on some physical properties of bone tissue. *Acta Anat (Basel)*, Vol.34, No.3, pp. 161-186.

Arlot, M. ; Meunier, P. J. ; Boivin, G.; Haddock, L.; Tamayo, J.; Correa-Rotter, R.; Jasqui, S.; Donley, D. W.; Dalsky, G. P.; Martin, J. S. & Eriksen, E. F. (2005). Differential effects of teriparatide and alendronate on bone remodeling in postmenopausal women assessed by histomorphometric parameters. *J Bone Miner Res*, Vol.20, No.7, pp. 1244-1253.

Bala, Y.; Depalle, B.; Douillard, T.; Meille, S.; Clément, P.; Follet, H.; Chevalier, J. & Boivin, G. (2011b). Respective roles of organic and mineral components of human cortical bone matrix in micromechanical behavior: An instrumented indentation study. *J Mech behav biomed materials*, Vol.4, pp. 1473-1482.

Bala, Y.; Farlay, D.; Chapurlat, R. & Boivin, G. (2011a). Modifications of bone material properties in postmenopausal osteoporotic women long-term treated with alendronate. *Eur J Endocrinol*, Vol 165, No. 4, pp. 647-655

Bala, Y.; Farlay, D.; Delmas, P. D.; Meunier, P. J. & Boivin, G. (2010). Time sequence of secondary mineralization and microhardness in cortical and cancellous bone from ewes. *Bone*, Vol.46, No.4, pp. 1204-1212. Copyright (2011), with permission from Elsevier.

Balena, R.; Kleerekoper, M.; Foldes, J. A.; Shih, M. S.; Rao, D. S.; Schober, H. C. & Parfitt, A. M. (1998). Effects of different regimens of sodium fluoride treatment for osteoporosis on the structure, remodeling and mineralization of bone. *Osteoporos Int*, Vol.8, No.5, pp. 428-435.

Barry, A. B.; Baig, A. A.; Miller, S. C. & Higuchi, W. I. (2002). Effect of age on rat bone solubility and crystallinity. *Calcif Tissue Int*, Vol.71, No.2, pp. 167-171.

Bertinetti, L.; Drouet, C.; Combes, C.; Rey, C.; Tampieri, A.; Coluccia, S. & Martra, G. (2009). Surface characteristics of nanocrystalline apatites: effect of mg surface enrichment on morphology, surface hydration species & cationic environments. *Langmuir*, Vol.25, No.10, pp. 5647-5654.

Bigi, A.; Foresti, E.; Gregorini, R.; Ripamonti, A.; Roveri, N. & Shah, J. S. (1992). The role of magnesium on the structure of biological apatites. *Calcif Tissue Int*, Vol.50, No.5, pp. 439-444.

Blumenthal, N. (1990). The in vitro uptake of trace elements by hydroxyapatite. *In: Priest ND, Van de Vyver FL (eds) Trace Metals and Fluoride in Bones and Teeth*. Vol.CRC Press, Boca Raton, pp. 307-313.

Blumenthal, N. C.; Betts, F. & Posner, A. S. (1975). Effect of carbonate and biological macromolecules on formation and properties of hydroxyapatite. *Calcif Tissue Res*, Vol.18, No.2, pp. 81-90.

Blumenthal, N. C.; Betts, F. & Posner, A. S. (1977). Stabilization of amorphous calcium phosphate by Mg and ATP. *Calcif Tissue Res*, Vol.23, No.3, pp. 245-250.

Blumenthal, N. C. & Posner, A. S. (1984). In vitro model of aluminum-induced osteomalacia: inhibition of hydroxyapatite formation and growth. *Calcif Tissue Int*, Vol.36, No.4, pp. 439-441.

Boivin, G.; Bala, Y.; Doublier, A.; Farlay, D.; Ste-Marie, L. G.; Meunier, P. J. & Delmas, P. D. (2008). The role of mineralization and organic matrix in the microhardness of bone tissue from controls and osteoporotic patients. *Bone*, Vol.43, No.3, pp. 532-538.

Boivin, G.; Farlay, D.; Khebbab, M. T.; Jaurand, X.; Delmas, P. D. & Meunier, P. J. (2010). In osteoporotic women treated with strontium ranelate, strontium is located in bone formed during treatment with a maintained degree of mineralization. *Osteoporos Int*, Vol.21, No.4, pp. 667-677.

Boivin, G.; Lips, P.; Ott, S. M.; Harper, K. D.; Sarkar, S.; Pinette, K. V. & Meunier, P. J. (2003). Contribution of raloxifene and calcium and vitamin D3 supplementation to the increase of the degree of mineralization of bone in postmenopausal women. *J Clin Endocrinol Metab*, Vol.88, No.9, pp. 4199-4205.

Boivin, G. & Meunier, P. J. (2002). The degree of mineralization of bone tissue measured by computerized quantitative contact microradiography. *Calcif Tissue Int*, Vol.70, No.6, pp. 503-511.

Boivin, G. & Meunier, P. J. (2003). Methodological considerations in measurement of bone mineral content. *Osteoporos Int*, Vol.14 Suppl 5, pp. S22-7; discussion S27-28.

Boivin, G. Y.; Chavassieux, P. M.; Santora, A. C.; Yates, J. & Meunier, P. J. (2000). Alendronate increases bone strength by increasing the mean degree of mineralization of bone tissue in osteoporotic women. *Bone*, Vol.27, No.5, pp. 687-694.

Borah, B.; Dufresne, T. E.; Ritman, E. L.; Jorgensen, S. M.; Liu, S.; Chmielewski, P. A.; Phipps, R. J.; Zhou, X.; Sibonga, J. D. & Turner, R. T. (2006). Long-term risedronate treatment normalizes mineralization and continues to preserve trabecular architecture: sequential triple biopsy studies with micro-computed tomography. *Bone*, Vol.39, No.2, pp. 345-352.

Borah, B.; Ritman, E. L.; Dufresne, T. E.; Jorgensen, S. M.; Liu, S.; Sacha, J.; Phipps, R. J. & Turner, R. T. (2005). The effect of risedronate on bone mineralization as measured by micro-computed tomography with synchrotron radiation: correlation to histomorphometric indices of turnover. *Bone*, Vol.37, No.1, pp. 1-9.

Boskey, A. (2003). Bone mineral crystal size. *Osteoporos Int*, Vol.14 Suppl 5, pp. S16-20; discussion S20-1.

Boskey, A.; Maresca, M. & Appel, J. (1989). The effects of noncollagenous matrix proteins on hydroxyapatite formation and proliferation in a collagen gel system. *Connect Tissue Res*, Vol.21, No.1-4, pp. 171-176; discussion 177-8.

Boskey, A. L. (1989). Noncollagenous matrix proteins and their role in mineralization. *Bone Miner*, Vol.6, No.2, pp. 111-123.

Boskey, A. L.; DiCarlo, E.; Paschalis, E.; West, P. & Mendelsohn, R. (2005). Comparison of mineral quality and quantity in iliac crest biopsies from high- and low-turnover osteoporosis: an FT-IR microspectroscopic investigation. *Osteoporos Int*, Vol.16, No.12, pp. 2031-2038.

Boskey, A. L.; Gadaleta, S.; Gundberg, C.; Doty, S. B.; Ducy, P. & Karsenty, G. (1998). Fourier transform infrared microspectroscopic analysis of bones of osteocalcin-deficient mice provides insight into the function of osteocalcin. *Bone*, Vol.23, No.3, pp. 187-196.

Boskey, A. L.; Rimnac, C. M.; Bansal, M.; Federman, M.; Lian, J. & Boyan, B. D. (1992). Effect of short-term hypomagnesemia on the chemical and mechanical properties of rat bone. *J Orthop Res*, Vol.10, No.6, pp. 774-783.

Boskey, A. L.; Spevak, L. & Weinstein, R. S. (2009). Spectroscopic markers of bone quality in alendronate-treated postmenopausal women. *Osteoporos Int*, Vol.20, No.5, pp. 793-800.

Bousson, V.; Bergot, C.; Wu, Y.; Jolivet, E.; Zhou, L. Q. & Laredo, J. D. (2011). Greater tissue mineralization heterogeneity in femoral neck cortex from hip-fractured females than controls. A microradiographic study. *Bone*, Vol.48, No.6, pp. 1252-1259.

Bouxsein, M. L. (2005). Determinants of skeletal fragility. *Best Pract Res Clin Rheumatol*, Vol.19, No.6, pp. 897-911.

Carden, A. & Morris, M. D. (2000). Application of vibrational spectroscopy to the study of mineralized tissues (review). *J Biomed Opt*, Vol.5, No.3, pp. 259-268.

Carden, A.; Rajachar, R. M.; Morris, M. D. & Kohn, D. H. (2003). Ultrastructural changes accompanying the mechanical deformation of bone tissue: a Raman imaging study. *Calcif Tissue Int*, Vol.72, No.2, pp. 166-175.

Carlstrom, D. (1954). Micro-hardness measurements on single haversian systems in bone. *Experientia*, Vol.10, No.4, pp. 171-172.

Cazalbou, S.; Combes, C.; Eichert, D. & Rey, C. (2004a). Adaptive physico-chemistry of bio(related calcium phosphates. *J Mater Chem*, Vol.14, pp. 2148-2153.

Cazalbou, S.; Combes, C.; Eichert, D.; Rey, C. & Glimcher, M. J. (2004b). Poorly crystalline apatites: evolution and maturation in vitro and in vivo. *J Bone Miner Metab*, Vol.22, No.4, pp. 310-317.

Cho, G.; Wu, Y. & Ackerman, J. L. (2003). Detection of hydroxyl ions in bone mineral by solid-state NMR spectroscopy. *Science*, Vol.300, No.5622, pp. 1123-1127.

Currey, J. D. (2003). How well are bones designed to resist fracture? *J Bone Miner Res*, Vol.18, No.4, pp. 591-598.

Doublier, A.; Farlay, D.; Jaurand, X.; Vera, R. & Boivin, G. (2011b). Effects of strontium on the quality of bone apatite crystals. *33rd Annual meeting of American Society for Bone and Mineral Research, San Diego, California, USA, September 16-20, 2011.*

Doublier, A.; Farlay, D.; Khebbab, M. T.; Jaurand, X.; Meunier, P. J. & Boivin, G. (2011a). Distribution of Strontium and Mineralization in Iliac Bone Biopsies from Osteoporotic Women Long-Term Treated with Strontium Ranelate. *Eur J Endocrinol*, Vol 165, No 3, pp. 469-476.

Elliott, S. R. & Robinson, R. A. (1957). The water content of bone. I. The mass of water, inorganic crystals, organic matrix, and CO_2 space components in a unit volume of the dog bone. *J Bone Joint Surg Am*, Vol.39-A, No.1, pp. 167-88.

Faibish, D.; Gomes, A.; Boivin, G.; Binderman, I. & Boskey, A. (2005). Infrared imaging of calcified tissue in bone biopsies from adults with osteomalacia. *Bone*, Vol.36, No.1, pp. 6-12.

Farlay, D.; Bala, Y.; Burt-Pichat, B.; Chapurlat, R.; Boivin, G. & Follet, H. (2010a). Relationship Between Age, Mineral Characteristics, Mineralization, Microhardness, And Microcracks In Human Vertebral Trabecular Bone. *32nd annual meeting of American Society for Bone and Mineral Research*. Toronto, Canada, October 15-19, 2010.

Farlay, D.; Panczer, G.; Rey, C.; Delmas, P. D. & Boivin, G. (2006). New characteristics of bone mineral validated by infrared microspectroscopy. *28th annual meeting of American Society for Bone and Mineral Research*, Philadelphia, Pennsylvania, USA, September 19-22, 2006.

Farlay, D.; Panczer, G.; Rey, C.; Delmas, P. D. & Boivin, G. (2010b). Mineral maturity and crystallinity index are distinct characteristics of bone mineral. *J Bone Miner Metab*, Vol.28, No.4, pp. 433-445.

Follet, H.; Boivin, G.; Rumelhart, C. & Meunier, P. J. (2004). The degree of mineralization is a determinant of bone strength: a study on human calcanei. *Bone*, Vol.34, No.5, pp. 783-789.

Follet, H.; Viguet-Carrin, S.; Burt-Pichat, B.; Depalle, B.; Bala, Y.; Gineyts, E.; Munoz, F.; Arlot, M.; Boivin, G.; Chapurlat, R. D.; Delmas, P. D. & Bouxsein, M. L. (2010). Effects of preexisting microdamage, collagen cross-links, degree of mineralization, age, and architecture on compressive mechanical properties of elderly human vertebral trabecular bone. *J Orthop Res*, Vol.29, No.4, pp. 481-488.

Fratzl, P.; Fratzl-Zelman, N.; Klaushofer, K. (1993) Collagen packing and mineralization. An x-ray scattering investigation of turkey leg tendon. *Biophys J*, Vol.64, No 1, pp 260-266.

Fratzl, P.; Gupta, HS, Paschalis EP, Roschger P. (2004). Structure and mechanical quality of the mineral quality of the collagen-mineral nano-composite in bone. *J Mater Chem*, Vol.14, pp. 2115-2123.

Frost, H. M. (1969). Tetracycline-based histological analysis of bone remodeling. *Calcif Tissue Res*, Vol.3, No.3, pp. 211-237.

Fuchs, R. K.; Allen, M. R.; Ruppel, M. E.; Diab, T.; Phipps, R. J.; Miller, L. M. & Burr, D. B. (2008). In situ examination of the time-course for secondary mineralization of Haversian bone using synchrotron Fourier transform infrared microspectroscopy. *Matrix Biol*, Vol.27, No.1, pp. 34-41.

George, A. & Veis, A. (2008). Phosphorylated proteins and control over apatite nucleation, crystal growth, and inhibition. *Chem Rev*, Vol.108, No.11, pp. 4670-4693.

Glimcher, M. G. (1998). The nature of the mineral phase in bone: Biological and clinical implications. *Metabolic bone disease*, Vol.Chap. 2, pp. 23-50.

Glimcher, M. J. (2006). Bone: Nature of the calcium phosphate crystals and cellular, structural, and physical chemical mechanisms in their formation. . *Rev Mineral Geochem*, Vol.64, pp. 223-282.

Glimcher, M. J.; Hodge, A. J. & Schmitt, F. O. (1957). Macromolecular Aggregation States in Relation to Mineralization: the Collagen-Hydroxyapatite System as Studied in Vitro. *Proc Natl Acad Sci U S A*, Vol.43, No.10, pp. 860-867.

Glorieux, F. H.; Travers, R.; Taylor, A.; Bowen, J. R.; Rauch, F.; Norman, M. & Parfitt, A. M. (2000). Normative data for iliac bone histomorphometry in growing children. *Bone*, Vol.26, No.2, pp. 103-109.

Grynpas, M. D. & Marie, P. J. (1990). Effects of low doses of strontium on bone quality and quantity in rats. *Bone*, Vol.11, No.5, pp. 313-319.

Guggenbuhl, P.; Filmon, R.; Mabilleau, G.; Basle, M. F. & Chappard, D. (2008). Iron inhibits hydroxyapatite crystal growth in vitro. *Metabolism*, Vol.57, No.7, pp. 903-910.

Hanschin, R. G. & Stern, W. B. (1995). X-ray diffraction studies on the lattice perfection of human bone apatite (Crista iliaca). *Bone*, Vol.16, No.4 Suppl, pp. 355S-363S.

Höhling, H. L.; Barckhaus, R. H.; Krefting, E. R.; Althoff, J. & Quint, P. (1990). Collagen mineralization: Aspects of the structural relationships between collagen and the apatitic crystallites. *In "Ulltrastructure of skeletal tissues (E. Bonucci and P. M. Motta, Eds). Academic Press; San Diego.;* pp. 41-62.

Huang, R. Y.; Miller, L. M.; Carlson, C. S. & Chance, M. R. (2003). In situ chemistry of osteoporosis revealed by synchrotron infrared microspectroscopy. *Bone,* Vol.33, No.4, pp. 514-521.

Jager, C.; Welzel, T.; Meyer-Zaika, W. & Epple, M. (2006). A solid-state NMR investigation of the structure of nanocrystalline hydroxyapatite. *Magn Reson Chem,* Vol.44, No.6, pp. 573-580.

Jonsson, U.; Ranta, H. & Stromberg, L. (1985). Growth changes of collagen cross-linking, calcium, and water content in bone. *Arch Orthop Trauma Surg,* Vol.104, No.2, pp. 89-93.

Landis, W. J. (1995). The strength of a calcified tissue depends in part on the molecular structure and organization of its constituent mineral crystals in their organic matrix. *Bone,* Vol.16, No.5, pp. 533-544.

Landis, W. J.; Song, M. J.; Leith, A.; McEwen, L. & McEwen, B. F. (1993). Mineral and organic matrix interaction in normally calcifying tendon visualized in three dimensions by high-voltage electron microscopic tomography and graphic image reconstruction. *J Struct Biol,* Vol.110, No.1, pp. 39-54.

Le Bail, A. & Loüer, D. (1978). Smoothing and validity of crystallite size distributions from X-ray line prolfile analysis. *J Appl Crystallogr,* Vol.11, pp. 50-55.

Lees, S. (1987). Considerations regarding the structure of the mammalian mineralized osteoid from viewpoint of the generalized packing model. *Connect Tissue Res,* Vol.16, No.4, pp. 281-303.

LeGeros, R. Z. (1981). Apatites in biological systems. *Prog.Crystal Growth Charact.;* Vol.4, pp. 1-45.

LeGeros, R. Z.; Bonel, G. & Legros, R. (1978). Types of "H2O" in human enamel and in precipitated apatites. *Calcif Tissue Res,* Vol.26, No.2, pp. 111-118.

LeGeros, R. Z. & LeGeros, J. P. (1983). Carbonate analysis of synthetic mineral and biological apatites. *J Dent Res,* Vol.62, pp. 259.

LeGeros, R. Z.; Trautz, O. R.; Legeros, J. P. & Klein, E. (1968). Carbonate substitution in the apatitic structure. *Bull Soc Chim Fr,* Vol.4, pp. 1712-1718.

Li, C.; Paris, O.; Siegel, S.; Roschger, P.; Paschalis, E. P.; Klaushofer, K. & Fratzl, P. (2010a). Strontium is incorporated into mineral crystals only in newly formed bone during strontium ranelate treatment. *J Bone Miner Res,* Vol.25, No.5, pp. 968-975.

Li, X.; Hu, C.; Zhu, Y.; Sun, H.; Li, Y. & Zhang, Z. (2010b). Effects of Aluminum Exposure on Bone Mineral Density, Mineral & Trace Elements in Rats. *Biol Trace Elem Res.* doi 10.2007/s12011-010-8861-4.

Li, Z. Y.; Lam, W. M.; Yang, C.; Xu, B.; Ni, G. X.; Abbah, S. A.; Cheung, K. M.; Luk, K. D. & Lu, W. W. (2007). Chemical composition, crystal size and lattice structural changes after incorporation of strontium into biomimetic apatite. *Biomaterials,* Vol.28, No.7, pp. 1452-1460. Copyright (2011), with permission from Elsevier.

Loong, C. K.; Rey, C.; Kuhn, L. T.; Combes, C.; Wu, Y.; Chen, S. & Glimcher, M. J. (2000). Evidence of hydroxyl-ion deficiency in bone apatites: an inelastic neutron-scattering study. *Bone,* Vol.26, No.6, pp. 599-602.

Magne, D.; Pilet, P.; Weiss, P. & Daculsi, G. (2001). Fourier transform infrared microspectroscopic investigation of the maturation of nonstoichiometric apatites in mineralized tissues: a horse dentin study. *Bone,* Vol.29, No.6, pp. 547-552.

Malaval, L.; Wade-Gueye, N. M.; Boudiffa, M.; Fei, J.; Zirngibl, R.; Chen, F.; Laroche, N.; Roux, J. P.; Burt-Pichat, B.; Duboeuf, F.; Boivin, G.; Jurdic, P.; Lafage-Proust, M. H.; Amedee, J.; Vico, L.; Rossant, J. & Aubin, J. E. (2008). Bone sialoprotein plays a functional role in bone formation and osteoclastogenesis. *J Exp Med*, Vol.205, No.5, pp. 1145-1153.

Marie, P. J.; Hott, M.; Modrowski, D.; De Pollak, C.; Guillemain, J.; Deloffre, P. & Tsouderos, Y. (1993). An uncoupling agent containing strontium prevents bone loss by depressing bone resorption and maintaining bone formation in estrogen-deficient rats. *J Bone Miner Res*, Vol.8, No.5, pp. 607-615.

Meunier, P. J. & Boivin, G. (1997). Bone mineral density reflects bone mass but also the degree of mineralization of bone: therapeutic implications. *Bone*, Vol.21, No.5, pp. 373-377.

Meunier, P. J.; Roux, C.; Seeman, E.; Ortolani, S.; Badurski, J. E.; Spector, T. D.; Cannata, J.; Balogh, A.; Lemmel, E. M.; Pors-Nielsen, S.; Rizzoli, R.; Genant, H. K. & Reginster, J. Y. (2004). The effects of strontium ranelate on the risk of vertebral fracture in women with postmenopausal osteoporosis. *N Engl J Med*, Vol.350, No.5, pp. 459-468.

Miller, L. M.; Little, W.; Schirmer, A.; Sheik, F.; Busa, B. & Judex, S. (2007). Accretion of bone quantity and quality in the developing mouse skeleton. *J Bone Miner Res*, Vol.22, No.7, pp. 1037-1045.

Miller, L. M.; Vairavamurthy, V.; Chance, M. R.; Mendelsohn, R.; Paschalis, E. P.; Betts, F. & Boskey, A. L. (2001). In situ analysis of mineral content and crystallinity in bone using infrared micro-spectroscopy of the nu(4) PO(4)(3-) vibration. *Biochim Biophys Acta*, Vol.1527, No.1-2, pp. 11-19.

Misof, B. M.; Roschger, P.; Cosman, F.; Kurland, E. S.; Tesch, W.; Messmer, P.; Dempster, D. W.; Nieves, J.; Shane, E.; Fratzl, P.; Klaushofer, K.; Bilezikian, J. & Lindsay, R. (2003). Effects of intermittent parathyroid hormone administration on bone mineralization density in iliac crest biopsies from patients with osteoporosis: a paired study before and after treatment. *J Clin Endocrinol Metab*, Vol.88, No.3, pp. 1150-1156.

Morris, M. D. & Mandair, G. S. (2011). Raman assessment of bone quality. *Clin Orthop Relat Res*, Vol.469, No.8, pp. 2160-2169.

Mueller, K. H.; Trias, A. & Ray, R. D. (1966). Bone density and compostiton. Age-related and pathological changes in water and mineral content. *J Bone Joint Surg Am*, Vol.48, No.1, pp. 140-148.

Myllyharju, J. & Kivirikko, K. I. (2004). Collagens, modifying enzymes and their mutations in humans, flies and worms. *Trends Genet*, Vol.20, No.1, pp. 33-43.

Naito, A.; Tuzi, S. & Saito, H. (1994). A high-resolution 15N solid-state NMR study of collagen and related polypeptides. The effect of hydration on formation of interchain hydrogen bonds as the primary source of stability of the collagen-type triple helix. *Eur J Biochem*, Vol.224, No.2, pp. 729-734.

Nalla, R. K.; Kinney, J. H. & Ritchie, R. O. (2003). Mechanistic fracture criteria for the failure of human cortical bone. *Nat Mater*, Vol.2, No.3, pp. 164-168.

Nuzzo, S.; Peyrin, F.; Cloetens, P.; Baruchel, J. & Boivin, G. (2002). Quantification of the degree of mineralization of bone in three dimensions using synchrotron radiation microtomography. *Med Phys*, Vol.29, No.11, pp. 2672-2681.

Nyman, J. S.; Roy, A.; Shen, X.; Acuna, R. L.; Tyler, J. H. & Wang, X. (2006). The influence of water removal on the strength and toughness of cortical bone. *J Biomech*, Vol.39, No.5, pp. 931-938.

Oliver, W. & Pharr, G. (1992). An improved technique for determining hardness and elastic modulus using load and displacement sensing indentation experiments. *J Mater Res*, Vol.7, No.6, pp. 1564-1593.

Omelon, S.; Georgiou, J.; Henneman, Z. J.; Wise, L. M.; Sukhu, B.; Hunt, T.; Wynnyckyj, C.; Holmyard, D.; Bielecki, R. & Grynpas, M. D. (2009). Control of vertebrate skeletal mineralization by polyphosphates. *PLoS One*, Vol.4, No.5, e5634.

Ou-Yang, H.; Paschalis, E. P.; Mayo, W. E.; Boskey, A. L. & Mendelsohn, R. (2001). Infrared microscopic imaging of bone: spatial distribution of CO3(2-). *J Bone Miner Res*, Vol.16, No.5, pp. 893-900.

Oyen, M. L. (2006). Nanoindentation hardness of mineralized tissues. *J Biomech*, Vol.39, No.14, pp. 2699-2702.

Paschalis, E. P.; Betts, F.; DiCarlo, E.; Mendelsohn, R. & Boskey, A. L. (1997a). FTIR microspectroscopic analysis of human iliac crest biopsies from untreated osteoporotic bone. *Calcif Tissue Int*, Vol.61, No.6, pp. 487-492.

Paschalis, E. P.; Betts, F.; DiCarlo, E.; Mendelsohn, R. & Boskey, A. L. (1997b). FTIR microspectroscopic analysis of normal human cortical and trabecular bone. *Calcif Tissue Int*, Vol.61, No.6, pp. 480-486.

Paschalis, E. P.; DiCarlo, E.; Betts, F.; Sherman, P.; Mendelsohn, R. & Boskey, A. L. (1996). FTIR microspectroscopic analysis of human osteonal bone. *Calcif Tissue Int*, Vol.59, No.6, pp. 480-487.

Paschalis, E. P. & Mendelsohn, R. (2000). Variations in the individual thick lamellar properties within osteons by nanodentation. *Bone*, Vol.26, No.5, pp. 545-546.

Pasteris, J. D.; Wopenka, B.; Freeman, J. J.; Rogers, K.; Valsami-Jones, E.; van der Houwen, J. A. & Silva, M. J. (2004). Lack of OH in nanocrystalline apatite as a function of degree of atomic order: implications for bone and biomaterials. *Biomaterials*, Vol.25, No.2, pp. 229-238.

Petra, M.; Anastassopoulou, J.; Theologis, T. & Theophanides, T. (2005). Synchrotron micro-FT-IR spectroscopic evaluation of normal paediatric human bone. *J Molec Struct*, Vol.733, No.101-110.

Pleshko, N.; Boskey, A. & Mendelsohn, R. (1991). Novel infrared spectroscopic method for the determination of crystallinity of hydroxyapatite minerals. *Biophys J*, Vol.60, No.4, pp. 786-793.

Posner, A. (1985). The structure of bone apatite surfaces. *J Biomed Materials Res* Vol.19, pp. 241-250.

Posner, A. S. (1969). Crystal chemistry of bone mineral. *Physiological reviews*, Vol.69, No.4, pp. 760-787.

Powder diffraction file (PDF), I. C. f. D. D.; 12 campus blvd, Newton square, PA 19073-3273, USA, http://www.idd.com.

Rauch, F. & Glorieux, F. H. (2004). Osteogenesis imperfecta. *Lancet*, Vol.363, No.9418, pp. 1377-1385.

Reginster, J. Y.; Seeman, E.; De Vernejoul, M. C.; Adami, S.; Compston, J.; Phenekos, C.; Devogelaer, J. P.; Curiel, M. D.; Sawicki, A.; Goemaere, S.; Sorensen, O. H.; Felsenberg, D. & Meunier, P. J. (2005). Strontium ranelate reduces the risk of nonvertebral fractures in postmenopausal women with osteoporosis: Treatment of Peripheral Osteoporosis (TROPOS) study. *J Clin Endocrinol Metab*, Vol.90, No.5, pp. 2816-2822.

Rey, C.; Collins, B.; Goehl, T.; Dickson, I. R. & Glimcher, M. J. (1989). The carbonate environment in bone mineral: a resolution-enhanced Fourier Transform Infrared Spectroscopy Study. *Calcif Tissue Int*, Vol.45, No.3, pp. 157-164.

Rey, C.; Combes, C.; Drouet, C. & Glimcher, M. J. (2009). Bone mineral: update on chemical composition and structure. *Osteoporos Int*, Vol.20, No.6, pp. 1013-1021.

Rey, C.; Hina, A.; Tofighi, A.; Glimcher M.J. (1995a). Maturation of poorly crystalline apatites: chemical and structural aspects in vivo and in vitro. *Cells and Mater.*; Vol.5, pp. 345-356.

Rey, C.; Miquel, J. L.; Facchini, L.; Legrand, A. P. & Glimcher, M. J. (1995b). Hydroxyl groups in bone mineral. *Bone*, Vol.16, No.5, pp. 583-586.

Rey, C.; Renugopalakrishnan, V.; Shimizu, M.; Collins, B. & Glimcher, M. J. (1991). A resolution-enhanced Fourier transform infrared spectroscopic study of the environment of the CO3(2-) ion in the mineral phase of enamel during its formation and maturation. *Calcif Tissue Int*, Vol.49, No.4, pp. 259-268.

Rey, C.; Shimizu, M.; Collins, B. & Glimcher, M. J. (1990). Resolution-enhanced Fourier transform infrared spectroscopy study of the environment of phosphate ions in the early deposits of a solid phase of calcium-phosphate in bone and enamel, and their evolution with age. I: Investigations in the upsilon 4 PO4 domain. *Calcif Tissue Int*, Vol.46, No.6, pp. 384-394.

Rietveld, H. (1969). A profile refinement method for nuclear and magnetic structure. *J Appl Crystallogr*, Vol.2, pp. 65-71.

Riggs, C. M.; Lanyon, L. E. & Boyde, A. (1993). Functional associations between collagen fibre orientation and locomotor strain direction in cortical bone of the equine radius. *Anat Embryol (Berl)*, Vol.187, No.3, pp. 231-238.

Robinson, R. A. (1975). Physiocochemical structure of bone. *Clin Orthop Relat Res*, No.112, pp. 263-315.

Roschger, P.; Fratzl, P.; Eschberger, J. & Klaushofer, K. (1998). Validation of quantitative backscattered electron imaging for the measurement of mineral density distribution in human bone biopsies. *Bone*, Vol.23, No.4, pp. 319-326.

Roschger, P.; Gupta, H. S.; Berzlanovich, A.; Ittner, G.; Dempster, D. W.; Fratzl, P.; Cosman, F.; Parisien, M.; Lindsay, R.; Nieves, J. W. & Klaushofer, K. (2003). Constant mineralization density distribution in cancellous human bone. *Bone*, Vol.32, No.3, pp. 316-323.

Roschger, P.; Plenk, H.; Jr.; Klaushofer, K. & Eschberger, J. (1995). A new scanning electron microscopy approach to the quantification of bone mineral distribution: backscattered electron image grey-levels correlated to calcium K alpha-line intensities. *Scanning Microsc*, Vol.9, No.1, pp. 75-86; discussion 86-8.

Ruffoni, D.; Fratzl, P.; Roschger, P.; Klaushofer, K. & Weinkamer, R. (2007). The bone mineralization density distribution as a fingerprint of the mineralization process. *Bone*, Vol.40, No.5, pp. 1308-1319.

Saito, H.; Yokoi, M. (1992) A 13C NMR study on collagens in the solid state: hydration/dehydration-induced conformational change of collagen and detection of internal motions. *J Biochem*, Vol. 111, No 3, pp 376-382.

Saito, H.; Tabeta, R.; Shoji, A.; Ozaki, T.; Ando, I.; Miyata, T. (1984) A high-resolution 13C-NMR study of collagenlike polypeptides and collagen fibrils in solid state studied by the cross-polarization-magic angle-spinning method. Manifestation of conformation-dependent 13C chemical shifts and application to conformational characterization. *Biopolymers*, Vol. 23, pp 2279-2297.

Saito, M. & Marumo, K. (2010). Collagen cross-links as a determinant of bone quality: a possible explanation for bone fragility in aging, osteoporosis, and diabetes mellitus. *Osteoporos Int*, Vol.21, No.2, pp. 195-214.

Seeman, E. & Delmas, P. D. (2006). Bone quality--the material and structural basis of bone strength and fragility. *N Engl J Med*, Vol.354, No.21, pp. 2250-2261.

Shemesh, A. (1990). Crystallinity and diagenesis of sedimentary apatites. *Geochimica et Cosmochimica Acta*, Vol.54, No.9, pp. 2433-2438.

Siris, E. S.; Brenneman, S. K.; Miller, P. D.; Barrett-Connor, E.; Chen, Y. T.; Sherwood, L. M. & Abbott, T. A. (2004). Predictive value of low BMD for 1-year fracture outcomes is similar for postmenopausal women ages 50-64 and 65 and Older: results from the National Osteoporosis Risk Assessment (NORA). *J Bone Miner Res*, Vol.19, No.8, pp. 1215-1220.

Sornay-Rendu, E.; Munoz, F.; Garnero, P.; Duboeuf, F. & Delmas, P. D. (2005). Identification of osteopenic women at high risk of fracture: the OFELY study. *J Bone Miner Res*, Vol.20, No.10, pp. 1813-1819.

Tarnowski, C. P.; Ignelzi, M. A.; Jr.; Wang, W.; Taboas, J. M.; Goldstein, S. A. & Morris, M. D. (2004). Earliest mineral and matrix changes in force-induced musculoskeletal disease as revealed by Raman microspectroscopic imaging. *J Bone Miner Res*, Vol.19, No.1, pp. 64-71.

Termine, J. D.; Eanes, E. D.; Greenfield, D. J.; Nylen, M. U. & Harper, R. A. (1973). Hydrazine-deproteinated bone mineral. Physical and chemical properties. *Calcif Tissue Res*, Vol.12, No.1, pp. 73-90.

Termine, J. D. & Posner, A. S. (1966). Infra-red determinaion of the percentage of crystallinity in apatitic calcium phosphates. *Nature*, Vol.211, No.5046, pp. 268-270.

Traub, W.; Arad, T. & Weiner, S. (1992). Origin of mineral crystal growth in collagen fibrils. *Matrix*, Vol.12, No.4, pp. 251-255.

Turner, C. H. & Burr, D. B. (1993). Basic biomechanical measurements of bone: a tutorial. *Bone*, Vol.14, No.4, pp. 595-608. Copyright (2011), with permission from Elsevier.

Vedi, S.; Compston, J. E.; Webb, A. & Tighe, J. R. (1983). Histomorphometric analysis of dynamic parameters of trabecular bone formation in the iliac crest of normal British subjects. *Metab Bone Dis Relat Res*, Vol.5, No.2, pp. 69-74.

Viguet-Carrin, S.; Garnero, P. & Delmas, P. D. (2006). The role of collagen in bone strength. *Osteoporos Int*, Vol.17, No.3, pp. 319-336.

Weaver, J. K. (1966). The microscopic hardness of bone. *J Bone Joint Surg Am*, Vol.48, No.2, pp. 273-288.

Wopenka, B. & Pasteris, J. D. (2005). A mineralogical perpective on the apatite in bone. *Mater. Sci. Eng. C*, Vol.25, pp. 131-143.

Yerramshetty, J. S.; Lind, C. & Akkus, O. (2006). The compositional and physicochemical homogeneity of male femoral cortex increases after the sixth decade. *Bone*, Vol.39, No.6, pp. 1236-1243.

Zhu, P.; Xu, J.; Sahar, N.; Morris, MD., Kohn, DH., Ramamoorthy, A. (2009) Time-resolved dehydration-induced structural changes in an intact bovine cortical bone revealed by solid-state NMR spectroscopy. *J Am Chem Soc*, Vol.131, No 7, pp 17064-17065.

Part 2

Public Health Data of Osteoporosis

4

Prevalence of Back Pain in Postmenopausal Osteoporosis and Associations with Multiple Spinal Factors

Naohisa Miyakoshi, Michio Hongo and Yoichi Shimada
Department of Orthopedic Surgery, Akita University Graduate School of Medicine
Japan

1. Introduction

Back pain is considered to be most prevalent musculoskeletal pain, particularly in elderly populations (Woo et al., 2009). The existing literature suggests a prevalence of chronic back pain among the elderly ranging from 7% to 58% (Edmond & Felson, 2000; Jacobs et al., 2006; Lavsky-Shulan et al., 1985; March et al., 1998), with differences attributable to a lack of concordance in terms of age stratification, definition, and methodology, but with consistently much higher rates in women than men (Jabobs et al., 2006; Woo et al., 2009). The reason why back pain is common among elderly women may be related to osteoporosis. As lower bone mineral density (BMD) and the rapid decline in BMD following menopause in women result in a greater prevalence of osteoporosis and vertebral fractures compared to men, osteoporosis is likely to represent a major cause of back pain among elderly women. However, although osteoporosis may be an underlying cause of back pain, especially in postmenopausal elderly women, the prevalence of back pain in this group has not been fully investigated.

Although back pain in osteoporosis is often attributed to vertebral fractures (Nevitt et al., 1998; Ulivieri, 2007), the intensity of pain is not always influenced by fracture status (Hübscher et al., 2010). Liu-Ambrose et al. demonstrated that osteoporotic women may experience back pain without a concomitant history of vertebral compression fractures (Liu-Ambrose et al., 2002). The cause of back pain in osteoporosis thus seems likely to be related to multiple factors.

Spinal alignment and mobility are important factors for spinal function and may be related to back pain. Loss of lumbar lordosis correlates well with the incidence of chronic low back pain in adults (Djurasovic & Glassman, 2007; Glassman et al., 2005). Patients with a less mobile spine may show more severe symptoms. In addition, we have previously demonstrated that back extensor strength is significantly associated with spinal mobility (Miyakoshi et al., 2005). However, to the best of our knowledge, simultaneous assessment of back pain and multiple spinal factors such as vertebral fractures, spinal alignment and mobility, as well as back extensor strength, has not yet been investigated in patients with osteoporosis.

The objectives of this study were thus: 1) to determine the prevalence of back pain in patients with postmenopausal osteoporosis who visited their practitioner; and 2) to evaluate associations of back pain and vertebral fractures, spinal alignment, mobility, and back extensor strength in these patients.

2. Materials and methods

2.1 Patients

A total of 174 consecutive women with postmenopausal osteoporosis aged 50 years and older who visited their practitioner (orthopedic clinic) were enrolled in the present study. All these patients were the same patients who enrolled in our previous study assessing back extensor strength and quality of life (QOL) (Miyakoshi et al., 2007). Osteoporosis was diagnosed according to the criteria proposed by the Japanese Society for Bone and Mineral Research (JSBMR) (Orimo et al., 2001). Briefly, patients with BMD less than 70% of the young adult mean BMD or with fragility fracture were diagnosed as having osteoporosis. All participants were asked whether they had clinically relevant back pain, and BMD, number of vertebral fractures, angle of kyphosis, range of motion (ROM) of the thoracic and lumbar spine, and back extensor strength were evaluated. These variables were compared between subjects with back pain (BP group) and those without back pain (non-BP group). In the BP group, associations between intensity of back pain and other measured variables were further evaluated.

Exclusion criteria were as follows: 1) women with a history of metabolic bone disease, malignancy, or recent antiosteoporotic treatment (with exception of calcium); 2) patients with hip fracture; 3) patients who could not lie in a prone position; 4) chronic use of glucocorticoids; 5) a concomitant illness that would substantially influence the daily living (e.g., chronic pulmonary disease, asthma, angina, chronic congestive heart failure, stroke, blindness, etc.); 6) other diseases that might cause back pain (e.g., scoliosis, lumbar spondylolisthesis, lumbar disc disease, etc.); and 7) patients with documented vertebral fracture within the last 6 months. Patients enrolled in the present study thus showed chronic back pain that was not attributable to a fresh vertebral fracture.

2.2 Definition of clinically relevant back pain

Back pain was considered clinically relevant if the participant answered that pain had been moderately to severely bothersome, or if the participant needed any medical treatment (Miyakoshi et al., 2010; Nevitt et al., 1998). In this study, the definition of back was not limited to the narrow sense of the upper and middle back, and low back was also included, as patients with osteoporosis often complain of pain affecting both definitions and differentiating between these seems difficult (Satoh et al., 1988).

2.3 Evaluation of back pain intensity

Intensity of back pain was evaluated using the pain domain score of the Japanese Osteoporosis QOL Questionnaire (JOQOL) (Table 1) (Kumamoto et al., 2010; Takahashi et al., 2000); as all questions for this score are limited to back pain, all domain scores show significant correlations on test and retest (Kendall's τ = 0.691-0.818) (Kumamoto et al., 2010) and the score can be used as a continuous variable to evaluate correlations with other measured variables. The pain domain score of JOQOL contains 5 questions. Scores for each item range from 0 to 4, for a full score of 20. Pain intensity indicated in this study was calculated as 20 – estimated pain domain score of JOQOL. The pain intensity evaluated in this study thus ranged from 0 (no pain) to 20 (worst pain).

Question	Score (points)
How often have you had back or low back pain in the last week?	
Never	4
1. 1 day per week or less	3
2. 2-3 days per week	2
3. 4-6 days per week	1
4. Every day	0
If you have had back pain or low back pain, for how long did you have it in the daytime?	
1. No pain	4
2. 1-2 hours	3
3. 3-5 hours	2
4. 6-10 hours	1
5. All day	0
While you kept still, how severe was your back or low back pain?	
1. No pain	4
2. Mild	3
3. Moderate	2
4. Severe	1
5. Unbearable	0
When you moved, how severe was your back or low back pain?	
1. No pain	4
2. Mild	3
3. Moderate	2
4. Severe	1
5. Unbearable	0
Has the back or low back pain disturbed your sleep in the last week?	
1. Never	4
2. Once	3
3. Twice	2
4. Every other night	1
5. Almost every night	0
Total	20

*Reference from Kumamoto et al., 2010.

Table 1. Pain domain questions of the Japanese Osteoporosis Quality of Life Questionnaire (JOQOL)*

2.4 Evaluation of vertebral fractures

X-rays of the thoracic and lumbar spine in lateral views with the patient in a neutral/lateral decubitus position were taken with a film-tube distance of 1 m. Thoracic films were centered on T8, while lumbar films were centered on L3 (Miyakoshi et al., 2003b). Anterior, central, and posterior heights of each vertebral body from T4 to L5 were measured using calipers (Miyakoshi et al., 2003b). Coefficient of variation for this measurement was 2-3% (Orimo et al., 1994). Vertebral fracture was considered present if at least one of the three height measurements (anterior, middle, or posterior) of one vertebral body had decreased by more than 20% compared with the height of the nearest uncompressed vertebral body (Orimo et al., 1994).

2.5 Measurement of spinal kyphosis angles and ROMs
Angles of kyphosis and ROM of the thoracic (T1-T12) and lumbar (L1-L5) spine were measured using a device for computerized measurement of surface curvature (SpinalMouse®; Idiag, Volkerswill, Switzerland) in an upright position and at maximum flexion and extension (Kasukawa et al., 2010; Miyakoshi et al., 2005). Details regarding this device have been provided elsewhere (Post & Leferink, 2004). The device consists of a mobile unit of 2 rolling wheels interfacing with a base station through telemetry. By sliding the mobile unit along the spinal curvature, sagittal spinal alignment is calculated and displayed on the computer monitor. Repeating this process with the patient in flexion and extension of the spine allows measurement of ROM (Post & Leferink, 2004). SpinalMouse® delivers consistently reliable values for standing curvatures and ROM (Mannion et al., 2004; Post & Leferink, 2004). Post and Leferink (Post & Leferink, 2004) reported that interrater intraclass correlation coefficients (ICCs) for curvature measurement with SpinalMouse® were greater than 0.92. Mannion et al. (Mannion et al., 2004) reported that intrarater ICCs ranged from 0.82 to 0.83, while interrater ICCs ranged from 0.81 to 0.86. In addition, our previous studies have shown that thoracic and lumbar angles of kyphosis and spinal ROM measured using the SpinalMouse® correlate strongly with those measured on spinal radiography (r=0.804, r=0.863, and r=0.783, respectively; p<0.0001) (Miyakoshi et al., 2004).

2.6 Measurement of BMD
BMD was measured by dual-energy X-ray absorptiometry (QDR-4500; Hologic, Bedford, MA). Measurements were obtained from anteroposterior projections of the second to fourth lumbar vertebrae, the femoral neck, and the whole body. The coefficient of variation for these variables in 5 corresponding measurements from 5 normal volunteers was less than 1.5% (Miyakoshi et al., 2007).

2.7 Measurement of back extensor strength
Isometric back extensor strength in prone position was measured using a strain-gauge dynamometer (Digital Force Gauge DPU-1000N; IMADA, Toyohashi, Japan) as previously described (Hongo et al., 2007; Limburg et al., 1991; Miyakoshi et al., 2005). Subjects were allowed one warm-up trial, followed by three successive maximal effort trials separated by 60-s rest periods (Hongo et al., 2007). Maximal force among the three trials was selected and documented. Coefficient of variation for this measurement was 2.3% (Limburg et al., 1991).

2.8 Data analysis
All data are presented as mean and standard deviation (SD). Statistical analysis was performed using StatView version 5.0 software (Abacus Concepts, Berkeley, CA). Statistical

differences between groups were compared using an unpaired t-test. Logistic regression analysis was used for analyzing significant risk factors for back pain. Correlations between pain intensity and other measured variables were analyzed using Pearson's correlation coefficient and simple regression analysis. Further analyses using multiple regression were conducted to determine which variables best correlated with back pain. Values of P<0.05 were considered statistically significant.

3. Results

In this study, among 174 patients with postmenopausal osteoporosis, 159 patients (91.4%) complained of back pain. Mean values for age and measured variables in the BP and non-BP groups are listed in Table 2. No significant differences were apparent between BP and non-BP groups with regard to age, BMDs, number of vertebral fractures, angles of thoracic and lumbar kyphosis, and thoracic and lumbar ROMs. However, back extensor strength was significantly lower in the BP group than in the non-BP group. Similarly, when univariate logistic regression analysis was performed with the presence of back pain as a dependent variable and the other estimated variables as independent variables, only back extensor strength was identified as an index significantly associated with the presence of back pain (Table 3).

In patients with back pain, correlations between pain intensity and measured variables were evaluated. Pain intensity showed a significant positive correlation with the number of vertebral fractures, and negative correlations with lumbar spinal ROM and back extensor strength (Table 4). However, no significant correlations were observed between pain intensity and age, BMDs of all measured sites, angles of thoracic and lumbar kyphosis, or thoracic spinal ROM. Based on these results, number of vertebral fractures, lumbar spinal ROM, and back extensor strength were selected as independent variables for multiple regression modeling of pain intensity. Multiple regression analysis for pain intensity revealed lumbar spinal ROM and back extensor strength as significantly associated with pain intensity (Table 5).

	BP (n=159)	Non-BP (n=15)	P
Age (years)	67.8±6.5	65.5±7.0	0.1819
Lumbar spine BMD (g/cm²)	0.696±0.111	0.687±0.103	0.7757
Femoral neck BMD (g/cm²)	0.550±0.087	0.542±0.070	0.7105
Whole-body BMD (g/cm²)	0.818±0.075	0.812±0.047	0.7556
No. of vertebral fractures	1.2±1.7	0.3±0.5	0.0637
Thoracic kyphosis angle (degrees)	44.2±14.1	42.9±12.3	0.7326
Lumbar kyphosis angle (degrees)	-15.5±18.2	-23.7±16.8	0.0977
Thoracic spinal ROM (degrees)	17.5±12.8	19.7±19.7	0.5499
Lumbar spinal ROM (degrees)	51.3±17.6	57.3±14.6	0.2025
Back extensor strength (kg)	12.9±6.3	17.3±6.6	0.0130

Values represent mean ± SD. BP, patients with back pain; non-BP, patients without back pain; BMD, bone mineral density; ROM, range of motion.

Table 2. Comparison of estimated variables between osteoporotic patients with and without back pain.

	OR	95% CI	P
Age (years)	1.052	0.976-1.134	0.1845
Lumbar spine BMD (g/cm²)	2.044	0.015-269.925	0.7741
Femoral neck BMD (g/cm²)	3.289	0.006-1695.221	0.7086
Whole body BMD (g/cm²)	3.275	0.002-5461.831	0.7540
No. of vertebral fractures	2.107	0.949-4.680	0.0670
Thoracic kyphosis angle (degrees)	1.007	0.969-1.046	0.7308
Lumbar kyphosis angle (degrees)	1.033	0.994-1.074	0.0958
Thoracic spinal ROM (degrees)	0.988	0.951-1.027	0.5475
Lumbar spinal ROM (degrees)	0.980	0.951-1.011	0.2033
Back extensor strength (kg)	0.906	0.835-0.982	0.0166

OR, odds ratio; CI, confidence interval; BMD, bone mineral density; ROM, range of motion.

Table 3. Univariate logistic regression analysis for back pain in patients with osteoporosis (n=174).

	Correlation coefficient (r)	P
Age (years)	0.118	0.1391
Lumbar spine BMD (g/cm²)	-0.089	0.2643
Femoral neck BMD (g/cm²)	-0.090	0.2583
Whole body BMD (g/cm²)	-0.097	0.2258
No. of vertebral fractures	0.171	0.0312
Thoracic kyphosis angle (degree)	-0.043	0.5892
Lumbar kyphosis angle (degree)	0.139	0.0803
Thoracic spinal ROM (degree)	-0.109	0.1707
Lumbar spinal ROM (degree)	-0.264	0.0007
Back extensor strength (kg)	-0.268	0.0006

*Pain intensity ranged from 0 (no pain) to 20 (worst pain) was calculated from 20 minus estimated pain domain score of JOQOL. BMD, bone mineral density; ROM, range of motion.

Table 4. Correlations between pain intensity* and estimated variables in patients with osteoporosis and back pain (n=159).

	Coefficient (r)	P
Intercept	11.238	<0.0001
No. of vertebral fractures	0.132	0.4517
Lumbar spinal ROM (degrees)	-0.041	0.0179
Back extensor strength (kg)	-0.116	0.0142

*Pain intensity ranged from 0 (no pain) to 20 (worst pain), calculated as 20 minus the estimated pain domain score of JOQOL. ROM, range of motion.

Table 5. Multiple regression analysis for pain intensity* in patients with osteoporosis and back pain (n=159).

4. Discussion

4.1 Prevalence of back pain

Back pain is a major source of morbidity among patients with osteoporosis. Osteoporotic vertebral fractures usually cause acute, disabling, painful episodes at the fracture site. Such acute back pain subsides with fracture healing. However, after the fracture heals, the resulting increase in spinal kyphosis is likely to cause chronic back pain (Francis et al., 2008; Satoh et al., 1988). Increased spinal kyphosis is likely to induce abnormal stress on the supporting structures of the spinal column and may cause chronic back pain that usually develops while standing, walking, or doing other normal daily activities (Satoh et al., 1988). The back pain evaluated in the present study was considered to be chronic, because patients with documented vertebral fracture within the preceding 6 months were not included.

The prevalence of back pain, particularly chronic back pain, in patients with osteoporosis has not been fully investigated. Cockerill et al. (Cockerill et al., 2000) reported that the prevalence of back pain in the current and past year for women aged 50 years and over was significantly higher in women with single lumbar vertebral deformities (51.4% and 72.6%, respectively) than in women without vertebral deformity (39% and 60.6%, respectively) (p<0.05). Jacobs et al. (Jacobs et al., 2006) undertook a longitudinal study of 277 elderly subjects, finding that the prevalence of chronic back pain increased from 44% to 58% at ages 70 and 77 years, respectively, and this pain was associated with female sex at age 70 years and osteoporosis at age 77 years. More recently, Kuroda et al. (Kuroda et al., 2009) reported that back pain was observed in 28% of 818 Japanese postmenopausal women aged over 40 years (mean, 62.1 years) who visited their practitioner, and this back pain was associated with osteoporosis and vertebral fractures. In the present study, the prevalence of clinically relevant back pain was 91.4%. This percentage is higher than previously reported prevalences of back pain in osteoporosis (28-72.6%) (Cockerill et al., 2000; Jacobs et al., 2006; Kuroda et al., 2009), probably because all patients enrolled in the present study were visitors to an orthopedic clinic and might have had more musculoskeletal symptoms.

4.2 Factors associated with back pain and pain intensity

Previous studies have shown that vertebral fractures are associated with back pain and disability, with the strength of these associations increasing with the number and severity of fractures (Ettinger et al., 1992; Huang et al., 1996; Matthis et al., 1998). Increased spinal kyphosis caused by vertebral fractures is also known to induce back pain and disability in patients with osteoporosis (Miyakoshi et al., 2003a). In the present study, the number of vertebral fractures and angles of lumbar kyphosis tended to be higher in patients with back pain than in those without back pain, but no significant differences were identified (p=0.0637 and p=0.0977, respectively). However, in patients with back pain, the present study also showed a significant positive correlation between number of vertebral fractures and pain intensity (r=0.171, p=0.0312).

An important association between back pain and back extensor strength in patients with osteoporosis is indicated from the present study. Back extensor strength was significantly lower in patients with back pain compared to those without back pain, but other factors we evaluated showed no significant differences between groups. In addition, among patients with back pain, multiple regression analysis for pain intensity revealed back extensor strength and lumbar spinal ROM as significantly associated with pain intensity. Decreased back extensor strength may thus represent the most important factor contributing to back pain and pain intensity in patients with osteoporosis. Subjects on acute back pain due to fresh vertebral fractures maybe could not perform the back extensor strength tests as good as non-acute pain subjects. However, because the back pain evaluated in the present study was considered to be chronic, all the patients could perform the strength tests without increasing the pain. Thus, we concluded that the weakness of back extensor is a very important factor for chronic back pain in patients with osteoporosis.

Back extensor strength reportedly shows a significant relation with spinal mobility (Miyakoshi et al., 2005), and decreased mobility of the spine is thought to lead to increased kyphosis and weakness of the paravertebral muscles, as well as the development of impaired physical function (Burger et al., 1997). Decreased back extensor strength may thus reduce mobility of the lumbar spine, and a less mobile lumbar spine may cause stiffness of the back muscles, resulting in back pain. As muscle strength is determined largely by muscle mass, particularly the cross-sectional area of muscle (Maughan, 2005), and because the muscle cross-sectional area of back extensor muscles (the erector spinae group) is larger at the lumbar spine level than at the thoracic spine level (Marras et al., 2001), total back extensor strength is largely influenced by lumbar extensor muscles rather than thoracic extensor muscles. The results of the present study are not inconsistent with this anatomical background. Weakness of the back extensor muscles, particularly the lumbar extensor muscles, is thought to be responsible for lumbar spinal mobility.

4.3 Other possible factors contributing to back pain in osteoporosis

The present study focused on back pain and multiple spinal factors in patients with osteoporosis. However, the etiology of back pain is more complex and more multifactorial than could be examined in this study. Prevalence of musculoskeletal pain is also known to be associated with various measures of socio-economic status, as well as comorbidities (Thomas et al., 1999; Woo et al., 2009). Severity of pain may also be influenced by psychological factors (Woo et al., 2009). In addition, elderly patients with osteoporosis sometimes show other painful spinal disorders such as spondylosis to varying extents (Miyakoshi et al., 2003b). Findings in the present study might also have been influenced, at least in part, by factors other than osteoporosis.

4.4 Study limitations

Limitations of the present study should be noted. First, the number of subjects in the present study was much smaller than in previous studies evaluating the prevalence of back pain (Cockerill et al., 2000; Jacobs et al., 2006; Kuroda et al., 2009). However, we would like to emphasize that this is the first study to simultaneously evaluate back pain and multiple spinal factors in patients with osteoporosis. Second, data could not be obtained from severely kyphotic patients with established osteoporosis who were too disabled to lie in a prone position because of increased back pain in this position. This was because the dynamometer for measuring back extensor strength in the present study needed the patient to lie in a prone position. Therefore, the results of the present study might be considered for patients with mild or moderate spinal deformity.

5. Conclusions

In conclusion, the prevalence of back pain among patients with postmenopausal osteoporosis ≥50 years old who visited their practitioner was 91.4%. Back extensor strength was significantly lower in patients with back pain compared to those without back pain. Among subjects with back pain, intensity of back pain showed significant relationships with decreased back extensor strength and limited lumbar spinal mobility.

6. Acknowledgement

We wish to thank all the staff of Joto Orthopedic Clinic for their valuable assistance in conducting the study.

7. References

Burger, H.; Van Daele, P.L.; Grashuis, K.; Hofman, A.; Grobbee, D.E.; Schütte, H.E.; Birkenhäger, J.C. & Pols, H.A. (1997). Vertebral deformities and functional impairment in men and women. *Journal of Bone and Mineral Research*, Vol.12, No.1, (January 1997), pp.152-157, ISSN 0884-0431

Cockerill, W.; Ismail, A.A.; Cooper, C.; Matthis, C.; Raspe, H.; Silman, A.J. & O'Neill, T.W. (2000). Does location of vertebral deformity within the spine influence back pain and disability? European Vertebral Osteoporosis Study (EVOS) Group. *Annals of the Rheumatic Diseases*, Vol.59, No.5, (May 2000), pp.368-371, ISSN 0003-4967

Djurasovic. M. & Glassman, S.D. (2007). Correlation of radiographic and clinical findings in spinal deformities. *Neurosurgery Clinics of North America*, Vol.18, No.2, (April 2007), pp.223-227, ISSN 1042-3680

Edmond, S.L. & Felson, D.T. (2000). Prevalence of back symptoms in elders. *The Journal of Rheumatology*, Vol.27, No.1, (January 2000), pp.220-225, ISSN 0315-162X

Ettinger, B.; Black, D.M.; Nevitt, M.C.; Rundle, A.C.; Cauley, J.A.; Cummings, S.R. & Genant, H.K. (1992). Contribution of vertebral deformities to chronic back pain and disability. The Study of Osteoporotic Fractures Research Group. *J Bone Miner Res*, Vol.7, No.4, (April 1992), pp.449-456, ISSN 0884-0431

Francis, R.M.; Aspray, T.J.; Hide, G.; Sutcliffe, A.M. & Wilkinson, P. (2008). Back pain in osteoporotic vertebral fractures. *Osteoporosis International*, Vol.19, No.7, (July 2008), pp.895-903, ISSN 0937-941X

Glassman, S.D.; Bridwell, K.; Dimar, J.R.; Horton, W.; Berven, S. & Schwab F. (2005). The impact of positive sagittal balance in adult spinal deformity. *Spine (Phila Pa 1976)*, Vol.30, No.18, (September 2005), 2024-2029, ISSN 0362-2436

Hongo, M.; Itoi, E.; Sinaki, M.; Miyakoshi, N.; Shimada, Y.; Maekawa, S.; Okada, K. & Mizutani, Y. (2007). Effect of low-intensity back exercise on quality of life and back extensor strength in patients with osteoporosis: a randomized controlled trial. *Osteoporosis International*, Vol.18, No.10, (October 2007), pp.1389-1395, ISSN 0937-941X

Huang, C.; Ross, P.D, & Wasnich, R.D. (1996). Vertebral fractures and other predictors of back pain among older women. *Journal of Bone and Mineral Research*, Vol.11, No.7, (July 1996), pp.1026-1032, ISSN 0884-0431

Hübscher, M.; Vogt, L.; Schmidt. K.; Fink, M. & Banzer, W. (2010). Perceived pain, fear of falling and physical function in women with osteoporosis. *Gait & Posture*, Vol.32, No.3, (July 2010), pp.383-385, ISSN 0966-6362

Jacobs, J.M.; Hammerman-Rozenberg, R.; Cohen, A. & Stessman, J. (2006). Chronic back pain among the elderly: prevalence, associations, and predictors. *Spine (Phila Pa 1976)*, Vol.31, No.7, (April 2006), pp.E203-207, ISSN 0362-2436

Kasukawa, Y.; Miyakoshi, N.; Hongo, M.; Ishikawa, Y.; Noguchi, H.; Kamo, K.; Sasaki, H.; Murata, K. & Shimada, Y. (2010). Relationships between falls, spinal curvature, spinal mobility and back extensor strength in elderly people. *Journal of Bone and Mineral Metabolism*, Vol.28, No.1, (January 2010), pp.82-87, ISSN 0914-8779

Kumamoto, K.; Nakamura, T.; Suzuki, T.; Gorai, I.; Fujinawa, O.; Ohta, H.; Shiraki, M.; Yoh, K.; Fujiwara, S.; Endo, N. & Matsumoto, T. (2010). Validation of the Japanese Osteoporosis Quality of Life Questionnaire. *Journal of Bone and Mineral Metabolism*, Vol.28, No.1, (January 2010), pp.1-7, ISSN 0914-8779

Kuroda, T.; Shiraki, M.; Tanaka, S.; Shiraki, Y.; Narusawa, K. & Nakamura, T. (2009). The relationship between back pain and future vertebral fracture in postmenopausal women. *Spine (Phila Pa 1976)*, Vol.34, No.18, (August 2009), pp.1984-1989 , ISSN 0362-2436

Lavsky-Shulan, M.; Wallace, R.B.; Kohout, F.J.; Lemke, J.H.; Morris, M.C. & Smith, I.M. (1985). Prevalence and functional correlates of low back pain in the elderly: the Iowa 65+ Rural Health Study. *Journal of the American Geriatrics Society*, Vol.33, No.1, (January 1985), pp.23-28, ISSN 0002-8614

Limburg, P.J.; Sinaki, M.; Rogers, J.W.; Caskey, P.E. & Pierskalla, B.K. (1991). A useful technique for measurement of back strength in osteoporotic and elderly patients. *Mayo Clinic Proceedings*, Vol.66, No.1, (January 1991), pp.39-44, ISSN 0025-6196

Liu-Ambrose, T.; Eng, J.J.; Khan, K.M.; Mallinson, A.; Carter, N.D. & McKay, H.A. (2002). The influence of back pain on balance and functional mobility in 65- to 75-year-old women with osteoporosis. *Osteoporosis International*, Vol.13, No.11, (November 2002), pp. 868-873, ISSN 0937-941X

Mannion, A.F.; Knecht, K.; Balaban, G.; Dvorak, J. & Grob, D. (2004). A new skin-surface device for measuring the curvature and global and segmental ranges of motion of the spine: reliability of measurements and comparison with data reviewed from the literature. *European Spine Journal*, Vol.13, No.2, (March 2004), pp.122-136, ISSN 0940-6719

March, L.M.; Brnabic, A.J.; Skinner, J.C.; Schwarz, J.M.; Finnegan, T.; Druce, J. & Brooks, P.M. (1998). Musculoskeletal disability among elderly people in the community. *The Medical Journal of Australia*, Vol.168, No.9, (May 1998), pp.439-442, ISSN 0025-729X

Marras, W.S.; Jorgensen, M.J.; Granata, K.P. & Wiand, B. (2001). Female and male trunk geometry: size and prediction of the spine loading trunk muscles derived from MRI. *Clinical Biomechanics (Bristol, Avon)*, Vol.16, No.1, (January 2001), pp.38-46, ISSN 0268-0033

Matthis, C.; Weber, U.; O'Neill, T.W. & Raspe, H. (1998). Health impact associated with vertebral deformities: results from the European Vertebral Osteoporosis Study (EVOS). *Osteoporosis International*, Vol.8, No.4, (August 1998), pp.364-372, ISSN 0937-941X

Maughan, R.J. (2005). The limits of human athletic performance. *Annals of Transplantation*, Vol.10, No.4, (October-December 2005), pp.52-54, ISSN 1425-9524

Miyakoshi, N.; Hongo, M.; Maekawa, S.; Ishikawa, Y.; Shimada, Y. & Itoi, E. (2007) Back extensor strength and lumbar spinal mobility are predictors of quality of life in patients with postmenopausal osteoporosis. *Osteoporosis International,* Vol.18, No.10, (October 2007), pp. 1397-1403, ISSN 0937-941X

Miyakoshi, N.; Hongo, M.; Maekawa, S.; Ishikawa, Y.; Shimada, Y.; Okada, K. & Itoi, E. (2005). Factors related to spinal mobility in patients with postmenopausal osteoporosis. *Osteoporosis International,* Vol.16, No.12, (December 2005), pp.1871-1874, ISSN 0937-941X

Miyakoshi, N.; Hongo, M.; Tani, T.; Maekawa, S.; Shimada, Y. & Itoi, E. (2004). Relationship between spinal mobility and quality of life in patients with osteoporosis. *Osteoporosis Japan,* Vol.12, No.1, (January 2004), pp.143-146, ISSN 0919-6307 (in Japanese)

Miyakoshi, N.; Itoi, E.; Kobayashi, M. & Kodama, H. (2003a). Impact of postural deformities and spinal mobility on quality of life in postmenopausal osteoporosis. *Osteoporosis International,* Vol.14, No.12, (December 2003), pp.1007-1012, ISSN 0937-941X

Miyakoshi, N.; Itoi, E.; Murai, H.; Wakabayashi, I.; Ito, H. & Minato, T. (2003b). Inverse relation between osteoporosis and spondylosis in postmenopausal women as evaluated by bone mineral density and semiquantitative scoring of spinal degeneration. *Spine (Phila Pa 1976),* Vol.28, No.5, (March 2003), pp.492-495, ISSN 0362-2436

Miyakoshi, N.; Kasukawa, Y.; Ishikawa, Y.; Nozaka, K. & Shimada, Y. (2010). Spinal alignment and mobility in subjects with chronic low back pain with walking disturbance: a community-dwelling study. *The Tohoku Journal of Experimental Medicine,* Vol.221, No.1, (January 2010), pp.53-59, ISSN 0040-8727

Nevitt, M.C.; Ettinger, B.; Black, D.M.; Stone, K.; Jamal, S.A.; Ensrud, K.; Segal, M.; Genant, H.K. & Cummings, S.R. (1998). The association of radiographically detected vertebral fractures with back pain and function: a prospective study. *Annals of internal medicine,* Vol.128, No.10, (May 1998), pp. 793-800, ISSN 0003-4819

Orimo, H.; Hayashi, Y.; Fukunaga, M.; Sone, T.; Fujiwara, S.; Shiraki, M.; Kushida, K.; Miyamoto, S.; Soen, S.; Nishimura, J.; Oh-Hashi, Y.; Hosoi, T.; Gorai, I.; Tanaka, H.; Igai, T. & Kishimoto, H. (2001). Diagnostic criteria for primary osteoporosis: year 2000 revision. *Journal of Bone and Mineral Metabolism,* Vol.19, No.6, (September 2001), pp.331-337, ISSN 0914-8779.

Orimo, H.; Shiraki, M.; Hayashi, Y.; Hoshino, T.; Onaya, T.; Miyazaki, S.; Kurosawa, H.; Nakamura, T. & Ogawa, N. (1994). Effects of 1 alpha-hydroxyvitamin D3 on lumbar bone mineral density and vertebral fractures in patients with postmenopausal osteoporosis. *Calcified Tissue International,* Vol.54, No.5, (May 1994), pp.370-376, ISSN 0171-967X

Post, R.B. & Leferink, V.J. (2004). Spinal mobility: sagittal range of motion measured with the SpinalMouse, a new non-invasive device. *Archives of Orthopaedic and Trauma Surgery,* Vol.124, No.3, (April 2004), pp.187-192. ISSN 0936-8051

Satoh, K.; Kasama, F.; Itoi, E.; Tanuma, S. & Wakamatsu, E. (1988). Clinical features of spinal osteoporosis: spinal deformity and pertinent back pain. *Contemporary Orthopaedics,* Vol.16, No.3 , (March 1988), pp.23-30, ISSN 0194-8458

Takahashi, H.; Iwaya, C.; Iba, K.; Gorai, I., Suzuki, T.; Hayashi, Y.; Fujinawa, S.; Yamazaki, K. & Endo, N (2001). The Japanese Osteoporosis QOL Questionnaire (JOQOL): 2000 edition. *Journal of Japanese Society for Bone and Mineral Research*, Vol.18, No.3, (January 2001), pp.85-101, ISSN 0910-0067 (in Japanese)

Thomas, E.; Silman, A.J.; Croft, P.R.; Papageorgiou, A.C.; Jayson, M.I. & Macfarlane, G.J. (1999). Predicting who develops chronic low back pain in primary care: a prospective study. *British Medical Journal*, Vol.318, No.7199, (June 1999), pp.1662-1667, ISSN 0959-8138

Ulivieri, FM. (2007). Back pain treatment in post-menopausal osteoporosis with vertebral fractures. *Aging Clinical and Experimental Research*, Vol.19, No.3 Suppl., (June 2007), pp.21-23, ISSN 1594-0667

Woo, J.; Leung, J. & Lau, E. (2009). Prevalence and correlates of musculoskeletal pain in Chinese elderly and the impact on 4-year physical function and quality of life. *Public Health*, Vol.123, No.8, (August 2009), pp.549-556, ISSN 0033-3506

5

Self-Reported Prevalence of Osteoporosis in Australia

Tiffany K. Gill[1], Anne W. Taylor[1],
Julie Black[2] and Catherine L. Hill[1]
[1]University of Adelaide,
[2]Arthritis SA
Australia

1. Introduction

"Self-report" is generally the only method of determining the prevalence of non-registry based chronic diseases (Bergmann et al., 2004). However, there are difficulties in "case definition" associated with self-report and often the most effective means of identifying the presence of disease is to determine whether the chronic condition in question has been diagnosed by the doctor. Chronic conditions such as osteoporosis are often difficult to identify as they do not generally manifest themselves until after a bone fracture occurs. The aim of this chapter is to determine the self-reported prevalence of osteoporosis and associated demographic factors from a community dwelling sample aged 15 years and over across a 16 year period and compare this prevalence with that obtained from a biomedical study. Associated risk and demographic factors can be examined using these data. The issues around the use of self-reported, doctor-diagnosed osteoporosis to determine disease prevalence will also be discussed.

2. Background

Osteoporosis is a hidden condition. Bone loss due to osteoporosis is subtle but as there are no overt symptoms, it is generally not until a fracture occurs that osteoporosis may be identified (Australian Institute of Health and Welfare [AIHW] 2011; Rachner et al., 2011; Sànchez-Riera et al., 2010). However, with an ageing population, the related medical issues and socioeconomic impact will only increase (Rachner et al., 2011). Osteoporosis is a condition which affects both men and women although the greatest focus has generally been on post menopausal women (Cawthon, 2011). A meta-analysis identified that there was a five to eight fold increase in the risk of mortality due to all causes within the first three months following a hip fracture (Haentjens et al., 2010), which is a common fracture type associated with osteoporosis (Cooper, 1997). An increased annual mortality remains over time and it is generally higher for men compared to women (Center et al., 2011; Haentjens et al., 2010). Fractures consequently are a significant health issue which lead to not only premature mortality but also an increased level of disability and risk of future fracture (Center et al., 2007; Center et al., 2011; Cooper, 1997).

Dual x-ray absorptiometry (DXA) is considered to be the gold standard for the diagnosis of osteoporosis (Keen, 2007). Guidelines have been developed and implemented to address effectively screening for osteoporosis (Rachner et al., 2011). In Australia, the guideline focuses on post menopausal women and older men (Royal Australian College of General Practitioners, 2010), as do other international guidelines (Compston et al., 2009; Hodgson et al., 2003). The guideline does not, however, come into effect until there has been a minimal trauma fracture (Royal Australian College of General Practitioners, 2010). Risk assessment tools have also been developed which combine clinical risk factors and DXA measurements (Borgström & Kanis, 2008; Unnanuntana et al., 2010). Thus DXA scans are only provided to those considered at risk of osteoporosis or in response to a minimal trauma fracture. Bone density screening is not provided to the population in a similar manner to breast cancer screening, as it is not considered cost effective, due to the cost of providing scans and limited availability (Davis et al., 2011).

A variety of data sources are used to determine the characteristics of osteoporosis within the Australian population and estimating the population prevalence can be difficult. Self-reported, doctor diagnosis of a condition is generally used in population surveys but these estimates do not generally reflect the true prevalence. This discrepancy with true prevalence has been demonstrated (Sacks et al., 2005) using arthritis information collected as part of the Behavioural Risk Factor Surveillance System (BRFSS) which is undertaken across the United States. In terms of osteoporosis, the prevalence is underestimated due to the absence of obvious symptoms until a diagnosis may occur following a minimal trauma fracture (AIHW, 2011; Werner, 2003). But even after a minimal trauma fracture, those with osteoporosis may be untreated or undiagnosed (Eisman et al., 2004) or the underlying disease may not be appropriately investigated (Elliot-Gibson et al., 2004).

Osteoporosis contributes to the global burden of disease. Chronic conditions (including osteoporosis), whether they are physical or mental, reduce quality living time, with the subsequent morbidity significantly impacting the population (McQueen, 2003). Regular surveillance allows the monitoring of health, demographic and other related data to assess trends and prevalence and also provide an explanation of demographic and exposure differences, the use of health services and evaluate if there is a response to health promotion and public health interventions (McQueen, 2003; Wilson, 2003). A system that monitors chronic disease and related risk factors does have some specific features which characterise it as "surveillance" (Campostrini, 2003). These include:

- Time, which is a essential element of the data collection,
- There is a focus on chronic or non-communicable diseases and related factors, and
- Attention is also focused on the data management, collection, analysis, use and interpretation (Campostrini, 2003).

While it is considered most ideal to collect data across short timeframes (e.g. a day, a week or a month) in order to simulate as closely as possible a continuous data collection, this is not always practical or feasible (Campostrini, 2003; McQueen, 2003). However, if questions and methodology remain stable over time so that changes or trends that occur can be attributed to true population changes and not questionnaire changes, and data are collected at regular intervals (McQueen, 2003); the information provided is extremely powerful.

Developing a systematic approach to surveillance addresses many needs. These include: an estimation of the size of the problem, the geographic distribution, detection of an epidemic or definition of a problem, stimulation of research and research hypotheses, monitoring changes in disease patterns and providing assistance to planning. Population-based information related to economic, social, cultural and physical factors which are relevant to health can be provided. These factors can then be associated with the effects of public health and health promotion interventions and targeted campaigns. Data on health risk factors can also be obtained and support afforded to health related legislative programs and disease prevention actions, and regular surveillance can also evaluate the long term effects of health promotion campaigns. Also, future trends, the use of health resources and the emergence of any new health issues can be recognised (International Union for Health Promotion and Education World Alliance for Risk Factor Surveillance Global Working Group [IUHPE WARFS GWG], 2011).

Thus, while self-report underestimates osteoporosis prevalences, use of this method of data collection can improve the understanding and knowledge of the disease, in addition to assisting the identification of high risk groups (Werner, 2003). Self-report has been used in population surveys in South Australia (SA), Australia for approximately 20 years, with osteoporosis data being collected since 1995. Questions have been asked in the same way, using the same methodology annually, and while this timeframe is considered to be infrequent in terms of the surveillance timeframe spectrum (IUHPE WARFS GWG, 2011), aggregated data from these surveys possess the characteristics of a more regular surveillance system. Aggregation of these data provides the ability to analyse data over time and enables an assessment of changes in prevalence over the period of time under examination. It also provides evidence for the development of policy and an investigation of the impact of these policies over time.

3. Methods

The data presented in this chapter are derived from two different sources. The first is a face-to-face survey and the second, a telephone survey and clinical assessment conducted as part of a longitudinal cohort study.

3.1 Health Omnibus Survey (HOS)

The self-reported prevalence of osteoporosis has been collected in SA since 1995, using the SA Health Omnibus Survey (SAHOS) which is conducted annually, with data collection between September and December each year (spring to summer in Australia). Key uses of the survey are:

- gaining information on knowledge, attitudes and behaviours;
- gaining information on perceptions towards, and acceptability of, services and programs or organisations;
- provision of prevalence or incidence data;
- explaining population perspectives, attitudes, values and behaviours associated with issues under investigation;
- allowing the segmentation of problems and related issues;
- identifying target groups for interventions and campaigns;
- monitoring changes in health problems and disease trends;
- gaining information on the acceptability and uptake of new initiatives and programs;
- obtaining information on the aetiology of specific health problems;
- obtaining data to test hypotheses; and
- evaluating interventions and programs.

Questions to be included in each survey are reviewed by a quality control committee, both before and after pilot testing, for appropriate wording and design. Approximately ten background demographic questions are included within the survey. SAHOS is a face-to-face survey, which is the original method and consequently the "gold standard" of interview techniques (Dillman, 1999; Dillman et al., 2009; Schonlau et al., 2002). Participation is voluntary. Interviewers read out the questions to participants and, if necessary, prompt cards are used to ensure that respondents remember all of the response categories. The questionnaire is designed to take approximately 30 to 40 minutes for respondents to complete. Prior to the main survey, a pilot study of 50 interviews is conducted to test questions, validate the survey instrument and assess survey procedures.

3.1.1 Sample size
The survey sample is a clustered, multi-stage, systematic, self-weighting, area sample. Each of these key sampling concepts is described in more detail below. Each survey usually samples 5,200 households. The SAHOS has been in operation since 1991 and since that time the observed response rate has generally ranged between approximately 60-70%, usually resulting in a minimum of 3,000 interviews being completed each year. This large sample size facilitates a high level of confidence that the results and trends obtained in response to the survey questions can be extrapolated to the South Australian population as a whole.

3.1.2 Clustered sample
Seventy-five percent of the sample is selected from from the metropolitan area of the capital, Adelaide, with the remaining sample being drawn from those country areas with a population of 1,000 or more (based on Australian Bureau of Statistics (ABS) Census information which is collected every five years in Australia). Country towns with smaller populations are not included within the sample frame because of the additional cost of interviewing people living in these remote areas. Within the selected metropolitan and country areas, the ABS Collection Districts (CDs) are the basis of the sample frame. A CD is a geographical area comprising approximately 200 dwellings. By using a cluster sampling technique, some, but not all, of these CDs are included in the sample. To achieve a sample of 5,200 households, 10 households are selected from each of 520 CDs.

Stage 1 - Selection of CDs

Based on ABS population estimates, 400 CDs are selected in metropolitan Adelaide, and 120 CDs from the selected country areas. All cities/towns in country SA with a population size of 10,000 or more are selected automatically with the balance of the country sample chosen from centres with a population of 1,000 or more. A randomly selected starting point and a fixed skip interval are used to determine which CDs are chosen from the sample frame. The skip interval is calculated as the number of households in metropolitan Adelaide (or country SA) divided by the number of CDs required for the metropolitan (or country) sector.

The process of selection is as follows. Firstly, all CDs in the sample frame are listed in numerical code order, along with the number of dwellings in that individual CD and the "cumulative number of dwellings" for that CD. The cumulative number of dwellings is defined as the total number of dwellings for a particular CD and all previously listed CDs. A random number between one and the skip number is chosen as the starting point for selections and the skip interval is then used to determine which CDs are selected. If, for example, the starting point is 80 and the skip interval is 100, then the CDs which contain the 80th, 180th and 280th cumulative dwelling will be the first three CDs to be selected. Thus, once the skip interval has been determined, selection of an individual CD is dependent on the number of dwellings within that CD. In some cases, larger CDs may, in theory, be selected more than once.

Stage 2 - Selection of households within CDs

The selection process of households is similar to the selection of CDs. Ten households per selected CD are chosen using a fixed skip interval from a random starting point.

Stage 3 - Selection of individuals within households

Within households, the person who was last to have a birthday (aged 15 years or over) is selected to participate in the survey. The sample is a non-replacement sample, thus, if the selected person is not available, interviews are not conducted with any other household members. Generally up to six visits are made to each household to interview the selected participant, before the selected individual is classified as a non-contact, however in some cases more visits may be conducted. Selections that occur in hotels, motels, hospitals, nursing homes and other institutions are excluded from the survey.

3.1.3 Systematic sample

The randomly selected starting points and the skip intervals between selected CDs and selected households within CDs produce a systematic even spread of households across the population.

3.1.4 Self weighting sample

The self-weighting sampling procedure of HOS ensures that every household within each of the two strata (metropolitan Adelaide and the major country towns) have the same probability of being selected even though different probabilities of selection exist at each stage of the sampling process.

The probability of selecting a household equals the probability of selecting a CD (i.e. the cumulative number of dwellings in the CD divided by the skip interval) multiplied by the probability of selecting a household, given that the CD was selected (i.e. the number of households required in each CD divided by the cumulative number of households in the CD).

3.1.5 Approach letter

In line with other epidemiologically-based surveillance systems, a letter introducing SAHOS is sent to each selected household including a brochure outlining how the information is used. It has been shown that sending a letter informing a person of a survey can increase response rates (Frey, 1989; Robertson et al., 2000). If respondents have any questions about the survey, they are able to call a free call telephone number listed in the approach letter.

3.1.6 Validation

Ten percent of all respondents are re-contacted and re-interviewed using selected questions to ensure the validity of the original responses. Data entry is fully verified using a double entry technique to ensure the accuracy of the final data.

3.1.7 Weighting

All SAHOS data are weighted by age, sex, area of residence and the inverse of the probability of selection in the household to the most recent ABS Census or Estimated Residential Population data for SA.

3.1.8 Ethics approval

Ethics approval for the methodology of the survey is provided by the Human Research Ethics Committee of the University of Adelaide and ethics approval for questions may be provided through the individual users' institutions, or if users do not have access to a committee, by the University of Adelaide.

3.1.9 Questions related to osteoporosis prevalence

The methodology of the SAHOS has remained consistent over time and questions relating to self-reported, doctor diagnosed osteoporosis have been included since 1995, which enables examination of prevalence changes over time.

Questions within the SAHOS include demographic characteristics:

- Sex;
- Age;
- Country of birth;
- Marital status;
- Income (gross annual household income before tax in Australian dollars);
- Work status;
- Area of residence; and
- Year of survey.

The question used to determine osteoporosis prevalence is "Have you ever been told by a doctor that you have osteoporosis? "

3.2 North West Adelaide Health Study

The North West Adelaide Health Study (NWAHS) is a longitudinal cohort study of over 4,000 participants located in the northwest suburbs of Adelaide, SA, Australia.

The study focuses on priority health conditions and risk factors that have been identified due to the significant burden that is placed on the community in terms of social, health, quality of life and economic factors. By identifying and describing specific population groups at risk of chronic conditions, the effectiveness of strategies for the prevention, early detection, and management of chronic conditions may be maximised (Grant et al., 2006; Grant et al., 2009).

Participants were recruited to Stage 1 of the study between 2000 and 2003, and undertook a second assessment between 2004 and 2006. The initial objective of the study was to establish both baseline self-reported and biomedically measured information on chronic diseases and risk factors, in terms of those who may be at risk of these conditions, those who already had these conditions but had not been diagnosed, and those who had previously been diagnosed with the conditions. Identifying those categories of disease along a chronic disease continuum provides a view of disease burden and presents opportunities for effective interventions, improved health service use and development of health policy (Grant et al., 2006; Grant et al., 2009). When specifically considering osteoporosis, the chronic disease continuum can be described as presented in Figure 1.

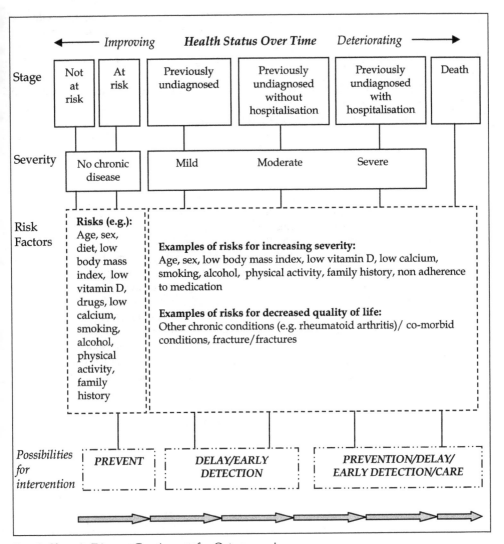

Fig. 1. Chronic Disease Continuum for Osteoporosis

3.2.1 Stage one

All households in the northern and western areas of Adelaide, SA, with a telephone connected and a telephone number listed in the Electronic White Pages were eligible for selection in the NWAHS. Households were randomly selected and sent an approach letter and brochure informing them about the study. The person who was last to have their birthday within each household and aged 18 years and over was selected for interview. Interviews were conducted using Computer Assisted Telephone Interview (CATI) technology.

During the telephone interview respondents were asked a range of health-related and demographic questions, and were invited to attend an assessment clinic for a 45 minute appointment at either of two local hospitals in Adelaide, one in the western suburbs and one in the northern suburbs. All study participants who agreed to attend the clinic were sent an information pack about the study, including a self-report questionnaire which examined other chronic conditions and health-related risk factors that were not included in the telephone interview.

During the clinic visit, the tests included: height, weight, waist and hip circumference, and blood pressure. Lung function was calculated and a fasting blood sample was taken to measure glucose, tryglycerides, total cholesterol, high density lipid (HDL), low density lipid (LDL), and glycated haemoglobin (HbA1c). The response rate for attending the clinic in Stage 1 was 49.4% with a final sample of n=4056.

3.2.2 Stage two

All participants that could be contacted, were invited to attend the clinic for Stage 2 using a telephone interview that also obtained demographic and health-related information. Of the original living cohort, over 90% provided some Stage 2 information, and 3,205 (over 81.0%) attended the clinic assessment between 2004 and 2006 for the second time. The minimum age of participants in Stage 2 was 20 years. In addition to the measurements taken at Stage 1 (which concentrated on the chronic conditions diabetes, chronic obstructive pulmonary disease and asthma), renal function and musculoskeletal conditions were also assessed. The musculoskeletal conditions included both arthritis and osteoporosis and a range of questions related to specific joint pain. Participants aged 50 years and over were offered a DXA scan to measure their bone density, and fat and lean body mass.

The longitudinal nature of the cohort study means that following Stage 2, valuable information was obtained relating to the number of people who had developed chronic conditions over the timeframe of the study and the factors that may have contributed to their risk of developing chronic disease. Stage 3 of the study has recently been completed with all respondents who could be contacted again being asked to attend the clinic for assessment and information relating to musculoskeletal conditions again included in the study. However the results in this chapter are limited to Stage 2 data only.

3.2.3 Weighting

Weighting was used to correct for the disproportionality of the original sample with respect to the population of interest. The data were weighted for age, sex, probability of selection in the household and area of residence. These weights reflect any unequal sample inclusion probabilities and compensate for differential non-response. The data were weighted using the ABS Census data so that the health estimates calculated would be representative of the adult populations of the north west area of Adelaide. Subsequently, each stage of the study is weighted with the initial sample weight as the foundation figure.

3.2.4 Ethics approval

Ethics approval for the each stage of the NWAHS has been granted by the Ethics of Human Research Committee of The Queen Elizabeth Hospital, Adelaide, SA.

3.2.5 Questions related to osteoporosis prevalence

Data collection methods for the NWAHS are a CATI, a self-complete questionnaire and a clinic assessment. Questions incorporated within the NWAHS include demographic characteristics:

- Sex;
- Age;
- Country of birth;
- Marital status;
- Income (gross annual household income before tax in Australian dollars);
- Work status; and
- Area of residence.

The question used to determine osteoporosis prevalence is "Have you ever been told by a doctor that you have osteoporosis?" This information is collected as part of the CATI in Stage 2. Other information collected as part of the CATI was the self-reported occurrence of fractures following a fall from a standing height or less in the past year and self-reported types of arthritis, including rheumatoid and osteoarthritis (that is, "Have you ever been told by a doctor that you have arthritis?"). Those who responded in the affirmative were then asked what type of arthritis they had.

Other variables that are collected as part of the NWAHS were: family history of osteoporosis (mother, father, sister, brother, grandparent, other), self-reported smoking (which is categorised as current, ex- or non-smoker) and alcohol intake. Regarding alcohol intake, participants were asked how often they drank alcohol, and if they drank, on a day when they drank alcohol, how many drinks they usually had. They were then classified according to their level of risk of harm from alcohol, as non-drinkers or no risk, low alcohol risk, and intermediate to very high alcohol risk (National Heart Foundation of Australia, 1989). Physical activity level was also determined, respondents were asked about the amount of walking, moderate and vigorous activity they had undertaken in the past two weeks. These questions were the same as those used in the Australian National Health Survey in 2001 and 2004 (ABS, 2003, 2006), and the responses were classified into four activity levels (sedentary, low, moderate and high). All of these variables were obtained from the self-completed questionnaire.

Height and weight were measured as part of the clinic assessment to calculate body mass index and DXA scans were provided to those aged 50 years and over who consented to the scan and respondents were classified as having osteoporosis (T score $\leq$ -2.5) or osteopenia (-1.0 < T score > -2.5) using the World Health Organization (WHO) definition of osteoporosis (WHO, 1994). Overall 75.7% of eligible participants undertook a DXA scan.

3.3 Data analysis
Analyses were conducted using SPSS Version 18 (IBM SPSS Statistics, New York, NY, USA) and STATA Version 11.2 (StataCorp, College Station, TX, USA).

4. Results

4.1 Prevalence of osteoporosis (SAHOS)
The self-reported prevalence of osteoporosis has been collected every year in SAHOS between 1995 and 2010 except in 1996 and 2000. Thus there are fourteen years of data available. The aggregated sample size was n=41,487. Overall, 49% of respondents were male and 51.0% female, with a mean age of 45.0 years (SD 18.85, range 15-102). The aggregated prevalence of self-reported osteoporosis among those aged 15 years and over, between 1995 and 2010, was 4.8% (95% CI 4.6-5.0).

The self-reported prevalence from SAHOS was then age and sex standardised to the 2006 Australian Census (ABS, 2007) to enable prevalence comparisons between years and the results are presented in Figure 2. Data points for 1996 and 2000 are not available as these years had missing data.

As the data were aggregated, autocorrelation may occur which violates the assumptions of linear analysis. A Durbin-Watson test was undertaken to determine if first order autocorrelation of the residuals of the annual prevalence estimates had occurred. The value was 1.73, close to 2 indicating that there was not excessive autocorrelation of the data (Chatfield, 2004; Yaffee & McGee, 2000).

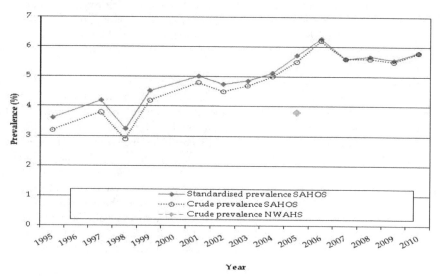

Fig. 2. Prevalence of self-reported osteoporosis from SAHOS and NWAHS

The data were examined to determine if a deviation from a linear trend existed. The regression coefficients were graphed and demonstrated an approximate straight line and a Box-Tidwell regression model was undertaken (Box & Tidwell, 1962), which also indicated that the nonlinear deviation was not significant (p=0.09). A chi-square test for trend was then conducted, which indicated that there had been a significant change in the self-reported osteoporosis prevalence over time (p<0.001).

4.2 Prevalence of osteoporosis (NWAHS)

Participants in Stage 2 of the NWAHS undertook one, two or all three of the data collection methods (CATI, self-complete questionnaire, clinic assessment) depending on their time constraints and desired level of participation. There were n=3500 respondents to the CATI questionnaire (49.1% male and 50.9% female; mean age 47.42, SD 17.57, range 20-93), n=3259 responded to the self-complete questionnaire (49.1% male and 50.9% female; mean age 47.59, SD 17.51, range 20-95) and n=3205 attended the clinic (49.1% male and 50.9% female; mean age 47.58, SD 17.52, range 20-95). The self-reported prevalence of osteoporosis among participants in the NWAHS aged 20 years and over during Stage 2 (2004 to 2006) was 3.8% (95% CI 3.2-4.5). The crude prevalence of osteoporosis obtained from the NWAHS is shown in Figure 2.

4.3 Logistic regression analyses

Logistic regression analysis of the aggregated SAHOS data set was then undertaken in order to determine the demographic characteristics most likely to be associated with self-reporting the presence of osteoporosis. Data for these analyses were restricted to respondents aged 20 years and over to enable comparisons with the NWAHS data. The variables included in the analysis were: age, sex, country of birth, income, education, marital status and work status. Area of residence was not included as SAHOS is a state wide sample and NWAHS is a metropolitan sample. Bivariate and then multivariate logistic regression analyses were conducted to identify the best sets of explanatory variables associated with osteoporosis, with variables that were significant at $p<0.25$ in the bivariate analysis included in the multivariate model, as these may still be candidates for model predictors - they can continue to be a good fit when other variables are included in the model (Hosmer & Lemeshow, 2000). Then the non-significant variables at $p≥0.05$ were removed until all remaining variables were significant. Finally, all models were tested for "goodness of fit" using the Hosmer and Lemeshow goodness of fit test (Hosmer & Lemeshow, 2000).

Analysis of the demographic variables associated with self-reported osteoporosis for the SAHOS and NWAHS produced similar factors, with increasing age, sex (female) and work status (unemployed, retired and "other") significant for both datasets (Table 1). In the SAHOS, those who reported that they undertook home duties were also significantly more likely to report that they had osteoporosis. Those earning between $12,001 and $50,000, were also significantly more likely to self-report osteoporosis in the SAHOS, whereas this variable was not significant for those self-reporting osteoporosis in the NWAHS.

A model was then created for the SAHOS data only, to examine the impact of time. The variables associated with self-reporting osteoporosis were: increasing age, sex (female), work status (unemployed, retired and "other", home duties), income (up to $50,000 and not stated) and year, with more recent years associated with higher self-reported prevalence of osteoporosis (data not shown).

The self-reported prevalences collected as part of the SAHOS and the NWAHS were then compared to the prevalence of osteoporosis and osteopenia as defined in the NWAHS using DXA scans. DXA scans were only undertaken on those aged 50 years and over, thus the analysis is limited to this age group. The aggregated prevalence of self-reported osteoporosis among those aged 50 years and over in SAHOS was 10.7% (95% CI 10.3-11.2) compared to 8.8% (95% CI 7.5-10.3) for self-report in NWAHS and 18.7% (95% CI 16.6-20.9) for those classified with osteoporosis and osteopenia combined as defined by DXA scans (osteoporosis 3.6% (95% CI 2.6-4.9) and osteopenia 15.1% (95% CI 13.2-17.1)). It was considered appropriate to combine the categories of osteoporosis and osteopenia as both are indicators of abnormal bone density.

Bivariate and multivariate analyses were then undertaken for all participants aged 50 years and over. This second group of models included all of the demographic characteristics collected as part of both studies and examined the variables associated with self-report and clinically defined osteoporosis (Table 2). Increasing age and female sex were significant for all three models and again for SAHOS and self-reported osteoporosis from NWAHS, work status (unemployed and retired) was significant. Income was also significantly associated with self-reporting osteoporosis in SAHOS, while marital status (never married) was significantly associated with low bone density as defined by DXA scans.

Group One	SAHOS self-report		NWAHS self-report	
	OR	p-value	OR	p-value
Sex				
Male	1.00		1.00	
Female	3.76	**<0.001**	5.55	**<0.001**
Age	1.06	**<0.001**	1.06	**<0.001**
Work status				
Full time	1.00		1.00	
Part time	1.13	0.432	1.48	0.430
Home duties	1.47	**0.009**	1.16	0.866
Unemployed	2.05	**0.024**	3.25	**0.015**
Retired	1.44	**0.015**	2.95	**0.037**
Student	1.40	0.436	-	-
Other	5.65	**<0.001**	4.43	**0.020**
Not stated	-	-	4.84	0.108
Income				
$80,001 and more	1.00			
$60,001 - $80,000	1.41	0.108		
$50,001 - $60,000	1.23	0.362		
$40,001 - $50,000	1.80	**0.004**		
$30,001 - $40,000	1.61	**0.022**		
$20,001 - $30,000	1.68	**0.006**		
$12,001 - $20,000	1.72	**0.004**		
Up to $12,000	1.33	0.129		
Not stated	1.31	0.146		

Table 1. Logistic regression analysis of self-report osteoporosis, SAHOS and NWAHS, age 20 years and over

A model was also constructed for those aged 50 years and over using SAHOS data only, which examined the demographic characteristics associated with self-reported osteoporosis and included year within the model. Increasing age, female sex, increasing years, work status (home duties, retired, student, other) and income (up to $50,000) were all significant and associated with self-reporting osteoporosis (data not shown).

A third group of models was then created using NWAHS data and examining other factors associated with osteoporosis. Variables examined at a bivariate level were alcohol risk, smoking, family history, body mass index, physical activity, fracture as a result of a fall from a standing height or less over the last year and self-reported rheumatoid arthritis. The results of the multivariate analysis are in Table 3.

Group two	SAHOS self-report		NWAHS self-report		NWAHS DXA	
	OR	p-value	OR	p-value	OR	p-value
Sex						
Male	1.00		1.00		1.00	
Female	4.44	**<0.001**	5.50	**<0.001**	1.94	**<0.001**
Age	1.04	**<0.001**	1.03	**0.020**	1.09	**<0.001**
Work status						
Full time	1.00		1.00			
Part time	1.16	0.46	1.12	0.823		
Home duties	1.72	**0.003**	0.93	0.934		
Unemployed	2.05	**0.035**	3.04	**0.015**		
Retired	1.75	**0.002**	2.67	**0.034**		
Student	3.25	**0.018**	-	-		
Other	6.08	**<0.001**	2.57	0.180		
Not stated	-	-	4.69	0.081		
Income						
$80,001 and more	1.00					
$60,001 - $80,000	1.31	0.295				
$50,001 - $60,000	1.14	0.632				
$40,001 - $50,000	1.87	**0.012**				
$30,001 - $40,000	1.50	0.106				
$20,001 - $30,000	1.55	0.051				
$12,001 - $20,000	1.60	**0.038**				
Up to $12,000	1.28	0.272				
Not stated	1.18	0.465				
Martial status						
Married/de facto					1.00	
Separated/divorced					0.80	0.345
Widowed					1.28	0.253
Never married					1.90	**0.043**
Not stated					0.86	0.903

Table 2. Logistic regression analysis of osteoporosis prevalence, SAHOS and NWAHS self-report and NWAHS DXA, age 50 years and over

For both self-report and DXA, non-smokers were more likely to have osteoporosis. Those with a low to high risk of harm from alcohol and with a first degree relative with osteoporosis were more likely to self-report that they had osteoporosis whereas those undertaking lower levels of activity were more likely to have low bone density. Those with a higher body mass index were less likely to have a low bone density (Table 3).

	NWAHS self-report		NWAHS DXA	
Group three	OR	p-value	OR	p-value
BMI			0.82	**<0.001**
Alcohol risk				
Non drinker/no risk	1.00			
Low to high risk	1.54	**0.025**		
Not stated	1.34	0.593		
Smoking				
Current smoker	1.00		1.00	
Ex smoker	1.21	0.629	1.13	0.637
Non smoker	2.37	**0.026**	1.80	**0.020**
Family history of osteoporosis				
No	1.00		1.00	
First degree relative	3.66	**<0.001**	1.43	0.095
Don't know	2.73	**<0.001**	1.45	**0.037**
Not stated	1.13	0.851	2.20	0.124
Physical activity				
High exercise			1.00	
Moderate exercise			1.71	0.144
Low exercise			2.07	**0.042**
Sedentary			2.15	**0.034**
Not stated			2.40	**0.027**

Table 3. Logistic regression analysis of other factors associated with osteoporosis, NWAHS self-report and DXA, age 50 years and over

Finally a fourth set of models combined both demographic and other relevant factors associated with osteoporosis, for the data obtained from the NWAHS. Increasing age and female sex remained significant for both models, while those with a higher body mass index were less likely to have a lower bone density and those with self-reported osteoporosis were more likely to have family members with the condition. The work status categories, unemployed and retired, also remained significant for self-reported osteoporosis (Table 4).

	NWAHS self-report		NWAHS DXA	
Group four	OR	p-value	OR	p-value
Sex				
Male	1.00		1.00	
Female	4.71	**<0.001**	2.13	**<0.001**
Age	1.03	**0.013**	1.10	**<0.001**
BMI			0.82	**<0.001**
Work status				
Full time	1.00			
Part time	1.05	0.922		
Home duties	0.78	0.775		
Unemployed	2.85	**0.023**		
Retired	2.55	**0.044**		
Student	-	-		
Other	2.19	0.275		
Not stated	6.22	**0.023**		
Family history				
No	1.00			
First degree relative	3.24	**<0.001**		
Don't know	2.17	**0.001**		
Not stated	0.97	0.962		

Table 4. Overall models demographic and other factors associated with osteoporosis, NWAHS, age 50 years and over

5. Discussion

The results of this analysis indicate that while determining the population prevalence of osteoporosis remains a difficult issue, there is a role for self-report to play in the monitoring of osteoporosis prevalence over time. At this time, DXA scans are not available to the general population as a screening tool (Davis et al., 2011) and other means of assessing osteoporosis in the population are required. However, it is likely, as this study has shown, that self-reported prevalence will differ from that obtained from bone density assessment. In this study, the prevalence of osteoporosis as measured by DXA among those 50 years and over was lower than the self-reported prevalence but when combined with osteopenia was higher. Sample differences and self-selection to undertake a DXA scan are likely to have contributed to this.

Data from the SAHOS indicate that there has been a significant increase in the self-reported prevalence of osteoporosis over time. It is however difficult to assess whether this is a true increase. Other factors such as a greater awareness of the condition due to marketing campaigns in Australia, particularly in relation to over the counter supplements such as vitamin D and calcium, may have played a role in increasing the awareness of the condition. Nevertheless, it can also be argued that this improved awareness, even if it impacts estimates of true prevalence, may still assist in the prevention or management of the condition. Nayak et al. (2010) demonstrated that belief in being susceptible to osteoporosis among older adults, those most at risk of osteoporosis, is low, and the older the respondents were, the less likely they were to believe that osteoporosis is a severe condition. Thus any information or advertising may assist patient education. It is also of interest that the results of DXA scans are not immune to errors in self-report with Cadarette et al. (2007) demonstrating that while there was minimal error in self-reporting that a DXA scan had been undertaken, the self-reporting of results was poor, again providing an underestimate of osteoporosis prevalence. The understanding of these results could however be improved by providing them in writing (Brask-Lindemann et al., 2011). This again highlights issues of patient knowledge and understanding of the condition.

Consequently, in recent years, there has been an increased focus on functional health literacy of the population, which is considered to be the ability of people to read, analyse and take action with regard to both oral and written information obtained in the health care setting (Nielsen-Bohlman et al. 2004). It has been acknowledged that those with low or limited functional health literacy are more likely to have adverse health outcomes, not undertake preventive health behaviours, have premature mortality and higher health-care costs. In addition, people with lower functional health literacy are less likely to undertake active management of their condition (Berkman et al., 2004; De Walt et al., 2005). Unpublished analysis of other data obtained using the SAHOS has indicated that 70% of those with doctor-diagnosed osteoporosis had a low health literacy, further supporting the view that despite the method used to assess osteoporosis prevalence, inaccuracies in the reporting of the condition may occur, which has implications for management of the condition.

While understanding of the condition and reporting of prevalence is variable, it is of note that there remained a general consistency in the variables that were associated with osteoporosis prevalence, and these are supported by previous work. Genetic factors have been shown to contribute to osteoporosis (Harvey & Cooper, 2003; Marini & Brandi, 2010; Recker & Deng, 2002), thus family history of osteoporosis is an important factor. Sex and age are also significant covariates (Cawthon, 2011; Keen, 2007; Werner, 2003) and these variables are strongly evident during multivariate modelling. Varenna et al. (1999) determined that higher levels of education were associated with a lower risk of osteoporosis and lower income levels and unemployment have been associated with a greater risk of hip fracture (Farahmand et al., 2000). Low body mass index, previous low trauma fracture, rheumatoid arthritis, physical activity, smoking and excessive alcohol consumption have all been identified as risk factors for osteoporosis (Keen, 2007). Despite the fact that many of these variables were self-report, the associations with osteoporosis all occurred in the expected manner, except for smoking, where non-smokers were more likely to have a lower bone density and to self-report osteoporosis. Smokers are more likely to be from lower socioeconomic groups (Scollo & Winstanley, 2008) which are also groups with a lower level of health literacy (Barber et al., 2009). Thus this group may be less likely to undergo a DXA scan and self-report osteoporosis, as they have a poorer understanding of the condition.

The consequences of osteoporosis in terms of fracture also need to be considered. The overall lack of awareness of osteoporosis within the population also extends to a lack of understanding of the risk of a prior fracture in relation to the occurrence of subsequent fractures (Center et al., 2007). Targeted self-management courses for osteoporosis have demonstrated an improved understanding of osteoporosis and related behaviours in the short term (Francis et al., 2009; Laslett et al., 2011) and in Australia, approximately 40% of those with osteoporosis are more likely to use complementary and alternative medicines, which includes vitamin D and calcium (Armstrong el al., 2011). But despite public campaigns promoting better nutrition and increasing the awareness of osteoporosis, Pasco et al. (2000) demonstrated that women did not achieve the required calcium intake and Czernichow et al. (2010) have shown that the vitamin D intake among postmenopausal women with osteoporosis in France is significantly lower than recommended doses.

As highlighted in this study, similar factors were associated with osteoporosis prevalence, notwithstanding the method of data collection. Thus, surveillance can play a role in the ability to target information, identify at-risk groups and evaluate the impact of health promotion programs. It is however evident that there is a continued need to further explore means of adequately ascertaining the prevalence of osteoporosis and to improve the understanding of the condition in the population.

6. Conclusion

While prevalence estimates of osteoporosis vary within the population according to data collection method, generally there are consistent covariates associated with osteoporosis, which are important for the targeting of health promotion campaigns. In the absence of clinical testing, the monitoring of the prevalence of osteoporosis using self-report has a role to play in the prevention and management of the condition.

7. Acknowledgment

The authors would like to acknowledge all of the SAHOS participants over the past 16 years and all of the participants in the NWAHS.
Tiffany Gill is currently a National Health and Medical Research Council Early Career fellow to Fellow (Australian Public Health, ID 1013552).

8. References

Armstrong, A.R., Thiébaut, S.P., Brown, L.J. & Nepal, B. (2011). Australian Adults Use Complementary and Alternative Medicine in the Treatment of Chronic Illness: A National Study. *Australian and New Zealand Journal of Public Health*, Vol. 35, No. 4, pp. 384-390, ISSN 1326-0200

Australian Bureau of Statistics. (2003). *National Health Survey: Users Guide, 2001*. Cat no 4363.0.55.001, ABS, Canberra, Australia, Retrieved from http://www.abs.gov.au/AUSSTATS/abs@.nsf/Lookup/4363.0.55.001Main+Featu res12001?OpenDocument

Australian Bureau of Statistics. (2006). *National Health Survey: Users Guide, 2004-05*. Cat no 4363.0.55.001, ABS, Canberra, Australia, Retrieved from http://www.ausstats.abs.gov.au/ausstats/subscriber.nsf/0/A58E031838C37F81C A257141000F1AAF/$File/4363055001_2004-05.pdf

Australian Bureau of Statistics. (2007). *2006 Census of Population and Housing, South Australia.* Cat no 2068.0 – 2006 Census Tables, Australian Bureau of Statistics, Retrieved from http://www.abs.gov.au

Australian Institute of Health and Welfare. (2011). *A Snapshot of Osteoporosis in Australia.* Arthritis series no. 15. Cat. No. PHE 137. AIHW, ISBN 978-1-74249-131-8, Canberra, Australia

Barber, M.N., Staples, M., Osborne, R.H., Clerehan, R., Elder, C. & Buchbinder, R. (2009). Up to a Quarter of the Australian Population May Have Suboptimal Health Literacy Depending Upon the Measurement Tool: Results From a Population-Based Survey. *Health Promotion International*, Vol. 24, No. 3, pp. 252-261, ISSN 0957-4824

Bergmann, M.M., Jacobs, E.J., Hoffmann, K. & Boeing, H. (2004): Agreement of Self-reported Medical History: Comparison of an In-person Interview with Self-administered Questionnaire. *European Journal of Epidemiology*, Vol. 19, No. 5, pp. 411-416, ISSN 0393-2990

Berkman, N.D., DeWalt, D.A., Pignone, M.P., Sheridan, S.L., Lohr, K.N., Lux, L., Sutton, S.F., Swinson, T. & Bonito, A.J. (2004). *Literacy and Health Outcomes.* AHRQ Publication No. 04-E007-1, Agency for Healthcare Research and Quality, ISBN 1-58763-142-3, Rockville, Md, USA

Borgström F. & Kanis, J.A. (2008). Health Economics of Osteoporosis. *Best Practice & Research Clinical Endocrinology & Metabolism*, Vol. 22, No. 5, pp. 885-900, ISSN 1521-690X

Box, G.E.P. & Tidwell, P.W. (1962). Transformation of the independent variables. *Technometrics*, Vol. 4, No. 4, pp. 531-550, ISSN 0040-1706

Brask-Lindemann, D., Cadarette, S.M., Eskildsen, P. & Abrahamsen, B. (2011). Osteoporosis Pharmacotherapy Following Bone Densitometry: Importance of Patient Beliefs and Understanding of DXA Results. *Osteoporosis International*, Vol. 22, No. 5, pp. 1493-1501, ISSN 0937-941X

Cadarette, S.M., Beaton, D.E., Gignac, M.A., Jaglal, S.B., Dickson, L. & Hawker, G.A. (2007). Minimal Error in Self-report of Having Had DXA, But Self-Report of its Results Was Poor. *Journal of Clinical Epidemiology*, Vol. 60, No. 12, pp. 1306-1311, ISSN 0895-4356

Campostrini, S. (2003). Surveillance Systems and Data Analysis: Continuously Collected Behavioural Data. British and American Examples, In: *Global Behavioral Risk Factor Surveillance*, D. McQueen & P. Puska, (Eds.), 47-56, Kluwer Academic, ISBN 0-306-47777-7, New York, USA

Cawthon, P. (2011). Gender Differences in Osteoporosis and Fractures. *Clinical Orthopaedics and Related Research*, Vol. 469, No. 7, pp. 1900-1905, ISSN 0009-921X

Center, J.R., Bliuc, D., Nguyen, N.D., Nguyen, T.V. & Eisman, J.A. (2011). Osteoporosis Medication and Reduced Mortality Risk in Elderly Women and Men. *Journal of Clinical Endocrinology and Metabolism*, Vol. 96, No. 4, pp. 1006-1014, ISSN 0021-972X

Center, J.R., Bliuc, D., Nguyen, T.V. & Eisman, J.A. (2007). Risk of Subsequent Fracture After Low-Trauma Fracture in Men and Women. *Journal of the American Medical Association*, Vol. 297, No. 4, pp.387-394, ISSN 0098-7484

Chatfield, C. (2004). The Analysis of Time Series. An Introduction. 6th ed., Chapman & Hall/CRC, ISBN 1-58488-317-0, Boca Raton, Florida

Compston, J., Cooper, A., Cooper, C., Francis, R., Kanis, J.A., Marsh, D., McCloskey, E.V., Reid, D.M., Selby, P., Wilkins, M., on behalf of the   National Osteoporosis Guideline Group (NOGG). (2009). Guidelines for the Diagnosis and Management of Osteoporosis in Postmenopausal Women and Men from the age of 50 years in the UK. *Maturitas*, Vol. 62, No. 2, pp. 105-108, ISSN 0378-5122

Cooper, C. (1997). The Crippling Consequences of Fractures and Their Impact on Quality of Life. *American Journal of Medicine*, Vol. 103, No. 2A, pp.12S-19S, ISSN 0002-9343

Czernichow, S., Fan, T., Nocea, G. & Sen, S.S. (2010). Calcium and Vitamin D Intake by Postmenopausal Women with Osteoporosis in France. *Current Medical Research & Opinion*, Vol. 26, No 7, pp. 1667-1674, ISSN 0300-7995

Davis, S.R., Kirby, C., Weekes, A., Lanzafame, A. & Piterman, L. (2011). Simplifying Screening for Osteoporosis in Australian Primary Care: the Prospective Screening for Osteoporosis; Australian Primary Care Evaluation of Clinical Tests (PROSPECT) Study. *Menopause*, Vol. 18, No. 1, pp. 53-59, ISSN 1072-3714

De Walt, D.A., Berkman, N.D., Sheridan, S., Lohr, K.N. & Pignone, M.P. (2005). Literacy and health outcomes: a systematic review of the literature, *Journal of General Internal Medicine*, Vol. 19, No. 12, pp.1228-1239, ISSN 0884-8734

Dillman, D.A. (1999). Mail and Other Self-administered Surveys in the 21st Century: the Beginning of a New Era. *The Gallup Research Journal*, Vol. 2, No. 1, pp. 121-140

Dillman, D.A., Smyth, J.D. & Christian, L.M. (2009). *Internet, Mail and Mixed-mode Surveys. The Tailored Design Method.* 3rd ed. John Wiley and Sons, ISBN 978-0-471-69868-5, New Jersey, USA

Eisman, J.A., Clapham, S. & Kehoe, L., Australian Bone Care Study (2004). Osteoporosis Prevalence and Levels of Treatment in Primary Care: the Australian BoneCare Study. *Journal of Bone and Mineral Research*, Vol. 19, No. 12, pp. 1969-1975, ISSN 0884-0431

Elliot-Gibson, V., Bogoch, E.R., Jamal, S.A. & Beaton, D.E. (2004). Practice Patterns in the Diagnosis and Treatment of Osteoporosis After a Fragility Fracture: A Systematic Review. *Osteoporosis International*, Vol. 15, No. 10, pp. 767-778, ISSN 0937-941X

Farahmand, B., Persson, P.-G., Michaelsson, K., Baron, J., Parker, M., Ljunghall, S., Swedish Hip Fracture Group. (2000). Socio-economic Status, Marital Status and Hip Fracture Risk: A Population-Based Case-Control Study. *Osteoporosis International*, Vol. 11, No. 9, pp. 803-808, ISSN 0937-941X

Francis, K.L., Matthews, B.L., Van Mechelen, W., Bennell, K.L. & Osborne, R.H. (2009). Effectiveness of a Community-Based Osteoporosis Education and Self-management Course: A Wait List Controlled Trial. *Osteoporosis International*, Vol. 20, No. 9, pp. 1563-1570, ISSN 0937-941X

Frey, J. H. (1989). *Survey Research by Telephone.* Sage Publications, ISBN 978-0803929852 Beverly Hills, USA

Grant, J.F., Taylor, A.W., Ruffin, R.E., Wilson, D.H., Phillips, P.J., Adams, R.J.T., Price, K., & the North West Adelaide Health Study Team. (2009). Cohort Profile: The North West Adelaide Health Study (NWAHS). *International Journal of Epidemiology*, Vol. 38, No. 9, pp. 1479-1486, ISSN 0300-5771

Grant, J.F., Chittleborough, C.R., Taylor, A.W., Dal Grande, E., Wilson, D.H., Phillips, P.J., Adams, R.J., Cheek, J.A., Price, K., Gill T., Ruffin, R.E., & the North West Adelaide

Health Study Team. (2006). The North West Adelaide Health Study: Detailed Methods and Baseline Segmentation of a Cohort for Selected Chronic Diseases. *Epidemiologic Perspectives & Innovations*, Vol. 3, (April 12 2006), pp. 4. ISSN 1742-5573

Haentjens, P., Magaziner, J., Colón-Emeric, C.S., Vanderschueren, D., Milisen, K., Velkeniers, B. & Boonen, S. (2010). Meta-analysis: Excess Mortality After Hip Fracture Among Older Men and Women. *Annals of Internal Medicine*, Vol. 152, No. 6, pp. 380-390, ISSN 0003-4819

Harvey, N. & Cooper, C. (2003). Determinants of Fracture Risk in Osteoporosis. *Current Rheumatology Reports*, Vol. 5, No. 1, pp. 75-81, ISSN 1523-3774

Hodgson, S.F., Watts, N.B., Bilezikian, J.P., Clarke, B.L., Gray, T.K., Harris, D.W., Johnston, C.C. Jr., Kleerekoper, M., Lindsay, R., Luckey, M.M., McClung, M.R., Nankin, H.R., Petak S.M., Recker, R.R., AACE Osteoporosis Task Force. (2003). American Association of Clinical Endocrinologists Medical Guidelines for Clinical Practice for the Prevention and Treatment of Postmenopausal Osteoporosis: 2001 Edition, With Selected Updates for 2003. *Endocrine Practice*, Vol. 9, No. 6, pp. 544-564, ISSN 1530-891X

Hosmer, D.W. & Lemeshow, S. (2000). *Applied Logistic Regression*, 2nd ed., J Wiley and Sons, ISBN 0-471-35632-8, New York, USA

International Union for Health Promotion and Education World Alliance for Risk Factor Surveillance Global Working Group. (2011). *White Paper on Surveillance and Health Promotion*, International Union for Health Promotion and Education, Geneva, Switzerland, Retrieved from http://www.iuhpe.org/uploaded/Activities/Scientific_Affairs/GWG/WARFS_white_paper_draft_may_2011.pdf

Keen, R. (2007). Osteoporosis: Strategies for Prevention and Management. *Best Practice & Research Clinical Rheumatology*, Vol. 21, No. 1, pp. 109-122, ISSN 1521-6942

Laslett, L.L., Lynch, J., Sullivan, T.R. & McNeil, J.D. (2011). Osteoporosis Education Improves Osteoporosis Knowledge and Dietary Calcium: Comparison of a 4 Week and a One-Session Education Course. *International Journal of the Rheumatic Diseases*, Vol. 14, No. 3, pp. 239-247, ISSN 1756-1841

Marini, F. & Brandi, M.L. (2010). Genetic Determinants of Osteoporosis: Common Basis to Cardiovascular Disease. *International Journal of Hypertension*, Mar 25, doi:10.4061/2010/394579, ISSN 2090-0392

McQueen, D.V. (2003). Perspectives on Global Risk Factor Surveillance. Lessons Learned and Challenges Ahead, In: *Global Behavioral Risk Factor Surveillance*, D. McQueen & P. Puska, (Eds.), pp. 233-245, Kluwer Academic, ISBN 0-306-47777-7, New York, USA

National Heart Foundation of Australia. (1989). *Risk Factor Prevalence Study. Survey No. 3 - 1989*. National Hearth Foundation, ISBN 978 0 909 47527 7, Canberra, Australia

Nayak, S., Roberts, M.S., Chang C-C.H. & Greenspan, S.L. (2010). Health Beliefs About Osteoporosis and Osteoporosis Screening in Older Women and Men. *Health Education Journal*, Vol. 69, No. 3, pp. 267-276, ISSN 0017-8969

Nielsen-Bohlman, L., Panzer, A. & Kindig D. (Eds.). (2011). *Committee on Health Literacy. A prescription to end confusion*, ISBN 0-309-52926-3, National Academies Press, Washington, DC, USA

Pasco, J.A., Sanders, K.M., Henry, M.J., Nicholson, G.C., Seeman, E. & Kotowicz, M.A. (2000). Calcium Intakes among Australian Women: Geelong Osteoporosis Study. *Australian and New Zealand Journal of Medicine*, Vol. 30, No. 1, pp.21-27, ISSN 0004-8291

Rachner, P.D., Khosla, S. & Hofbauer, L.C. (2011). Osteoporosis: Now and the Future. *Lancet*, Vol. 377, No. 9773, pp. 1276-1287, ISSN 0140-6736

Recker, R.R. & Deng, H.W. (2002). Role of Genetics in Osteoporosis. *Endocrine Journal*, Vol. 17, No. 1, pp. 55-66, ISSN 1355-008X

Royal Australian College of General Practitioners. (2010). *Clinical Guideline for the Prevention and Treatment of Osteoporosis in Postmenopausal Women and Older Men. February 2010*, Royal Australian College of General Practitioners, ISBN 978-0-86906-306-4, Melbourne, Australia

Robertson, B., Sinclair, M., Forbes, A., Kirk, M., & Fairley, C. K. (2000). The Effect of an Introductory Letter on Participation Rates Using Telephone Recruitment. *Australian and New Zealand Journal of Public Health*, Vol. 24, No. 5, pp. 552, ISSN 1326-0200

Sacks, J.J., Harrold, L.R., Helmick, C.G., Gurwitz, J.H., Emani, S. & Yood, R.A. (2005). Validation of a Surveillance Case Definition for Arthritis. *Journal of Rheumatology*, Vol. 32, No. 2, pp. 340-347, ISSN 0315-162X

Sànchez-Riera, L., Wilson, N., Nolla J.M., Macara, M., Chen, J.S., Sambrook, P.N., Hernández, C.S. & March, L. (2010). Osteoporosis and Fragility Fractures. *Best Practice and Research Clinical Rheumatology*, Vol. 24, No. 6, pp. 793-810, ISSN 1521-6942

Schonlau, M., Fricker, R.D., Elliott, M.N. (2002*). Conducting Research Surveys via Email and the Web*, Rand, ISBN 978-0833031105, New York, USA

Scollo, M.M. & Winstanley, M.H. (Eds.). (2008). *Tobacco in Australia: Facts and Issues*. 3rd ed. Cancer Council Victoria, Melbourne, Australia, Retrieved from http://www.tobaccoinaustralia.org.au

Unnanuntana, A., Gladnik, B.P., Donnelly, E., & Lane, J.M. (2010). The Assessment of Fracture Risk. *Journal of Bone and Joint Surgery. American Volume*, Vol. 92, No. 3, pp. 743-753, ISSN 0021-9355

Varenna, M., Binelli, L., Zucchi, F., Ghringhelli, D., Gallazzi, M., & Sinigaglia, L. (1999). Prevalence of Osteoporosis by Educational Level in a Cohort of Post-menopausal Women. *Osteoporosis International*, Vol. 9, No. 3, pp. 236-241, ISSN 0937-941X

Werner, P. (2003). Self Reported Prevalence and Correlates of Osteoporosis: Results from a Representative Study in Israel. *Archives of Gerontology and Geriatrics*, Vol. 37, No. 3 pp. 277-292, ISSN 0167-4943

Wilson, D.H. (2003). Comparison of Surveillance Data on Metropolitan and Rural Health. Diabetes in Southern Australia as an Example, In: *Global Behavioral Risk Factor Surveillance*, D. McQueen & P. Puska, (Eds.), 95-117, Kluwer Academic, ISBN 0-306-47777-7, New York, USA

World Health Organization. (1994). *Assessment of Fracture Risk and its Application to Screening for Postmenopausal Osteoporosis*. Technical Report Series 843, WHO, ISBN 92-4-1208430, Geneva, Switzerland

Yaffee, R. & McGee, M. (2000). *Introduction to Time Series Analysis and Forecasting With Applications of SAS and SPSS*, Academic Press, ISBN 978-0-12-767870-2, San Diego, USA

Part 3

The Diagnosis and Assessment of Osteoporosis and Fractures Risk

6

The Diagnosis and Workup of Patients for Osteoporosis or Osteopenia (Low Bone Mass)

Frank Bonura

St. Catherine of Siena Medical Center, Smithtown, NY
USA

1. Introduction

The rate of screening and treatment for osteoporosis remains low. Osteoporosis affects approximately 200 million women worldwide and two thirds of women 80 or older have this disease. It causes more than 1.6 million hip fractures worldwide. (International Osteoporosis Foundation, 2006) In the United States, more than 10 million Americans have osteoporosis and 3.6 million have low bone mineral density of the hip. In 2005 in the United States, there were more than 2 million osteoporotic fractures in men and women. These fractures caused more than 432,000 hospitalist admissions, 2.5 million physician office visits and about 180,000 nursing home admissions yearly in the United States. In 2005, the cost of osteoporotic fractures was approximately 17 billion dollars. (U.S. Department of Health and Human Services, 2004) Osteoporosis is responsible for approximately 90% of all spine and hip fractures in Caucasian females age 65-84 in the United States.

Fifty percent of women and twenty-five percent of men greater than age 50 will experience an osteoporotic fracture in their remaining lifetime. (National Osteoporosis Foundation, Feb. 2008) Less that 5 percent of patients with a clinical low trauma fragility fracture are referred for medical evaluation and treatment. (Bonura, 2009) In 2005, a population based study reported that the proportion of women screened and treated for osteoporosis after a fragility fracture was 10.2 percent and 12.9 percent respectfully. In males, studies indicate that a low proportion of men are evaluated for osteoporosis or receive anti-resorptive therapy after a fragility fracture. (Feldstein, 2005) Most patients with hip fractures receive no pharmacologic treatment for osteoporosis.

Physician frequently fail to diagnose and treat osteoporosis, even in the elderly patients who have suffered a fractures. (Bonura, 2009) Less then 20 percent of women with wrist fractures are screened for osteoporosis, and only 12.9 percent are treated for osteoporosis after a facture. (Cuddihy, 2002) In a clinical study the majority of patients with clinical vertebral fractures (80 percent) did not receive osteoporosis therapy. (Lindsay, 2005) A prior osteoporotic fracture increases the risk of future fractures. A forearm fracture is associated with a two fold increased risk of fractures. Radiographic vertebral fractures are associated with a higher risk of subsequent hip and other fractures. In the year following a vertebral fracture, 26 percent of patients will fracture a hip, pelvis, vertebrae, wrist, humerus, or leg. (Klotzbuecher, 2000)

Following a hip fracture in women, the mortality ranges between 20-24% within one year. 25% of patients are admitted to a long term healthcare facility and only 40% are able to obtain their pre-fracture level of independence. Worldwide, one-third of hip fractures occur in men and more men than women die after a hip fracture with a mortality rate of about 37.5%. (Jiang, 2005) The most common of all the osteoporotic fractures are vertebral fractures. They are usually painless, but can cause back pain, height loss, deformity, reeducated respiratory function, disability, and a reduced quality of life. There is also an increase in mortality in women of about 23% over 8 years and they can cause an increase in future vertebral and non vertebral fractures. (Kado, 1999)

Prior Fracture	Relative Risk of Future Fractures		
	Wrist	Vertebral	Hip
Wrist	3.3	1.7	1.9
Vertebral	1.4	4.4	2.3
Hip	Not Available	2.5	2.3

Table 1. Prior Fracture as a Predictor of Fracture Risk (Klotzbuecher, 2000))

2. Evaluation

Postmenopausal women and men after age 50 should be evaluated for their risk factors for osteoporosis and fracture, and their risk factors of falling. This evaluation includes a history and a physical exam, including a height measurement and, if necessary diagnostic testing. Several clinical risk factors for osteoporosis have been indentified and should be evaluated. Non-modifiable risk factors include advancing age, female sex, Asian or Caucasian ethnicity, history of a fracture as an adult, family history of a fracture in a first degree relative (maternal or paternal history of a hip fracture) and rheumatoid arthritis. Modifiable risk factors comprise low body weight, hormone deficiency, long term use of medications that affect bone homeostasis (e.g., glucocorticoids), causes of secondary osteoporosis, smoking, excessive alcohol consumption, an inactive lifestyle, and a lifetime diet low in calcium and vitamin D. The more risk factor that a patient has, the greater the risk of a fracture. (Bonura, 2009)

The most important of all these risk factors are age (65 or greater in women and 70 or greater in men) and the occurrence of a low trauma fracture after age 40. Other risk factors of importance are bone mineral density, genetics, menopause, BMI, and lifestyle.

As a woman ages, their fracture risk increases. After age 50, their fracture risk doubles every 7 or 8 years. The average age of a hip fracture in women is 82 years and in men 50% of their hip fractures occur before age 80. Vertebral fractures usually occur in women and men in their seventies. (Chang, 2004) A prior osteoporotic fracture increases the risk of future osteoporotic fracture risk. If a postmenopausal female sustains an osteoporotic fracture, she has approximately a two fold increase of sustaining another osteoporotic fracture in her lifetime.

Bone mineral density also is a risk factor for future fractures. Bone mineral density affects fracture risk. The lower the bone mineral density (BMD), the higher the risk for fractures. A decrease of 1 standard deviation of bone mineral density (BMD) represents a 10-12% decrease in BMD and can increase fracture risk by 1.5 to 2.6 times. (Marshall, 1996) Genetics plays a role in osteoporosis and future fracture risk. Daughters of women who have had an osteoporotic fracture, and daughters of first degree relatives (mother or sisters) or have osteoporosis have lower bone mineral density (BMD) for their age. Also a history of an

Lifestyle Factors		
Low calcium intake	Vitamin D insufficiency	Excess vitamin A
High caffeine intake	High salt intake	Aluminum (in antacids)
Alcohol (3 or more drinks/d)	Inadequate physical activity	Immobilization
Smoking (active or passive)	Falling	Thinness
Hypogonadal States		
Androgen insensitivity	Hyperprolactinemia	Premature ovarian failure
Anorexia nervosa and bulimia	Panhypopituitarism	Turner's & Klinefelter's syndromes
Athletic amenorrhea		
Endocrine Disorders		
Adrenal insufficiency	Diabetes mellitus	Thyrotoxicosis
Cushing's syndrome	Hyperparathyroidism	
Gastrointestinal Disorders		
Celiac disease	Inflammatory bowel disease	Pancreatic disease
Gastric bypass	Malabsorption	Primary biliary cirrhosis
GI surgery		
Genetic Factors		
Cystic fibrosis	Homocystinuria	Osteogenesis imperfecta
Ehlers-Danlos	Hypophosphatasia	Parental history of hip fracture
Gaucher's disease	Idiopathic hypercalciuria	Porphyria
Glycogen storage diseases	Marfan syndrome	Riley-Day syndrome
Hemochromatosis	Menkes steely hair syndrome	
Hematologic Disorders		
Hemophilia	Multiple myeloma	Systemic mastocytosis
Leukemia and lymphomas	Sickle cell diseases	Thalassemia
Rheumatic and Autoimmune Diseases		
Ankylosing spondylitis	Lupus	Rheumatoid arthritis
Miscellaneous Conditions and Diseases		
Alcoholism	Emphysema	Muscular dystrophy
Amlyloidosis	End stage renal disease	Parenteral nutrition
Chronic metabolic acidosis	Epilepsy	Post-transplant bone disease
Congestive heart failure	Idiopathic scoliosis	Prior fracture as an adult
Depression	Multiple sclerosis	Sarcoidosis
Medications		
Anticoagulants (heparin)	Cancer chemotherapeutic drugs	Glucocorticoids (≥ 5 mg/d of prednisone or equivalent for $\geq$ 3 mo)
Anticonvulsants	Cyclosporine A and tacrolimus	Gonadotropin releasing hormone agonists
Aromatase inhibitors	Depo-medroxyprogesterone	Lithium
Barbiturates		

Table 2. Conditions, Diseases and Medications That Cause or Contribute to Osteoporosis and Fractures (National Osteoporosis Foundation, 2008)

osteoporotic fracture in a first degree relative increases an individual's risk of osteoporotic fractures. (Seaman, 1989) During the late menopausal transition (2-3 years before menopause) and during menopause, there is an increase in bone resorption due to a decrease in estrogen production. Women lose approximately 2% of BMD annually for about 5 years during menopause. After which they lose 1-2% per year. They can lose 10.5% in their spine and 5.3% in their hip over this 5-7 year period in this time. (Recker, 2000) In men bone loss increases after age 70 and it is more common in men who are deficient in testosterone or estradiol. (Fink, 2006)

If a woman is thin, a weight of less than 127 pounds, it is a risk factor for a low BMD and a high risk for fracture, A high BMI may be protective. In older women, low BMI is associated with a higher fracture risk. (Van Der Voort, 2001)

The lifestyle factors that are associated with low bone mass and fracture risk are cigarette smoking, alcoholism, poor nutrition, and lack of physical activity, There are also secondary causes of low bone mineral density, including medications, genetic disorders, and various disease states.

Also, in all menopausal women and men after age 50, their risk for falls should be evaluated. About one-third of men and women age 65 years of age or older fall each year. They should be questioned about their history of falls, muscle weakness, dizziness, difficulty walking, impaired vision, balance problems, or medications that affect balance (e.g., sedatives, narcotics, anti-hypertensives). Some of the medications that have the highest association with falls are the serotonin-reuptake inhibitors, antiarrhythmic drugs, tricyclic antidepressants, neuroleptic agents, benzodiazepines, and the anticonvulsants. (Leipzig, 1999) Ten percent of these falls result in hip fractures and 90% of hip fractures are due to falls. An excellent screening test is the "Get Up and Go" test. Have a senior patient get up from a chair, without using their arms, and then have them walk and observe for unsteadiness. (Mathias, 1986) The more number of risk factors of falling, the greater risk of falls.

Medical Risk Factors		
Age	Medications causing over-sedation (narcotic analgesics, anticonvulsants, psychotropics)	
Anxiety and agitation	Orthostatic hypotension	
Arrhythmias	Poor vision and use of bifocals	
Dehydration	Previous fall	
Depression	Reduced problem solving and mental acuity and diminished cognitive skills	
Female gender	Urgent urinary incontinence	
Impaired transfer and mobility	Vitamin D insufficiency [serum 25-hydroxyvitamin D (25(OH)D) < 30 ng/ml (75 nmol/L)]	
Malnutrition		
Environmental Risk Factors	Neuro and Musculoskeletal Risk Factors	Other Risk Factors
Lack of assistive devices in bathrooms	Kyphosis	Fear of falling
Loose throw rugs	Poor balance	
Low level lighting	Reduced proprioception	
Obstacles in the walking path	Weak muscles	
Slippery outdoor conditions		

Table 3. Risk Factors for Falls (National Osteoporosis Foundation, 2008)

During a patient's examination, height measurement may be useful to indicate occult vertebral compression fractures, which are indicative of osteoporosis. They are the most common osteoporotic fractures in postmenopausal women, and two-thirds of these fractures are not clinically recognized. (Cauley, 2007) The loss of height, kyphosis, and back pain may be signs of vertebral fractures. Normally after achieving maximal height, women can lose up to 1.0 - 1.5 inches (2.0 - 3.8 cm) of height as part of the normal aging process, due to degenerative arthritis and shrinkage of intervertebral disks. Height loss of greater than 1.5 inches (3.8 cm) increases the risk of a vertebral fracture. One must suspect a vertebral fracture in postmenopausal women with a historical height loss greater than 4 cm (1.6 in.) or a prospective height loss greater than 2 cm (0.8 in.). In men, a historical height loss greater than 6 cm (2.4 in.) or a prospective height loss greater than 3 cm (1.2 in.). Vertebral fractures are associated with an increase of vertebral and nonvertebral fractures in the future. Nineteen percent of patients who have a vertebral fracture will sustain another fracture within one year. (Laster, 2007) Across a range of BMD, prevalent vertebral fractures increase fracture risk by up to 12 times. Risk assessments based only on BMD may overestimate the risk of future fractures in patients without vertebral fractures and under estimate the risk of future fractures in patients with vertebral fractures. (Siris, 2007) When measuring height annually, it should be performed with a stadiometer or a wall mounted ruler. If there is a historical height loss of more than 1.5 inches (3.8 cm) in menopausal women or than 2.4 inches (6 cm) in men, an evaluation to rule out vertebral fractures should be performed. This can be accomplished by a vertebral fracture assessment (VFA) or by a lateral thoracolumbar radiograph. It is also important in patients who have acute or chronic back pain or kyphosis (to rule out vertebral fractures).

3. Bone mineral density assessment

The diagnosis of osteoporosis is made by BMD. The decision to assess bone density should be based on the skeletal health and risk profile of the individualized patient. Table 4 and 5 summarizes the Internal Society of Clinical Densitometry and the North American Menopausal Society indications for Bone Mineral Density (BMD).

Indications for Bone Mineral Density (BMD) Testing – ISCD	
Women aged 65 and older	Adults with a disease or condition associated with low bone mass or bone loss
Postmenopausal women under age 65 with risk factors for fracture	Adults taking medications associated with low bone mass or bone loss
Women during the menopausal transition with clinical risk factors for fracture, such as low body weight, prior fracture or high-risk medication use	Anyone being considered for pharmacologic therapy
Men aged 70 and older	Anyone being treated, to monitor treatment effect
Men under age 70 with clinical risk factors for fracture	Anyone not receiving therapy in whom evidence of bone loss would lead to treatment
Adults with a fragility fracture	Women discontinuing estrogen should be considered for bone density testing according to the indications listed above

Table 4. Indications for Bone Mineral Density (BMD) Testing - ISCD (Baim, 2008))

Indications for Bone Mineral Density (BMD) Testing - NAMS	
BMD Should Be Measured in the Following Populations:	Testing should be considered for postmenopausal women age 50 and over when one or more of the following risk factors for fracture have been identified
• All women age 65 and over regardless of clinical risk factors	• Fracture (other than skull, facial bone, ankle, finger, and toe) after menopause
• Postmenopausal women with medical causes of bone loss (eg, steroid use, hyperparathyroidism), regardless of age	• Thinness (body weight < 127 lbs. [57.7 kg] or BMI < 21 kg/m²)
• Post menopausal women age 50 and over with additional risk factors (see below)	• History of hip fracture in a parent
• Postmenopausal women with a fragility fracture (eg, fracture from a fall from standing height)	• Current smoker
	• Rheumatoid arthritis
	• Alcohol intake of more than two units per day (one unit is 12 oz. of beer, 4 oz. of wine, or 1 oz. of liquor)

Table 5. Indications for Bone Mineral Density (BMD) Testing of the North American Menopause Society (NAMS) (North American Menopause Society, 2010)

There are many techniques that measure BMD. The gold standard in diagnosis of osteoporosis is made by central DXA using dual energy absorptiometry. Using two different x-ray energies, a DXA device can record attenuation profiles at two different photon energies. At low energy (30-50 keV) bone attenuation is greater than soft tissue attenuation; where as high energy (greater than 70 keV) bone attenuation is similar to soft tissues attenuation. Thus, two types of tissue are distinguished: bone (hydroxyapatite) and soft tissue (everything else). (International Society of Clinical Densitometry, 2010) DXA measures areal BMD. The results are reported as grams of mineral per square centimeter (g/cm²).

The skeletal sites that are measured with central DXA are both the PA spine ($L_1 - L_4$) and the hip (femoral neck or total proximal femur of either hip). In certain circumstances when a hip or a spine cannot be measured then a forearm (33% radius or one third radius of the non dominant arm) should be measured (e.g., patients who are obese and whose weight is above the limit of the DXA table). Results of DXA are reported as a comparison of two norms. A T-score uses a Caucasian female 20-29 NHANES III database, for women of all ethnic groups. In men, a Caucasian male 20-29 NHANES III database is used in all ethnic groups. The difference between the patient's score is expressed in standard deviation above or below the norm. Also, a Z-score will be generated. The patient's BMD is compared to individuals of the same age, sex, and ethnicity. Z-scores should be population specific where adequate reference data exists (International Society for Clinical Densitometry, 2009).

The lower the BMD (T-score) the higher the fracture risk. A decrease of 1 standard deviation represents a 10 - 12% decrease in BMD and an increase in fracture risk by a factor of 1.5 to 2.6, depending on fracture type. The risks of spine and hip fracture increase 2.3 fold and 2.6 fold respectively, for each decrease of 1 standard deviation at the spine and hip. A Z-score of -2.0 or lower is defined as below expected range for age. A Z-score above -2.0 is within the expected range for age.

Peripheral Dual Energy X-Ray Absorptiometry (pDXA) measures areal bone density of the forearm, finger, or heel. It can indentify individuals at risk for fracture but this modality cannot be used for the diagnosis of osteoporosis or for follow up of patients. The measurement of peripheral sites are useful only in screening patients for the need of a central DXA, they are not useful for follow up in patients or in patients taking medications for osteoporosis. (Recker, 2000) Quantitative Computed Tomography (QCT) can measure spinal BMD and can predict vertebral fractures in women, but there is a lack of evidence of a prediction of vertebral fractures in men. There is no evidence that spine QCT can predict hip fractures in women or men. Peripheral Quantitative Computed Tomography (pQCT) of the ultra distal radius can predict hip fracture risk, but not spine fracture risk in postmenopausal women. Quantitative Ultrasound (QUS) can predict fragility fractures in postmenopausal women (hip and vertebral) and men over age 65 (hip and nonvertebral fractures). (Baim, 2008)

According to the World Health Organization (WHO) only the measurement of BMD by central DXA can be used for the diagnosis of osteoporosis, the follow up of individuals and the monitoring of treatment efficacy. (National Osteoporosis Foundation, 2008)

The WHO has defined low bone mass (Osteopenia) as a BMD between -1.0 and 2.5 SD below the normal for young healthy adults of the same sex (T-score < 1.0 and > -2.5), osteoporosis by a BMD of -2.5 SD or below (T-score ≤ -2.5) and severe osteoporosis with a T-score of ≤ -2.5 and a fragility fracture. (World Health Organization, 2003)

The World Health Organization has established the following definitions based on BMD measurement at the spine, hip, or forearm by DXA devices:		
Normal	Low Bone Mass (Osteopenia)	Osteoporosis
BMD is within 1 SD of a "young normal" adult (T-score at -1.0 and above.	BMD is between 1.0 and 2.5 SD below that of a "young normal" adult (T-score between -1.0 and -2.5).	BMD is 2.5 SD or more below that of a "young normal" adult (T-score at or below -2.5). Patients in this group who have already experienced one or more fracture are deemed to have severe or "established" osteoporosis."

Note: Although these definitions are necessary to establish the presence of osteoporosis, they should not be used as the sole determinant of treatment decisions.

Table 6. Defining Osteoporosis by BMD (Kanis, 1994)

In postmenopausal women and men age 50 and older, T-scores are preferred, using the WHO criteria. In women prior to menopause and in males younger than age 50, Z-scores, not T-scores are preferred. The WHO diagnostic criteria may be applied to women in the menopausal transition with risk factors for osteoporosis.

At the time of a central DXA, a vertebral fracture assessment (VFA) can be performed. It is a densitometric spine imaging than can detect vertebral fractures. (Schousboe, 2008) Most vertebral fractures are asymptomatic and if present can increase an individual's future risk of fracture. A Vertebral Fracture Assessment (VFA) is a diagnostic method in which low intensity or dual x-ray absorptiometry is used to examine the lateral spine (T_4-L_4), thereby identifying vertebral fractures. (Leipzig, 1999) There is much less radiation with a VFA in comparison to a lateral spine x-ray (3μSV for VFA versus 600μSV for a radiograph).

According to the International Society of Clinical Densitometry a vertebral fracture assessment should be performed in the following circumstances:

Consider VFA when results may influence management.	
Postmenopausal women with low bone mass (Osteopenia) by BMD criteria PLUS any one of the following:	**Men with low bone bass (Osteopenia) by BMD criteria, PLUS any one of the following:**
• Age greater than or equal to 70 years	• Age 80 years or older
• Historical height loss greater than 4 cm (1.6 in.)	• Historical height loss greater than 6 cm (2.4 in.)
• Prospective height loss greater than 2 cm (0.8 in.)	• Prospective height loss greater than 3 cm (1.2 in.)
• Self-reported vertebral fracture (not previously documented)	• Self-reported vertebral fracture (not previously documented)
• Two or more of the following:	• Two or more of the following:
• Age 60 to 69 years	• Age 70 to 79 years
• Self-reported prior non-vertebral fracture	• Self-reported prior non-vertebral fracture
• Historical height loss of 2 to 4 cm	• Historical height loss of 3 to 6 cm
• Chronic systemic diseases associated with increased risk of vertebral fractures (e.g., moderate to severe COPD or COAD, seropositive rheumatoid arthritis, Crohn's disease)	• Chronic systemic diseases associated with increased risk of vertebral fractures (e.g., moderate to several COPD or COAD, seropositive rheumatoid arthritis, Crohn's disease
	On pharmacologic androgen deprivation therapy or following orchiectomy
Women or men on Chronic Glucocorticoid therapy (equivalent to 5 mg or more of prednisone daily for three (3) months or longer).	**Postmenopausal women or men with osteoporosis by BMD criteria, if documentation of one or more vertebral fractures will alter clinical management.**

Table 7. Indications for VFA (Schousboe, 2008)

The VFA is interpreted using a semi-quantitative visual inspection with assignment of fracture grade by the radiologist or the clinician. Using Genant's method, the clinician determines if a vertebra is fractured or normal. The thoracic and lumbar spine is scanned for deformities and height loss exceeding twenty percent in the anterior, middle, or posterior dimensions. What the clinician determines visually using the semiquantitative method of Genant are morphological changes in the vertebrae. Clinicians should look for end plate deformities (horizontal edges), lack of parallelism of the end plates, buckling of the cortices (vertical edges) and loss of vertical continuity with the adjacent vertebrae. Clinicians then grade the fracture deformity. If a fracture is suspected, it is compared to a standard:

- Grade 1 (mild fracture) height loss 20-25%
- Grade 2 (moderate) height loss of 25-40%
- Grade 3 (severe) height loss of > 40%

Depending on where deformities are present in the vertebra, fractures are classified as wedge (loss of anterior height), crush (loss of posterior height) and biconcave (loss of middle height). (Genant, 1993)

In a study comparing VFA to spine radiographs, VFA had a sensitivity of 95% to detect vertebral fractures indentified by spine radiographs and a specificity of 82% to exclude fractures not visualized in a radiograph. (Vokes, 2003)

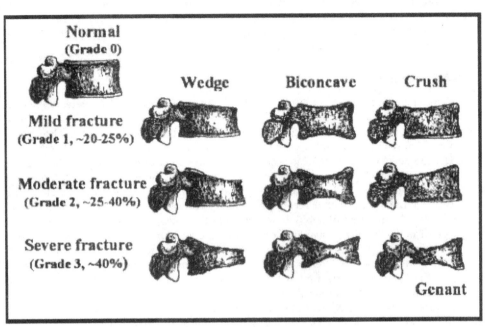

Fig. 1. Genant's Semiquantitative Analysis Grading of Fracture Deformity (Genant, 1993)

4. Follow up bone mineral density testing

Follow up DXA testing by central DXA should be performed every 2-5 years in untreated menopausal women and in men age 70 or older. In patients who are receiving osteoporosis therapy, BMD testing should be performed every 1-2 years. (Van Der Voort, 2001) In order to determine if the change in BMD over time is a real biological change and not to due to chance, a precision study must be performed. Each DXA facility should determine its precision error and calculate the least significant change (LSC), within a 95% statistical confidence. The precision error that is supplied by the manufacturer should not be used.

To perform a precision analysis, the technologist measures 15 patients 3 times or 30 patients 2 times, repositioning the patient after each scan. They then calculate the root mean square stand deviation and obtain the LSC at 95% confidence. This is a real biological change over time and is not due to chance. The minimum acceptable precision for an individual technologist is: lumbar spine 1.9% (LSC = 5.3%), total hip 1.8% (LSC = 5.0%), and femoral neck 2.5% (LSC = 6.9%). (International Society for Clinical Densitometry, 2007)

5. Evaluation for treatment

Within one year of a hip fracture 10-20% of patients die, 20% are placed in nursing homes, and only 40% regain independent functioning. (U.S. Department of Health and Human

Services, 2004) There are more low-trauma fractures in patients with low bone density (Osteopenia) than in those with a DXA diagnosis of osteoporosis. This occurs because there are more individuals with Osteopenia than osteoporosis. (Khosla, 2007) In the study of osteoporotic fractures (SOF), 54% of women with hip fractures did not have osteoporosis according to their BMD results. (Wainwright, 2005) Therefore, it is important to identify and treat individuals who have Osteopenia (low bone density) who have the highest chance of a fracture. Not all patients with low bone mass will fracture.

6. FRAX assessment tool

The WHO sponsored the development of the FRAX assessment tool to indentify which individuals with low bone mineral density have the greatest chance of fracture and which patients need to be treated. (Kanis, 2008) It identifies which patients, who have Osteopenia (low bone lass) who have a higher fracture risk and need to be treated. (Internal Society for Bone Densitometry Course) FRAX is based on an analysis of approximately 60,000 patients that were studied in Europe, North American, Asia, and Australia. The FRAX tool is for untreated individuals with low bone density and indentifies which individuals are at the highest risk of fracture. The NOF recommends the FRAX tool for untreated postmenopausal and men 50 or more years of age with a T-score in the osteopenic range (low bone mass). FRAX predicts the 10 year probability for hip fracture and for major osteoporotic fractures (hip, proximal humerus, distal forearm, and clinical vertebral fractures). FRAX uses clinical risk factors with or without femoral neck BMD. Economic modeling was performed to indentify the 10 year hip fracture risks above which is cost effective, from the societal perspective, to treat with pharmacological agents.

NOF criteria for using FRAX to assist with treatment decisions are:
a.   An untreated postmenopausal women or a man age 50 or older
b.   With low bone mass (T-score between -1.0 and -2.5)
c.   With no prior hip or vertebral fracture (clinical or morphometric)
d.   An evaluable hip for DXA study

Examples of "untreated" patients include:
a.   No ET/HT or estrogen agonist/antagonist (SERM) for the past one year
b.   No calcitonin for the past one year
c.   No PTH for the past one year
d.   No denosumab for the past one year
e.   No bisphosphonate for the past two years (unless it is an oral taken for < 2 months)

This model uses femoral neck BMD but, in women, if femoral neck BMD is unavailable, total hip BMD may be used. In men, only femoral neck BMD can be used in FRAX. (World Health Organization, 2003) Spine of peripheral BMD measurements should not be used in FRAX. (Kanis) There are multiple limitations of FRAX. It does not consider the other risk factors for fracture. These include a history of falls, patients with clinical vertebral fractures, doses of glucocorticoids, exposure dose of alcohol, nicotine, drugs which lower BMD (anticonvulsants, anticoagulants, antineoplastics, antiestrogenic or antiandrogenic agents), parental history of non hip fractures and lumbar spine BMD. This tool only recognizes a hip fracture of a parent. Spinal fractures of a parent due to osteoporosis also may increase fractures risk in the offspring. The therapeutic thresholds that are proposed in the FRAX tool are for clinical guidance and are not rules. They do not preclude clinicians from considering intervention strategies in patients who do not have osteoporosis, nor should they mandate treatment in patients with osteopenia. The decision to treat a patient must be made on a case by case basis.

Risk Factor	Type of Variable	Description
Age	Continuous	40-90 years. For ages below or above this range, the model computes fracture risks as of age 40 or 90.
Sex	Male/female	Model validated for men and women.
Weight	Continuous	Expressed in kilograms.
Height	Continuous	Expressed in centimeters. The modal calculates body mass index and uses it as a continuous variable.
Previous fracture	Yes/no	Includes adult fractures occurring spontaneously or with low trauma (e.g., osteoporosis-related fractures), including morphometric vertebral fractures.
Parental hip fracture	Yes/no	Any hip fracture affecting either parent.
Current smoking	Yes/no	Dose-dependence of fracture risk has been observed but is not reflected in the model.
Oral glucocorticoid use	Yes/no	Present or past exposure to doses equivalent to 5 mg/d prednisolone for ≥ 3 months. Dose-dependence of fracture risk has been observed but is not reflected in the model.
Rheumatoid arthritis	Yes/no	Only a confirmed diagnosis of rheumatoid arthritis should be scored.
Secondary osteoporosis	Yes/no	Secondary osteoporosis occurs in the presence of conditions including, but not limited to, insulin-dependent diabetes, adult osteogenesis imperfecta, uncontrolled hyperthyroidism, menopause at 45 years, hypogonadism, chronic malnutrition/malabsorption, or chronic liver disease.
Alcohol ≥ 3 units daily	Yes/no	1 unit is 285 mL beer, 120 mL wine, 60 mL aperitif, or 30 mL distilled spirits. Dose-dependence of fracture risk has been observed but is not reflected in the model.
Femoral neck BMD	Continuous	Enter BMD value and select DXA machine model used to obtain it, or enter T-score. Risk estimates can also be produced without BMD. If only total hip BMD is available, that can be used. Spinal or peripheral BMD are not to be used.
Clinical vertebral fractures and multiple osteoporosis-related fractures confer additional risk beyond what the model calculates; clinical judgment should be used.		
For a "yes" answer to smoking, alcohol, or glucocorticoid use, the model assumes average levels of exposure. With high exposures, facture risk may increase more than the model accounts for, and clinical judgment should be used.		
When a femoral neck T-score is entered into the online FRAX model, the secondary osteoporosis button becomes inactivated.		

Table 8. Risk Factors Included in the FRAX Algorithm (Siris, 2010)

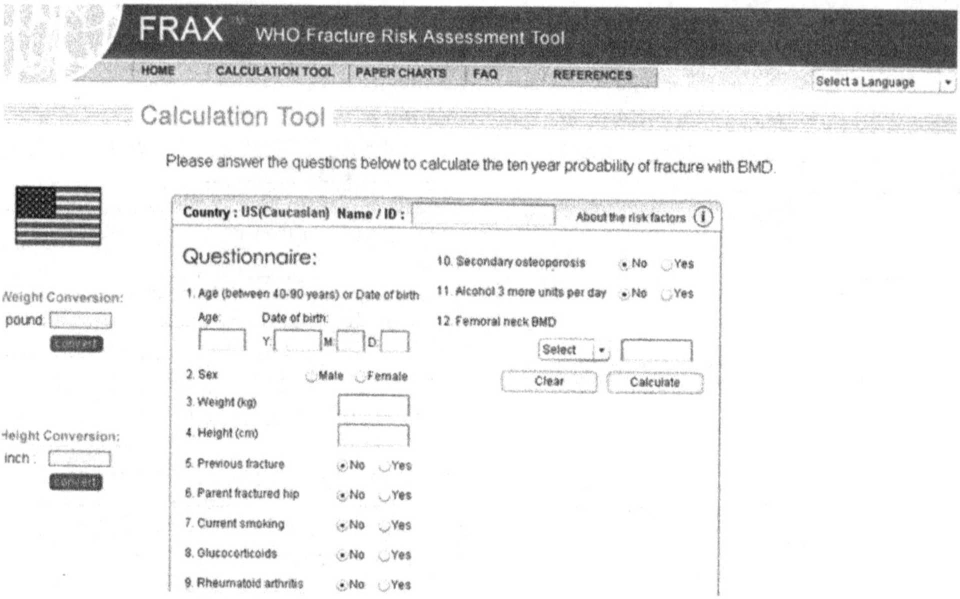

FRAX   WHO Fracture Risk Assessment Tool

HOME   CALCULATION TOOL   PAPER CHARTS   FAQ   REFERENCES   Select a Language ▼

Calculation Tool

Please answer the questions below to calculate the ten year probability of fracture with BMD.

Country : US(Caucasian) Name / ID :   About the risk factors ⓘ

Questionnaire:

10. Secondary osteoporosis   ● No   ○ Yes

1. Age (between 40-90 years) or Date of birth   11. Alcohol 3 more units per day   ● No   ○ Yes

Age: Date of birth: 12. Femoral neck BMD

Y: M: D: Select ▼

2. Sex   ○ Male ○ Female   Clear   Calculate

3. Weight (kg)

4. Height (cm)

5. Previous fracture   ● No   ○ Yes

6. Parent fractured hip   ● No   ○ Yes

7. Current smoking   ● No   ○ Yes

8. Glucocorticoids   ● No   ○ Yes

9. Rheumatoid arthritis   ● No   ○ Yes

Weight Conversion:
pound:
convert

Height Conversion:
inch:
convert

Fig. 2. FRAX Calculation Tool

7. Whom should we treat: NOF guidelines

Consider FDA approved medical therapies for patients with:

- A hip or vertebral (clinical or morphometric) fracture
- Osteoporosis diagnosed by a BMD T-score ≤ -2.5 (femoral neck or spine) after appropriate evaluation to exclude secondary causes of osteoporosis
- Low bone density (a BMD score between -1 and -2.5 at the femoral neck or spine) and a FRAX 10 year probability of hip fracture ≥ 3% or a major osteoporotic fracture (hip, wrist, proximal humerus, clinical vertebral fracture) of ≥ 20%

Physicians should use clinical judgment to treat patients at lower FRAX risk levels if additional risk factors for fracture are present.

Before developing a management plan, the clinician should rule out secondary causes of osteoporosis or bone loss. About 20% of postmenopausal women with osteoporosis and 40% of men with osteoporosis have a secondary cause that can be indentified and treated. (Fitzpatrick, 2002) Secondary osteoporosis can result from a variety of medical conditions including endocrine, hematopoietic or nutritional disorders, and vitamin D deficiency. Diseases such as celiac (malabsorption), liver and renal diseases, the use of glucocorticoids, aromatase inhibitors, antiandrogen therapy (GNRH) and chemotherapy can cause bone loss. These secondary causes must be ruled out before staring pharmacological therapy.

Some of the routine tests would be a complete blood count, serum levels of calcium and phosphate, 25-hydroxyvitamin D, bone specific alkaline phosphatase, creatinine and a 24-hour urine for calcium. Some of the specialized tests may include a thyroid stimulating hormone (TSH), serum levels of parathyroid hormone (PTH) to screen for hyperparathyroidism, a serum protein electrophoresis to indentify abnormal protein produced by multiple myeloma and antitissue transglutaminase antibodies for celiac disease. (Hodgson, 2003)

Test	Diagnostic Result	Possible Secondary Cause
Completed blood cell count	Anemia	Multiple myeloma
Serum calcium	Elevated	Hyperparathyroidism
	Low	Vitamin D deficiency, Gastrointestinal (GI) malabsorption
Serum phosphate	Elevated	Renal failure
	Low	Hyperparathyroidism
Serum 25-hydroxyvitamin D	Low	Undersupplemenataion, GI malabsorption, celiac disease
Serum albumin	Used to interpret serum calcium, nutritional deficiencies	
Serum alkaline phosphatase	Elevated	Vitamin D deficiency, GI malabsorption, hyperparathyroidism, Paget's disease, liver/biliary disease
Urinary calcium excretion	Elevated	Renal calcium leak, multiple myeloma, metastatic cancer involving bone, hyperparathyroidism, hyperthyroidism
	Low	GI malabsorption, inadequate intake of calcium and vitamin D
Thyroid-stimulating hormone (TSH)	Low	Hyperthyroidism (causes excess bone turnover)
	High	Hypothyroidism
Serum protein electrophoresis	Monoclonal band	Multiple myeloma
Tissue transglutaminase antibody (gluten enteropathy)	Elevated	Predictive of celiac disease
Creatinine	Elevated	Renal osteodystrophy, possible contraindication to bisphosphonates
PTH	Elevated	Hyperparathyroidism, vitamin D deficiency

Table 9. Laboratory Tests for Osteoporosis Evaluation (North American Menopause Society, 2010)

8. Bone turnover markers

Bone turnover markers are proteins that are produced by the activity of osteoclasts and by osteoblasts. The resorption markers of osteoclastic activity are the breakdown products of type I collagen (N-telopeptides, C-telopeptides, deoxypyridinolone). There are markers of osteoblastic synthesis of bone matrix (bone-specific alkaline phosphatates, osteocalcin, procollagen type I N-terminal propetide).

Suppression of biochemical markers of bone turnover occur 3-6 months of specific antiresorptive therapies and they increase after 1-3 months of anabolic therapies. The NOF recommends a baseline and a repeat bone resorption marker after initiation of therapy as a method of monitoring the therapeutic effect of an antiresportive agent.

The changes of bone turnover markers occur more rapidly than changes in BMD and they can also predict patient compliance or poor response to antiresorptive therapy. There is a high degree of biological and analytical variability in the measurement of biochemical markers. This variability can be reduced by obtaining samples in the early morning after an overnight fast. (National Osteoporosis Foundation, 2008)

9. Conclusion

In all senior men and in all postmenopausal women a history should be obtained to evaluate a patient's risk factors for osteoporosis and for fractures. As part of a patient's physical exam, a height measurement should be performed. This can indentify when there is a significant height loss or an asymptomatic vertebral fracture. When necessary, a central DXA and sometimes a Vertebral Fracture Assessment (VFA) may be performed. Clinicians should estimate a patient's 10-year probability of a hip or a major osteoporotic related fracture using FRAX. We should use the WHO criteria to determine who we should treat and which individuals whom we should not treat. Clinicians also must perform a laboratory workup on patients, to rule our secondary causes of osteoporosis, before starting a pharmacological treatment regimen.

10. References

Baim, S, et Al. (2008). Official Position of the International Society for Clinical Densitometry. *Journal of Clinical Densitometry*, 11, 1, (January 2008), pp. 6-16

Bonura, F. (2009). Prevention, Screening, and Management of Osteoporosis. *Postgraduate Medicine*, 121, 5, (July 2009), pp. 5-17

Cauleu, J et Al. (2007). Long Term Risk of Vertebral Fracture. *Journal of the American Medical Association*, 298, 23, (December 2007), pp. 2761-2767

Chang, K, et Al. (2004). Incidence of Hip and Other Osteoporotic Fractures in Elderly men and Women. *Journal of Bone Mineral Research*, 19, 4, (April 2004), pp. 532-536

Cuddihy, M, et Al. (2002). Osteoporosis Intervention Following Distal Forearm Fractures: A Missed Opportunity? *Archives of Internal Medicine*, 164, 4, (February 2002), pp. 421-426

Feldstein, AC, et Al. (2005). The Near Absence of Osteoporosis Treatment in Older Men with Fractures. *Osteoporosis International*, 16, 8, (August 2005), pp. 953-962

Fink, H, et Al. (2006). Association of Testosterone and Estradiol Deficiency with Osteoporosis and rapid Bone Loss in Older Men. *Journal of Clinical Endocrinology and Metabolism*, 91, 10, (October 2006), pp. 3908-3915

Fitzpatrick, L. (2002). Secondary Causes of Osteoporosis. *Mayo Clinic Proceedings*, 77, 5, (May 2002), pp. 453-468

Genant, H, et Al. (1993) Vertebral Fracture Assessment Using a Semiquantitative Technique. *Journal of Bone Mineral Research*, 8, 9, (September 1993), pp. 1137-1148

Hodgson, S, et Al. (2003). AACE Osteoporosis Task Force: AACE Medical Guidelines for Clinical Practice for the Prevention and Treatment of Postmenopausal Osteoporosis. *Endocrine Practice*, 9, 6, (November/December 2003), pp. 544-564

International Osteoporosis Foundation. (n.d.) Facts and Statistics about Osteoporosis and Its Impact, 12.09.2006, Available from: <http://www.iofbonehealth.org/facts-and-statistics.html>

International Society for Clinical Densitometry Course. (n.d.). *Basic Science of Bone Densitometry and Device Operating Principles*, (2010), pp. 24-35

International Society for Clinical Densitometry. (2007). ISCD Official Positions Brochure. *Densitometry*, 11, (January 2009), pp. 6-21.

Jiang, H, et Al. (2005). Development and Initial Validation of a Risk Score for Predicting In-Hospital and 1-Year Mortality in Patients with Hip Fractures. *Journal of Bone Mineral Research*, 20, 3, (March 2005), pp. 494-500

Kado, D, et Al. (1999). Vertebral Fractures and Mortality in Older Women. Study of Osteoporotic Fractures Research Group. *Archives of Internal Medicine*, 159, 11, (June 1999), pp. 1215-1220

Kanis, J. (n.d.) FRAX. *WHO Fracture Risk Assessment Tool*, 18.06.2009, Available from: <http://FRAX/index-htm>

Kanis, J, et Al. (1994). The Diagnosis of Osteoporosis. *Journal of Bone Mineral Research*, 9, 8, (August 1994), pp. 1137-1141

Kanis, J, et Al. (2008). FRAX and the Assessment of Fracture Probability in Men and Women from the UK. *Osteoporosis International*, 19, 4, (April 2008), pp. 385-397

Khosla, S, et Al. (2005). Study of Osteoporosis Fractures Group. *Journal of Clinical Endocrinology and Metabolism*, 90, 5, (May 2005), pp. 2787-2793

Khosla, S, et Al. (2007). Clinical Practice: Osteopenia. *New England Journal of Medicine*, 356, 22, (November 2007), pp. 2293-2300

Klotzbuecher, C, et Al. (2000). Patients with Prior Fracture Have an increased Risk of Future Fractures. *Journal of Bone Mineral Research*, 15, 4, (April 2000), pp. 721-739

Laster, J, et Al. (2007). Vertebra Fracture Assessment By Dual Energy X-Ray Absorptiometry. *Journal of Clinical Densitometry*, 10, 3, (July 2007), pp. 227-237

Leipzig, R, et Al. (1999). Drugs and Falls in Older People. *Journal of the American Geriatric Society*, 47, 1, (January 1999), pp. 30-39

Lindsay, R, et Al. (n.d.). Early Osteoporosis Treatment Reduced Fracture Risk Almost 50 Percent, *Proceedings of the American Society of Bone and Mineral Research Annual Meeting*, Nashville, TN, September 2005

Marshall , D, et Al. (1996). Meta-Analysis of How Well Measures of Bone Mineral Density Predict Occurrence of Osteoporotic Fractures. *British Medical Journal*, 312, 7041, (May 1996), pp. 1254-1259.

Mathis, S, et Al. (1986), Balance in Elderly Patients: The "Get Up and Go" Test. *Archives of Physical Medicine and Rehabilitation*, 67, 6, (June 1986), pp. 387-389

National Osteoporosis Foundation. (Feb. 2008). *Fast Facts on Osteoporosis*, National Osteoporosis Foundation, Washington, DC

National Osteoporosis Foundation. (2008). *Clinician's Guide to Prevention and Treatment of Osteoporosis*. National Osteoporosis Foundation, pp. 1-36

North American Menopause Society. 2010. Management of Osteopororsis in Postmenopausal Women: 2010 Position Statement of the North American Menopause Society. *Menopause*, 17, 1, (January 2010), pp. 23-54

Recker, R, et Al. (2000). Characterization of Perimenopausal Bone Loss: A Prospective Study. *Journal Bone Mineral Research*, 15, 10, (October 2000), pp. 1965-1973

Seaman, E, et Al. (1989) Reduced Bone Mass in Daughters of Women with Osteoporosis. *New England Journal of Medicine*, 320, 9, (March 1989), pp. 554-558

Schousboe, J, et Al. (2008), Vertebral Fracture Assessment: 2007 ISCD Official Positions. *Journal of Clinical Densitometry*, 11, 1, (January 2008), pp. 92-108

Siris, E, et Al. (2007). Enhanced Predication of Fracture Risk Combining Fracture Status and BMD. *Osteoporosis International*, 18, 6, (June 2007), pp. 761-770

Siris, E, et Al. (2010), Primary Care Use of FRAX: Absolute Fracture Risk Assessment in Postmenopausal Women and Older Men. *Postgraduate Medicine*, 122, 1, (January 2010), pp. 82-90

U.S. Department of Health and Human Services. (2004). *Bone Health and Osteoporosis: A Report of the Surgeon General*, Department of Health and Human Services, Office of the Surgeon General, Rockville, MD

Van Der Voort, D, et Al. (2001). Risk Factors for Osteoporosis Related to Their Outcomes. *Osteoporosis International*, 12, 8, (September 2001), pp. 630-638

Vokes, T, et Al. (2003). Clinical Utility of Dual Energy Vertebral Assessment (DVA). *Osteoporosis International*, 14, 11, (November 2003), pp. 871-878

World Health Organization. (2003). Prevention and Management of Osteoporosis. World Health Organization Technical Report Series, 921, (2003), pp. 1-64

7

Evolutionary Pathways of Diagnosis in Osteoporosis

Antonio Bazarra-Fernández
A Coruña University Hospital Trust
Spain

1. Introduction

Osteoporosis was formally identified as a disease by a group of World Health Organization (WHO) experts in 1994 resulting in publication of "Assessment of Fracture Risk and its Application to Screening for Postmenopausal Osteoporosis" (WHO Technical Report Series, 1994).

Osteoporosis is defined as a skeletal disorder characterized by compromised bone strength predisposing to an increased risk of fracture. Bone strength reflects the integration of two main features: bone density and bone quality. Bone density is expressed as grams of mineral per area or volume and in any given individual is determined by peak bone mass and amount of bone loss. Bone quality refers to architecture, turnover, damage accumulation and mineralization (NIH Consensus, 2001).

Osteoporosis occurs in all populations and at all ages and is a devastating disorder with significant physical, psychosocial and financial consequences. The WHO operationally defines osteoporosis as a bone density at least 2.5 standard deviations below the mean peak bone mass for healthy young adult white women, also referred to as a *T-score* of –2.5. Because of the difficulty in accurate measurement and standardization between instruments and sites, controversy exists among experts regarding the continued use of this diagnostic criterion. So different instruments have not the same performance in regard to a accurate bone density measurement.

The aims of this chapter are stated in table 1.

1.	Identify the technique, safety and limitations of dual energy X-ray absorptiometry (DEXA or DXA) scanning.
2.	Explain the value of utilizing bone densitometry to assess and monitor fracture risk.
3.	Incorporate clinical risk factors that predict future fracture.
4.	Explain the value of identifying the different components that make up the bone metabolism.
5.	Open new tracks for diagnosis of osteoporosis

Table 1. Statement of objectives

In the evolutionary pathways of diagnostics in bone loss the osteoporosis diagnosis is often performed by measuring bone mineral density (BMD) that measures the amount of calcium in different regions of the skeleton as femur neck or/and 1-4 lumbar vertebrae .

In establishing diagnosis of osteoporosis three parameters should be considered as stated in table 2.

1. The diagnosis of osteoporosis.
2. The diagnosis of bone metabolism components.

Table 2. Statement of objectives

2. Osteoporosis and fracture risk: Monitoring and assessment

Several methods are available to measure BMD. In general, the lower bone density the greater osteoporotic fracture risk. Unfortunately osteoporosis frequently remains undiagnosed until a fracture occurs. BMD methods involve DEXA or quantitative computer tomography scans (Osteo CT or QCT) of bones in the spine or femur. The most widely used technique is DXA.

2.1 Technique, safety and limitations of DXA scanning

Bone densitometry is the *gold standard method* for measuring BMD. Bone densitometry is the method used to determine the drug efficacy in recent large clinical trials and to characterize fracture risk in large epidemiological studies. DXA, previously DEXA, is a method of measuring BMD. A DXA scan uses low energy X-rays. A machine sends X-rays from two different sources through the bone being tested. Bone blocks a certain amount of the X-rays. The more dense the bone is, the fewer X-rays get through to the detector. By using two different X-ray sources rather than one it greatly improves the accuracy in measuring the bone density. The amount of X-rays that comes through the bone from each of the two X-ray sources is measured by a detector. This information is sent to a computer which calculates a score of the average density of the bone. A low score indicates that the bone is less dense than it should be, some material of the bone has been lost, and is more prone to fracture.

Older methods such as single photon absorptiometry(SPA) do not predict hip fractures as well as DXA.

But currently there is no accurate measure of overall bone strength. Osteoporosis is related to decreased bone strength, which encompasses both BMD and bone quality. Notwithstanding BMD assessed by DXA remains the *gold standard* for the diagnosis of osteoporosis.

DEXA is the most widely available method of bone densitometry. The measurement of BMD by DEXA has served as a fit surrogate for the measurement of bone strength and accounts for approximately 70 percent of bone strength, it was said. DEXA measures the BMD in the spine, hip or total body.

Based on the 1994 WHO report, osteoporosis is defined as a BMD value from at least -2.5 SD below the mean value of a young healthy population (T-score≤-2.5). Any bone can be affected, but of special concern are the fractures of the hip and spine.

Diagnosis of osteoporosis is generally on the basis of BMD assessment at the spine and proximal femur by DXA. Two X-ray beams with differing energy levels are targeted at the patient' s bones. But, there are other variables in addition to age which are suggested to confound the interpretation of BMD as measured by DXA. One important confounding variable is bone size. DXA has been shown to overestimate the bone mineral density of taller subjects and underestimate the bone mineral density of smaller subjects. This error is due to the way in which DXA calculates BMD. In DXA, bone mineral content, measured as the attenuation of the X-ray by the bones being scanned, is divided by the area, also measured by the machine, in the site being scanned.

Because of DXA calculates BMD using area (aBMD: areal Bone Mineral Density), it is not an accurate measurement of true bone mineral density, which is mass divided by a volume. In order to distinguish DXA BMD from volumetric bone-mineral density, researchers sometimes refer to DXA BMD as aBMD.

The National Osteoporosis Foundation's guidelines state that women over 65, younger post menopausal women who have any of the osteoporosis risk factors, as well as those with specific fractures should have this test. However, men are also at risk for osteoporosis as they age especially if they have some of the causes of osteopenia or osteoporosis

2.2 Other methods of osteoporosis diagnosis

The bone density test is performed using various methods. Some of these BMD tests are explained here briefly.

2.2.1 Quantitative ultrasound parameters

Quantitative Ultrasound (QUS) is the most basic bone density test performed. It can be the first step in order to diagnose any primary bone related problem. If the ultrasound test finds any defect in the bone density, then the DEXA test is recommended. QUS can be used to predict fracture risk, but it cannot be used for the diagnosis of osteoporosis or for monitoring the effects of treatment. Ultrasounds measure the BMD in the heel and uses sound waves of different frequencies through water or air, to perform the task. Bone density test is painless, fast and without harmful radiations. Ultrasounds are unable to detect complicated bone problems and hence there are other methods that are capable of detecting the more complicated ones.

Ultrasound axial transmission, a technique using propagation of ultrasound waves along the cortex of cortical bones, has been proposed as a diagnostic technique for the evaluation of fracture healing. Quantitative ultrasound parameters have been reported to be sensitive to callus changes during the regeneration process. The results suggest that the time of flight measured in axial transmission is affected by local changes of speed of sound induced by changes in local mineralization.

2.2.2 Quantitative computer tomography scan

Quantitative Computer Tomography Scan (QCT) is done to find true volumetric bone mineral content by measuring separately trabecular and three-dimensional cortical bone.

Image quality degradation due to subject motion is a common artefact affecting *in vivo* high-resolution peripheral quantitative computed tomography (HR-pQCT) of bones. These artefacts confound the accuracy and reproducibility of bone density, geometry, and cortical and trabecular structure measurements. Observer-based systems for grading image quality and criteria for deciding when to repeat an acquisition and post hoc data quality control remain highly subjective and non-standardized (Sodeab et al, 2011).

The QCT scan is a not so famous form of bone density test because it is expensive, utilizes a high amount of radiation and its accuracy is minimum.

The QCT measures BMD at spine or hip. Bone architecture, measured by CT, is a BMD-independent determinant of bone strength (Bauer & Link, 2009).

Because bone density can vary from one location in the body to another, a measurement taken at the heel usually is not as accurate a predictor of fracture risk as is a measurement taken at the spine or hip. That is why, if the test on a peripheral device is positive, DXA scan should be performed at the spine or hip to confirm the diagnosis. But what happen at the spine or hip is not what happen at the heel or wrist. So, the problem endures.

2.2.3 Bone fracture risk calculators

The fracture risk assessment tool (FRAX®) case finding algorithm has been developed to predict the 10-year risk of major and hip fractures based on clinical risk factors, with and without BMD. The Garvan fracture risk calculator is another tool that is available online to calculate the risk of fracture. The FORE Fracture Risk Calculator™ uses risk factors established by the W HO, such as alcohol use, family history of hip fractures, and certain chronic diseases.

FRAX and Garvan fracture risk calculators estimate the absolute risk of osteoporotic fractures. Garvan estimated higher absolute fracture risk than FRAX. None of the calculators provide better discrimination than models based on age and BMD, and their discriminative ability is only moderate, which may limit their clinical utility (Bolland et al., 2011).

The Framingham Osteoporosis Study, an ancillary study of the Framingham Heart Study, has contributed substantially to the understanding of risk factors for age-related bone loss and fractures in men and women. For the past fifteen years, this research program has been investigating a variety of risk factors for bone loss and fractures by assessing BMD using SPA, dual photon absorptiometry (DPA), DXA, QUS, and by ascertaining fracture incidence in the Framingham Study

The FRAX® tool has been developed by WHO to evaluate fracture risk of patients that integrate the risks associated with clinical risk factors as well as with or without BMD at the femoral neck. The FRAX® algorithms give the 10-year probability of fracture (Kanis et al., 2000).

The prediction of hip fracture and other osteoporotic fractures based on the assessment algorithms (FRAX™) which includes clinical risk factors alone, or the combination of clinical risk factors plus BMD is prediction, but Medicine is Medicine and future prediction is not Medicine and the important is not the statistics but if the human ill being who must be treated or not. In the evaluation of the FRAX and Garvan fracture risk calculators in older women it was found that Garvan calculator was well calibrated for osteoporotic fractures but overestimated hip fractures. FRAX with BMD underestimated osteoporotic and hip fractures. FRAX without BMD underestimated osteoporotic and overestimated hip fractures. In summary, none of the calculators provided better discrimination than models based on age and BMD, and their discriminative ability was only moderate, which may limit their clinical utility. The calibration varied, suggesting that the calculators should be validated in local cohorts before clinical use.

The probability is not certainty of fracture. It is statistics. That is science that deals with the collection, classification, analysis, and interpretation of numerical facts or data, and that, by use of mathematical theories of probability, imposes order and regularity on aggregates of more or less disparate elements. Is that the matter?. May be, but it is not medicine. And osteoporosis is a medical condition. And risk factors do not mean disease. The patient is the patient and not one year probability. On the other hand "the FRAX® assessment does not tell you who to treat which remains a matter of clinical judgement. In many countries, guidelines are provided that are based on expert opinion and/or on health economic grounds", what the question remain to be wonder what to do with?. That supposes one first principles answer. Level D evidence-based medicine according to the standards of the UK National Health Service or lower level if any existed in the evidence-based medicine.

2.2.3.1 The Bayes' theorem

Bayes' theorem deals with the role of new information in revising probability estimates. The theorem assumes that the probability of a hypothesis (the posterior probability) is a function of new evidence (the likelihood) and previous knowledge (prior probability).

Specific chart reminders to physicians combined with mailed patient education substantially increased the levels of bone density testing and could potentially be used to improve osteoporosis screening in primary care. Bayesian hierarchical analysis makes it possible to assess practice-level interventions when few practices are randomized (Levy BT et al. 2009).

In probability theory and applications, Bayes' theorem shows how to determine inverse probabilities: knowing the conditional probability of B given A, what is the conditional probability of A given B? This can be done, but also involves the so-called prior or unconditional probabilities of A and B.

This theorem is named for Thomas Bayes and often called Bayes' law or Bayes' rule. Bayes' theorem expresses the conditional probability, or "posterior probability", of a hypothesis H (its probability after evidence E is observed) in terms of the "prior probability" of H, the prior probability of E, and the conditional probability of E given H. It implies that evidence has a confirming effect if it is more likely given H than given not-H. Bayes' theorem is valid in all common interpretations of probability, and it is commonly applied in science and engineering. However, there is disagreement among statisticians regarding the question whether it can be used to reduce all statistical questions to problems of inverse probability. Can competing scientific hypotheses be assigned prior probabilities?

The key idea is that the probability of an event A given an event B depends not only on the relationship between events A and B but also on the marginal probability of occurrence of each event.

As a formal theorem, Bayes' theorem is valid in all common interpretations of probability. However, frequentist and Bayesian interpretations disagree on how (and to what) probabilities are assigned. In the Bayesian interpretation, probabilities are rationally coherent degrees of belief, or a degree of belief in a proposition given a body of well-specified information. Bayes' theorem can then be understood as specifying how an ideally rational person responds to evidence. In the frequentist interpretation, probabilities are the frequencies of occurrence of random events as proportions of a whole. Though his name has become associated with subjective probability, Bayes himself interpreted the theorem in an objective sense.

Bayes' theorem is often more easy to apply, and to generalize, when expressed in terms of odds. It is then usually referred to as Bayes' rule, which is expressed in words as posterior odds equals prior odds times likelihood ratio. The term Bayes factor is often used instead of likelihood ratio.

In statistics, the use of Bayes factors is a Bayesian alternative to classical hypothesis testing. Bayesian model comparison is a method of model selection based on Bayes factors.

The adoption of Bayes' theorem has led to the development of Bayesian methods for data analysis. Bayesian methods have been defined as "the explicit use of external evidence in the design, monitoring, analysis, interpretation and reporting" of studies (Spiegelhalter, 1999). The Bayesian approach to data analysis allows consideration of all possible sources of evidence in the determination of the posterior probability of an event. It is argued that this approach has more relevance to decision making than classical statistical inference, as it focuses on the transformation from initial knowledge to final opinion rather than on providing the "correct" inference.

In addition to its practical use in probability analysis, Bayes' theorem can be used as a normative model to assess how well people use empirical information to update the probability that a hypothesis is true.

The odds in favor of an event or a proposition are expressed as the ratio of a pair of integers, which is the ratio of the probability that an event will happen to the probability that it will not happen.

Frequency probability is the interpretation of probability that defines an event's probability as the limit of its relative frequency in a large number of trials. The development of the frequentist account was motivated by the problems and paradoxes of the previously dominant viewpoint, the classical interpretation. The shift from the classical view to the frequentist view represents a paradigm shift in the progression of statistical thought.

Frequentists talk about probabilities only when dealing with well-defined random experiments.The set of all possible outcomes of a random experiment is called the sample space of the experiment.

A paradigm is what members of a scientific community, and they alone, share. A paradigm shift (or revolutionary science) is, according to Thomas Kuhn in his influential book The Structure of Scientific Revolutions (1962), a change in the basic assumptions, or paradigms, within the ruling theory of science. It is in contrast to his idea of normal science. A proposition is true if it works. Thus, older occupants in motor-vehicle crashes are more likely to experience injury than younger occupants. Crash-injury data were used with Bayes' Theorem to estimate the conditional probability of AIS 3+ skeletal injury given that an occupant is osteoporotic for the injury to the head, spine, thorax, lower extremities, and upper extremities. It suggests that the increase in AIS 3+ injury risk with age for non-spine injuries is likely influenced by factors other than osteoporosis (Rupp et al., 2010).

2.2.4 The radiological assessment of vertebral osteoporosis

Vertebral fracture assessment (VFA) is recognized as the standard in fracture risk assessment. High definition instant vertebral assessment allows identifying spine fractures with one rapid, low dose, single energy image at double the resolution of previously available techniques. VFA differs from radiological detection of fractures, because VFA uses a lower radiation exposure and can detect only fractures, while traditional x-ray images can detect other bone and soft tissue abnormalities in addition to spinal fractures.

2.2.5 Some other methods

1. Morphometry. VFA may be referred to as DEXA or DXA or morphometric x-ray absorptiometry. Magnetic resonance imaging (MRI) is a new method of measuring bone density. MRI has made significant contributions to the diagnosis of acute hip joint disease in adults by enabling early differentiation between such conditions as idiopathic avascular femoral head necrosis, septic coxitis, degenerative disease, and tumors. MRI may provide information pertaining to bone density and structure as well as to occult fracture detection.

Quantitative methods such as morphometry or MRI have been developed over the past years and can be used to assess more precisely the features of vertebral fractures.

2. Single-energy X-ray absorptiometry (SXA) is a method of assessing bone mineral density using a single energy X-ray beam. This may be used to measure the wrist or heel bone density, but SXA is not used as often as DEXA. It is now widely considered inferior to dual-energy X-ray absorptiometry which uses a second energy beam to correct for absorption of X-ray energy by non-calcium containing tissues. Many previous studies of peripheral bone mineral density measurement for instance at the wrist, used SXA to assess bone mineral density.

3. Peripheral dual energy X-ray absorptiometry (PDEXA) is a type of DEXA test that measures the density of bones in the arms or legs, such as the wrist or a finger. It cannot measure the density of the bones most likely to break, such as the hip and spine. PDEXA is not as useful as DEXA for finding out how well medicine used to treat osteoporosis is working.

4. SPA is a method that uses a single-energy photon beam that is passed through bone and soft tissue to a detector. The amount of mineral in the path is then quantified.

5. Dual-photon absorptiometry (DPA) uses a photon beam that has two distinct energy peaks. One energy peak is absorbed more by the soft tissue. The other energy peak is absorbed more by bone. The soft-tissue component is subtracted to determine the BMD.

6. Radiographic absorptiometry (RA) uses an X-ray of the hand and a small metal wedge to calculate bone density. This is an approach that include different methods to significantly increase the proportion of eligible patients tested for low BMD, using a low-cost peripheral BMD system in the primary care physician's office or satellite facility to identify those patients who could receive further BMD assessment by central DXA.

2.3 The diagnosis of bone metabolism control

Bone metabolism control is performed inside and outside the bone. Through lab tests which may be carried out in blood and urine samples, bone metabolism becomes known. The results of these tests can help identify conditions that may be contributing to bone loss. The most common blood tests evaluate: blood calcium levels, blood vitamin D levels, liver function, kidney function tests: both creatinine and BUN are included on the common chemical profiles, thyroid function: TSH, T4, T3 tests , parathyroid hormone levels, estradiol levels in women, follicle stimulating hormone test to establish menopause status, testosterone levels in men, osteocalcin levels to measure bone formation.

A 24-hour urine collection can show if there is a problem with intestinal absorption of calcium (Ca) or leakage of calcium through the kidneys. Blood tests are done to check things such as blood chemistries, blood count, proteins, vitamin D level, thyroid function, and antibodies for celiac disease, a condition that may cause poor intestinal absorption of important nutrients. A simple urine specimen shows the bone metabolism or an important factor in determining bone density and bone strength. With this test, natural bone protein products such as N-telopeptide (NTX) are tested.

Dairy products constitute one of the most important types of functional food. And dairy products-calcium intake and its good intestinal absorption is basic. Renal Ca clearance is other parameter to be measured.

Essential hypertensive (EH) patients have a higher rate of urinary calcium excretion and, according to some reports, somewhat lower levels of serum ionized calcium. The mean renal calcium clearance is somewhat higher, but the difference from controls did not reach statistical significance. These data indicate an abnormal handling of a calcium load by patients with EH and raise the possibility that such abnormality may not be due simply to a renal defect but perhaps to an altered calcium distribution among different compartments in the body.

Altered regulation of serum calcium level was proposed to be associated with arterial hypertension and to be dependent on a renal Ca leak or altered Ca binding to plasma proteins and cell membrane described in human and experimental hypertension. Hypertensive patients have an altered regulation of serum Ca concentrations, probably due to a different body distribution of Ca, rather than to altered Ca binding to plasma proteins.

It has been reported that changes in salt loading influence parameters of calcium metabolism in hypertensive subjects. It was also reported that response of blood pressure to salt intake is related to salt-induced increase in intracellular calcium and decrease in intracellular magnesium concentrations. Several authors showed that salt-sensitive hypertensive subjects significantly decreased blood pressure after calcium intake which was emphasized by high salt intake.

It has been showed that during high salt intake regimen increase in blood pressure was followed with decrease in serum calcium level, this was explained by the fact that high salt intake stimulates the Ca uptake by cells. They also reported the following characteristics of hypertensive patients with additionally lower blood pressure as a response to Ca intake: salt-sensitive, low serum ionized Ca and plasma renin activity (PRA) values and high parathyroid hormonE (PTH) values and 1,25-(OH)2-D3 values.

A number of abnormalities in the extracellular and intracellular handling of Ca in arterial hypertension, namely an increased urinary Ca excretion, a reduced serum ionized Ca level and an enhanced intracellular free calcium concentration, have previously been reported. The total body Ca clearance, calculated from the area under the curve of the serum Ca concentrations, was enhanced in hypertensive patients (P less than 0.03). Although the renal Ca excretion is higher in hypertension, the renal calcium clearance account for only a minor fraction of the total body clearance, suggesting that the reduced serum Ca levels achieved by the hypertensive patients are not explained by the renal Ca leak. The enhanced total body Ca clearance found in hypertensive subjects is therefore due to an increased tissue Ca uptake. This finding provides indirect evidence of altered cell Ca handling in hypertension.

Ca metabolism has been investigated in patients with essential hypertension and normal renal function to evaluate the renal calcium handling and the reported increase in renal Ca loss. The results support the hypothesis of primary renal Ca leak in essential hypertension. Enhanced urinary calcium excretion rate may cause compensatory PTH overactivity.

Increased gut Ca absorption or reduced renal tubular Ca reabsorption have been alternatively reported in idiopathic hypercalciuria with kidney calculi. Although renal Ca excretion is higher in hypercalciurics, renal Ca clearance account for only a minor fraction of the total body clearance, suggesting that the reduced serum Ca levels found in the hypercalciurics could not be explained by the renal Ca leak. The enhanced total body Ca clearance found in hypercalciuric subjects is therefore due to an increased tissue Ca uptake. This finding provides indirect evidence of altered cell Ca handling in idiopathic hypercalciura with no difference between the so-called absorptives and renals in terms of the pathophysiologic mechanism.

2.3.1 Testing collagen in urine or blood
Laboratory tests that measure the amount of collagen in urine or blood samples can indicate bone loss. Lab tests may also be used in conjunction with DEXA or other methods of bone

densitometry to diagnose and monitor osteoporosis, such as beta-crosslap, a biochemical bone marker of bone resorption. Biochemical bone markers, such as the bone isoenzyme form of alkaline phosphatase, have been used to assess the bone formation phase of bone turnover in health and disease. Markers of biochemical bone remodeling can be used in assessing and managing osteoporis in conjunction with DEXA.

2.3.2 The active vitamin D

Chronic uremia is characterized by decreased levels of plasma 1,25-dihydroxyvitamin D3(1,25-(OH)2D3), a hormone with immunomodulatory properties, due to decreased renal 1-hydroxylase activity and by decreased renal phosphate excretion. The consequence is an increased synthesis and secretion of parathyroid hormone--secondary hyperparathyroidism--due to the low levels of plasma calcium, low levels of plasma 1,25(OH)2D3 and high levels of phosphate. The association between renal bone disease and chronic renal failure is well described. An association also exists between secondary hyperparathyroidism and increased mortality and cardiovascular calcifications in chronic uremic patients.

Calcium carbonate and calcium acetate were used as phosphate binders. Until recently, the most commonly used active vitamin D drug was either the natural 1,25(OH)2D3, or the 1 alpha-hydroxylated analog, 1alpha(OH)D3 which after 25-hydroxylation in the liver is converted to 1,25(OH)2D3. This increases the intestinal absorption of calcium and improves skeletal abnormalities. The combined treatment with calcium containing phosphate binders and active vitamin D induces an increase in plasma Ca and hypercalcemia became a clinical problem. It was demonstrated a direct suppressive effect of intravenous 1,25(OH)2D3 on plasma PTH.

The use of 1 alpha-hydroxyvitamin D3 (1 alpha(OH)D3) derivatives in a uremic patient is justified only in the treatment of hyperparathyroidism. The following prerequisites have however to be satisfied: a good vitamin D3 repletion should be secured by plasma 25-OH-D3 levels of 20-30 ng/ml, and phosphate retention and the consequent possible hyperphosphatemia should be prevented or corrected by the oral administration of alkaline salts of calcium given before the meals as phosphate binders without inducing hypercalcemia.

In X-linked hypophosphatemia, phosphate wasting results from increased circulating levels of fibroblast growth factor 23 (FGF-23). Administration of calcitonin causes a drop in serum levels of FGF-23. Calcitonin might have the same effect in patients with X-linked hypophosphatemia. Serum levels of 1,25-dihydroxyvitamin D rose similarly in untreated patients with X-linked hypophosphatemia and in controls after a single subcutaneous injection of 200 IU of salmon calcitonin in both groups for 21 hours but diverged thereafter (P=0.008). The rise in serum levels of 1,25-dihydroxyvitamin D is probably due to the direct stimulatory effect of calcitonin on renal 1α-hydroxylase. Both groups had slight and similar changes in serum levels of calcium and PTH. Serum phosphate levels rose after treatment.

Recently, it was reported that osteocytes express the calcitonin receptor and respond to calcitonin with an increase in sclerostin production. Sclerostin has an inhibitory effect on the lifetime of the osteoblast. Sclerostin production by osteocytes is inhibited by PTH.

2.3.3 The PTH, serum Ca, insulin and vitamin D

PTH is the most important endocrine regulator of Ca and phosphorus concentration in extracellular fluid. It enhances the release of Ca from the large reservoir contained in the bones. Bone resorption is the normal destruction of bone by osteoclasts, which are indirectly stimulated by PTH. Stimulation is indirect since osteoclasts do not have a receptor for PTH; rather, PTH binds to osteoblasts, the cells responsible for creating bone. In the kidney it enhances active reabsorption of Ca and magnesium from distal tubules and the thick ascending limb. It enhances the absorption of calcium in the intestine by increasing the production of activated vitamin D.

Patients with primary hyperparathyroidism have impaired glucose tolerance more often than do controls, and parathyroid resection sometimes improves this derangement. However, it is unclear whether serum Ca or PTH is more strongly related to impaired glucose metabolism in subjects without primary hyperparathyroidism. Multiple regression analyses showed that the significant and positive correlations between serum Ca vs fasting plasma glucose and homeostasis model assessment insulin resistance in men still remained after adjustment for intact PTH as well as age, body weight, height, creatinine, albumin, phosphate, bone metabolic markers, and estradiol (P < .05). Serum Ca level is positively associated with impaired glucose metabolism, independent of PTH or bone metabolism, in men with type 2 DM.

In the relationship between biochemical parameters, parathyroid adenoma volume, and bone mineral density with respect to intact parathyroid hormone (iPTH) levels in patients with primary hyperparathyroidism, it was found there was no correlation between iPTH, serum calcium levels and total T scores at the femur and lumbar spine. After excluding patients with 25-(OH)D3 insufficiency, there was still no correlation between serum iPTH and calcium levels. Parathyroid adenoma volume, serum iPTH and calcium levels were also not different between patients with and without 25-(OH)D3 insufficiency.

Primary hyperparathyroidism (PHPT) and vitamin D insufficiency are two very frequent conditions. Vitamin D treatment is recommended and may decrease PTH levels in PHPT. However, there is no randomized controlled trial to prove any beneficial effect. For safety reasons, it is recommended to monitor plasma and urinary Ca during treatment. Furthermore, the effect of vitamin D repletion on other outcomes like quality of life, muscle function and central nervous system symptoms should be assessed.

2.3.4 Ghrelin and bone mass density

Serum ghrelin is positively correlated with trabecular BMD in a cohort of elderly healthy Italian women. The fact that trabecular is more metabolically active than cortical bone and the larger number of females might explain this selective association.

Previously undetected contributors to secondary osteoporosis and metabolic bone diseases (SECOB) are frequently found in patients with osteoporosis, but the prevalence in patients at the time they present with a clinical fracture is unknown (Napoli et al. 2011). At presentation with a fracture, 26.5% of patients have previously unknown contributors to SECOB, as monoclonal proteinemia, renal insufficiency grade III or greater, primary and secondary hyperparathyroidism, hyperthyroidism, and hypogonadism in men. Newly diagnosed SECOBs, serum 25-hydroxyvitamin D less than 50 nmol/liter (in 63.9%), and dietary calcium intake less than 1200 mg/d were found at any age, in both sexes, after any fracture (except SECOB in men with finger and toe fractures) and at any level of bone mineral density, which are treatable or need follow-up, and more than 90% of patients have an inadequate vitamin D status and/or calcium intake. Systematic screening of patients with a recent fracture identifies those in whom potentially reversible contributors to SECOB and calcium and vitamin D deficiency are present (Bours et al., 2011).

2.3.5 Calcitonin and PTH

Calcitonin is a 32-amino acid linear polypeptide hormone that is produced in humans primarily by the parafollicular cells (also known as C-cells) of the thyroid, and in many other animals in the ultimobranchial body. It acts to reduce blood Ca, opposing the effects of PTH. The hormone participates in calcium Ca and phosphorus metabolism. In many ways, calcitonin counteracts PTH.

2.3.6 Environmental contaminants

Polybrominated diphenyl ethers (PBDEs) are flame retardants that have been widely used in manufacturing. They are major household and environmental contaminants that bioaccumulate. Humans are exposed primarily through dust inhalation and dietary ingestion of animal products. PBDEs increase rodent circulating T3 and T4 concentrations and gonadal osteopontin mRNA, and activate the osteopontin gene promoter. These changes may have clinical implications as others have shown associations between human exposure to PBDEs and subclinical hyperthyroidism (Blake et al., 2011).

2.3.7 Vitamin K_2 (menaquinone)

Vitamin K_2 (menaquinone), is itself a category of vitamin K that includes many types of vitamin K_2. The two subtypes of vitamin K_2 that have been most studied are menaquinone-4 (MK4) and menaquinone-7 (MK7). MK4 is produced via conversion of vitamin K_1 in the body, in the testes, pancreas and arterial walls. Studies demonstrate that the conversion of vitamin K1 to MK4, is not dependent on gut bacteria .

In contrast to MK4, MK7 is not produced by humans but is converted from phylloquinone in the intestines by gut bacteria. However, bacteria-derived menaquinones appear to contribute minimally to overall vitamin K status. MK4 has been approved for the prevention and treatment of osteoporosis, and it has been shown to decrease fractures up to 87%. MK4 has also been shown to prevent bone loss and/or fractures caused by corticosteroids, anorexia nervosa, cirrhosis of the liver and postmenopausal osteoporosis. MK7 has never been shown in any clinical trials to reduce fractures and is not approved by any government for the prevention or treatment of any disease. MK7 has been approved in the purpose of increasing bone mineral density.

3. Overture

BMD is only bone mineral density, risk factors for osteoporosis are only risk factors and the mixing of both parameters does not make quite more sense. It is not better than each one separately. BMD is a subrogate parameter for diagnosing bone strength that is good but it is not enough, because with a suitable BMD caused by sodium fluoride bone fragility is increased and some individuals with decreased BMD undergo quantitatively and objectively bone fractures and another different person does not suffer this bone condition. Bone risk factors are good for diagnosis but they do not mean necessarily one disease and nor are they sufficient to osteoporosis. With and without them there are persons with and without suitable bone strength and with and without fractures. It is important to understand that bone is not a hard and lifeless structure; it is, in fact, a complex, living tissue.

The confounding effect of differences in bone size is due to the missing depth value in the calculation of BMD. It should be noted that despite DXA technology' s problems in estimating volume, it is still a fairly accurate measure of BMD.

Methods to correct for this shortcoming include the calculation of a volume which is approximated from the projected area measure by DXA. DXA BMD results adjusted in this manner are referred to as the bone mineral apparent density (BMAD) and are a ratio of the bone mineral content versus a cuboidal estimation of the volume of bone. As aBMD, BMAD results do not accurately represent true bone mineral density, since they use approximations of the bone's volume.

It is important to get repeated BMD measurements done on the same machine each time, or at least a machine from the same manufacturer. Error between machines, or trying to convert measurements from one manufacturer's standard to another can introduce errors large enough to wipe out the sensitivity of the measurements.

It is possible to use a scaling system for pixels which has a one to one correspondence to the concentration of what you are studying. Sample concentrations can be determined using optical, electronic, and most importantly for our purposes, a computer based imaging technique. Densitometric science was described originally by Bouguer and Lambert who described loss of radiation (or light) in passing through a medium. Later, Beer found that the radiation loss in a media was a function of the substance's molarity or concentration.

According to Beer's law, concentration is proportional to optical density (OD). The logarithmic optical density scale, and net integral of density values for an object in an image is the proper measure for use in quantitation. By Beer's law, the density of a point is the log ratio of incident light upon it and transmitted light through it.

$OD = Log10(Io / I)$

When dealing with noisy data if there is a region of interest (ROI) or image area that is calibrated, such as is done during concentration calibrations, which method for calculation of a the calibrated mean is preferable?

1. Adding up a calibrated value for each pixel in terms of the calibrated unit, then finding the average calibrated unit value and calling this the calibrated mean.
    Calibrated mean = (sum(cvalue(P[i,j])) / N where cvalue(P[i,j]) is the calibrated value for each pixel in your ROI, and N is the total number of pixels in the ROI
2. Adding up all the pixel values in pixel intensity units, finding the mean pixel intensity value, finally finding the one calibrated value for the mean pixel intensity and calling this the calibrated mean.

Calibrated mean = cvalue(sum(P[i,j]) / N) where P[i,j] is each pixel intensity in the ROI, and N is the total number of pixels in the ROI. In an ideal world, it would not make any difference. Both methods would yield the same value. However in the real world, measurement and other types of error enter in, and we should think of the problem in a statistical context. If the errors (i.e. the standard deviation) are small, the method used does not matter much. But how small is small? What really matters is the relationship of the standard deviation to the curvature of the calibration curve.

If the calibration curve were truly linear, the order of operations would not matter (a property of linear functions). However, in the current context, the calibration curve is always nonlinear, at least in some regions.

The key question then becomes which of the two methods is appropriate on the data? The answer is: it depends. Some cases are clear cut others are in-between. It is safe to assume that, if there is a fairly uniform grey level region of interest, where the only variation is caused by the noise of the imaging process (all noises), method two produces a better estimation of the mean. In cases where the region contains two highly differing density regions included in one ROI (the variation is not caused by noise or the imaging process), then the method one produces a better estimation of mean.

The error of method one is directly proportional to the noise of the system used and becomes highest when data is measured nearest the asymptote of the curve fit used to calibrate the data. Most data unfortunately have some natural density variation and some variation caused by the imaging process (noise).

We are facing a big concern: Osteoporosis is a major public health threat. How can we treat it if we have not the adequate diagnosis tool?.

An expert technical assessment of the many factors that influence the risk of osteoporotic fracture in postmenopausal women need to be considered when planning the most effective public health interventions. In view of growing awareness of the need to prevent and treat postmenopausal osteoporosis, it is good to resolve several controversies concerning the usefulness of screening programmes, the appropriate target populations, the most effective methods for predicting fracture risk, techniques for assessment, and the comparative effectiveness of currently available preventive and therapeutic interventions. There are advantages and limitations of the methods for predicting future fracture risk: assessment of bone mass, assessment of bone loss, and clinical assessment of risk factors. It is needed information on non-invasive physical techniques for bone mass assessment. The aims and design of screening programmes are not clear.

By reason of the two-dimensional nature of DXA, assumptions must be made regarding the tridimensional nature of the bones involving a great deal to cope with. Therefore it is deduced, that this method seems to be very sensitive to error, and it is necessary to know how to deal with these errors, especially with the systematic errors introduced by using a parameterized model. Even though a high concordance between the densitometers was observed on a single measurement occasion, a significant discordance in longitudinal changes in BMD was observed.

Bone strength is comprised of many components, which include architecture, geometry, cortical porosity, and tissue mineralization density. These components are contained within the measurement of BMD but cannot be individually distinguished.

Bone strength is comprised of many components including, but not limited to bone architecture, geometry, cortical porosity and tissue mineralization density.

The exceptional mechanical properties of bones are not only the result of the amount and type of the micro-constituents, but also of their morphological organization at the different lower scales.

Mechanical properties of bone are determined not only by BMD, but also by tissue trabecular structure and organic composition. Direct measurement of these components of bone strength may result in improved fracture risk prediction or therapeutic monitoring than is currently possible using the surrogate measure of BMD.

In addition to loading in axial compression, long bones are also and, in fact, primarily loaded in bending. In linear coupled bending and extension of an unbalanced bonded repair the tensile forces are exerted on the bending-created convex surface, whereas compressive forces are exerted on the concave surface. This bending increases the stress intensity in the underlying crack and causes adhesive peel stresses and bending of the repair which can, relative to a repair that is restrained against bending, lead to early failure and certain assumptions must be made about the symmetry of the bone in cross-section at the different ROIs, which are not entirely accurate. Additionally, cortical thickness must be assumed to be uniform about the circumference of the cross-section. Many of these assumptions are necessitated by the 2-dimensional nature of DXA and may be addressed with 3-dimensional imaging.

The geometric parameters are predictive of fracture risk although they do not seem to be better predictors of risk than a conventional measurement of BMD. DXA measured *in vivo* "BMD" methodology shows to be an intrinsically flawed and misleading indicator of bone mineral status and an erroneous gauge of relative fracture risk.

DXA methodology to provide accurate, quantitative, and meaningful *in vivo* (not in cadaver) area bone mineral density ("aBMD") determinations have been proven to be unwarranted and misplaced. The underlying systematic of sizable, inherently unavoidable and un-correctable inaccuracies in the DXA output values of *in vivo* "BMD" have been shown to be quantitatively consistent with being the root cause of unreliable, misdirected, and misinterpreted aspects of consensual knowledge of bone fragility, osteoporotic diagnostics/prognostics, and remodelling therapies.

So, as said above, BMD is only BMD, risk factors to osteoporosis are only risk factors and mixing of both parameters does not make quite more sense. It is not best than each of them alone. Although spatial information is currently recorded in the form of a DXA image, this information is not utilised clinically. It should be noted that BMD assessment provides an areal density measure, where the cross-sectional scan area is known but not the tissue thickness, providing units of g/cm2.

Precise in vivo measurement of the trabecular bone mechanical properties is very important, being essential a method for quantitatively and objectively assessing bone mass and anisotropy and not only in a qualitative manner and with risks which sometimes are not. The cortical bone properties constitute another system with microsystems, isotropy and anisotropy and variety of cross-section of the long bone. But the mechanical properties of bones are not only the result of the amount and type of the micro-constituents, but also of their morphological organization at the different lower scales. Measurement of BMD has served as a fit surrogate for the measurement of bone strength. DXA is one osteoporosis imaging diagnosis testing. By reason of the two-dimensional nature of DXA, assumptions must be made regarding the tridimensional nature of the bones, dealing with an inference problem from a set of measurements. It is needed to make inference about certain parameters which help to make predictions of a certain fracture risk. The main limitation for a proper inference is that only 2d information is got from detectors, and therefore all 3d information is lost, as it is integrated out due to the nature of detector. It is necessary to be very careful when using models for data inference, because we obviously will never know the underlying truth contained in the data. Therefore, it is tried to regain some information about the third dimension by building a model of the bone, which assumes axial symmetry.

By using a model, to be arranged the parameter of this model in such a way that they best fit the data, so it is only gained information about how good the model can explain the data, but it is not gotten any information of how good this model actually is, and maybe there is a much better model, which we do not know it yet. It is very difficult to make good inference of the bone strength due to the noisy character of the data, and dealing with the errors of the apparatus is crucial for making inference.

Therefore it is deduced, that this method seems to be very sensitive to error, and it is necessary to know how to deal with these errors, especially with the systematic errors introduced by using a parameterized model.

There is concern that the additional 3d information which is gained in this inference process comes entirely from the model, which then would increase the systematic uncertainties about the quantities that are inferred from the data.

And there is an anisotropic problem, and therefore different inferences must be done making measurements from different directions. But we wonder should the anisotropies are really that bad problem.

It should be very easy to test the reliability of this method, by making inferences from datasets taken from different sides, and see to what degree they agree, this would give a simple estimate about some of the systematic errors introduced in the inference method, and how reliable the entire method is. If the reliability is sufficiently high for purposes to study then it would be say there is no use in making a more complicated model. A much deeper investigation of these effects can be carried out in the framework of Bayesian statistics, which is very well suited for problems like this.

But if the reliability is not within the desired range, then of course the only way to tackle this problem is to introduce more complexity to the model to also pick up effects coming from the anisotropies. Which would also means more data might be needed. Treating anisotropies in data inference is in general a very hard business, and a lot of work is going on at the moment to tackle this problems.

In this case we have good chances of attacking this problem, because the anisotropies which might occur are not so nasty, so it might be feasible to build a slightly more general model by allowing elliptic shapes, which introduces two parameters $a(x)$ and $b(x)$ for semi and major axis at each point x along the bone axis, or use other Kernel functions which can describe the shape more precisely.

3.1 The finite element method

The finite element method (FEM), its practical application often known as finite element analysis (FEA), is a numerical technique for finding approximate solutions of partial differential equations (PDE) as well as of integral equations. FEA was first developed in 1943 by R. Courant, who utilized the Ritz method of numerical analysis and minimization of variational calculus to obtain approximate solutions to vibration systems. FEA has been developed to an incredible precision. It consists of a computer model of a material or design that is stressed and analyzed for specific results. It is used in new product design, and existing product refinement. Modifying an existing product or structure is utilized to qualify the product or structure for a new service condition. In case of structural failure, FEA may be used to help determine the design modifications to meet the new condition.

FEA is a widely-used technique for the computer modelling of structures under mechanical loading. A finite element is an individual regular shape thathas a known stiffness so that any applied load will give a predictable corresponding displacement. Elements are joined together at nodes and along edges. Complex designs are created as an assembly of elements to which restraints and loads may be applied. During the computer analysis of the model, a series of simultaneous equations are established that represent the overall stiffness of the structure. The equations are then solved giving the nodal displacements resulting from the applied loads. For the analysis of bone structures, finite element analysis would therefore be dependent upon the density of each element, the arrangement of elements (eg trabecular structure), the composition (eg cortical shell or cancellous) and the external shape (eg length, angle and width of femoral neck).

FEA has previously been applied to computer modelling of several bioengineering situations incorporating bone including cellular remodelling, prosthetic loosening, fracture progression and fracture healing. Studies related to osteoporosis have tended to utilise the full 3D potential of FEA via incorporation of computed tomography data.

FEA predicts the mechanical behaviour (displacement or stress) of a structure under loading rather than the exact yield point (fracture); but since osteoporosis fracture risk assessment requires only a proportional, rather than exact, measure of fracture load, FEA derived stiffness (load / displacement) should have significant clinical potential. FEXI (finite element analysis of x-ray images) provides a thin plate computer simulation of a bone being mechanically tested.

Finite element analysis inherently offers dependence upon the external shape and internal structure of a bone and should, therefore, have the potential to provide a superior prediction of mechanical integrity than simple areal density (BMD). The novel feature of the FEXI approach is that a conventional mechanical compression test is simulated. An important aspect of the technique is that, being based upon conventional 2D DXA images or radiographs, it could be readily utilised into routine clinical practice.

Thus, bone microarchitecture and biomechanical properties in men have been investigated (Vilayphiou et al. 2011). Patient-specific finite element (PSFE) models based on QCT are generally used to predict the biomechanical response of human bones with the future goal to be applied in clinical decision-making (Trabelsi & Yosibash, 2011). The biomechanical mechanisms underlying sex-specific differences in age-related vertebral fracture rates are ill defined. To gain insight into this issue, we used finite element analysis of clinical CT scans of the vertebral bodies (Christiansen et al., 2011).

4. Conclusion

Therefore it is necessary to carry out more research and to open new tracks to have any further reliable tool in the diagnosis of osteoporosis. Precise *in vivo* measurement of the bone mechanical properties is very important, being essential a method for assessing quantitatively and objectively bone mass and anisotropy and not only in a qualitative way and with risks which sometimes are not. Thus, a mathematical, physical and physiological 5-dimensional model must be developed in order to gauge bone properties including geometry(2-dimensional DXA), space, time, motion and stress with some portable-computer-devices that uses the body space of the user as an interface with equipment and programs designed to communicate information from one system of computing devices and programs to anothers. Because the person is not one body died, and is more than one statistic sampling; he is not a 10-year probability of hip fracture; he is alive and not one lifeless inert element; and bones are not quite as strong as one compact material object without life; it is somewhat more flexible and this is useful in bones that are jointed performing its necessary task. Probability is good after the event but not before. It is unknown what is going to happen to one person as the justification is wholly independent of sense experience in *a priori* knowledge. The person to study can be the case who is no concluded from the probability. The probability is not the reality and the patient, to a greater or lesser extent, is not a probability that is to say it is one sophism: a plausible but fallacious argument or deceptive argumentation. This is one poor approach to diagnosis in osteoporosis. There is not any disease but one ill person and so must be considered irrespective of other philosophies including economic resources. These facts are essential in drawing up any test for diagnosis in osteoporosis.

5. References

Report of a WHO Study Group (1994). *Assessment of fracture risk and its application to screening for postmenopausal osteoporosis,* World Health Organ Tech Rep Ser.;843:1-129.

NIH Consensus Panel Addresses Osteoporosis Prevention, Diagnosis, and Therapy on osteoporosis prevention, diagnosis, and therapy (2001). *JAMA*;14;285(6):785-95.

Kanis, J.A.; Johnell, O.; Oden, A.; Jonsson, B,; Dawson, A.; Dere, W. (2000). Risk of hip fracture derived from relative risks: an analysis applied to the population of Sweden. *Osteoporosis International;* 11: 120-127.

Sodeab, M.; Burghardtb, A. J.; Pialatbcd, J.B.; Linkb, T. M.; Majumdarab, S. (2011) . Quantitative characterization of subject motion in HR-pQCT images of the distal radius and tibia. *Bone*, 48: 1291-1297.

Bauer, J.S.; & Link T.M. (2009). Advances in osteoporosis imaging. *Eur J Radiol.*, 71(3):440-9.

Bolland, M.J.; Siu, A.T.; Mason, B.H.; Horne, A.M.; Ames, R.W.; Grey, A,B.; Gamble, G.D.; Reid, I.R. (2011). Evaluation of the FRAX and Garvan fracture risk calculators in older women. *J Bone Miner Res*, 26:420-7.

Levy, B.T; Hartz, A; Woodworth, G; Xu, Y; Sinift, S. Interventions to improving osteoporosis screening: an Iowa Research Network (IRENE) study. (2009) *J Am Board Fam Med.* ;22(4):360-7.

Napoli, N.; Pedone; C.; Pozzilli, P.; Lauretani, F.; Bandinelli, S.; Ferrucci, L.; Incalzi, R.A. Effect of ghrelin on bone mass density: The InChianti study (2011). *Bone.*; Apr 9. [Epub ahead of print].

Bours, S.P.; van Geel T.A.; Geusens, P.P.; Janssen, M.J.; Janzing, H.M.; Hoffland, G.A.; Willems, P.C.; van den Bergh, J.P.(2011). Contributors to Secondary Osteoporosis and Metabolic Bone Diseases in Patients Presenting with a Clinical Fracture. *J Clin Endocrinol Metab,* Mar 16. [Epub ahead of print].

Rupp, J.D; Flannagan, C.A; Hoff, C.N; Cunningham, R.M.; Effects of osteoporosis on AIS 3+ injury risk in motor-vehicle crashes. (2010). *Accid Anal Prev.*; 42(6):2140-3.

Vilayphiou N, Boutroy S, Szulc P, van Rietbergen B, Munoz F, Delmas PD, Chapurlat R. Finite element analysis performed on radius and tibia HR-pQCT images and fragility fractures at all sites in men. J Bone Miner Res. (2011). *J Bone Miner Res.*;

Blake, C.A.; McCoy G.L.; Hui, Y.Y.; Lavoie, H.A. (2011). Perinatal exposure to low-dose DE-71 increases serum thyroid hormones and gonadal osteopontin gene expression. *Exp Biol Med (Maywood);* 236(4):445-55. Epub 2011 Mar 2.26(5):965-73.

Christiansen, B.A.; Kopperdahl, D.L.; Kiel, D.P.; Keaveny, T.M.; Bouxsein, M.L. Mechanical contributions of the cortical and trabecular compartments contribute to differences in age-related changes in vertebral body strength in men and women assessed by QCT-based finite element analysis. (2011). *J Bone Miner Res.*; 26(5):974-83.

Trabelsi, N.; Yosibash, Z. Patient-specific finite-element analyses of the proximal femur with orthotropic material properties validated by experiments. *J Biomech Eng.* 2011 Jun;133(6):061001.

8

Early Detection Techniques for Osteoporosis

Kanika Singh[1,2] and Kyung Chun Kim[2]
[1]*KHAN Co, Ltd, Aju-dong, Geoje-do,*
[2]*Pusan National University, Busan,*
Republic of Korea

1. Introduction

Osteoporosis (OP) is a serious disease and its early diagnosis is very important at the right time. These days, there are some conventional techniques of the diagnosis of this disease but these techniques have their limitations and reliable information is not obtained at the initial stage of the disease. Therefore, a new technique for the detection of OP at an early stage is required to be developed. In the present chapter, a new technique, based on Micro Electro Mechanical System (MEMS) technology, will be discussed to overcome the limitations of earlier techniques.

In the present chapter, main emphasis is placed on the early detection of OP. New types of OP detection techniques, based on the biomechanical, optical and electrochemical principles, will be explained and compared to achieve an improved detection methodology for OP. A new amperometric immunosensor using gold nanoparticles and a novel microfluidics BioMEMS chip as a point of care testing (POCT) technique will be introduced for design, fabrication and characterization.

The chapter covers the study which has been mainly divided into three parts: basic measurements on physical, biomechanical, optical and chemical properties of normal and OP bones and serum; and design and development of amperometric immunosensor and BioMEMS chip. (Ahn C.H et al., 2004, Arnaud C.D at al., 1996 Atkinson, P.J. 1964, Auroux, P.A et al., 2002, Bakker, E., 2006, Berthonnaud L, F., 2002, Bianchi, 2005, Ban C, 2004, Bal S.K, 2002)

An overview of OP research trends with the objectives of the research, and scope and significance of the study, is also presented. Causes and diagnostic techniques for OP will be reviewed in the beginning of the chapter.

2. OP detection & early detection of osteoporosis (EDO)

Since OP is most common among elder people, the overall costs to maintain the healthy body will most likely escalate in the near future. Hence to reduce the sufferings, the best solution is early detection (Bianchi, M.L., 2000, Blair, 2000). The early detection of disease states results in improved treatment outcomes, possibility of living longer a healthy life (Arnaud et al., 1996; Singh, 2006).

Early detection is possible by biomarkers or the "intervening phenotypes" in the biofluids like saliva, serum and urine which can be (a) surrogate measures of any malignancy in the bone;

(b) identifiers of inherited variations associated with disease susceptibility; or (c) "pre-disease" lesions that are highly predictive of subsequent disease(Becerra-Rojas & Jupari, 2001).

Diagnosis of OP at the right time can save from compressive treatments and immobility. Generally, in medical practice, identification of disease is based on recognition of symptoms and also testing specific features to confirm the presence of a particular disease. But for OP, it is hard to predict the disease as it silently creeps into the body with minimal symptoms of back pain, toothache and some hunch-over, etc. These initial symptoms point to the old age also and hence the unaware patient realizes this only after having a fracture in the bone. The unaware human when realizes about the disease due to some bone-fractures. In the hospital, anteroposterior and lateral X-rays of the special bone site are obtained to assess the presence of fractures, using the BMD measurements. Finally, they realize the presence of OP then the treatment becomes unaffordable and the patient becomes bed-ridden as shown in Fig. 2. Hence early detection of OP (EDO) is extremely necessary (see Table 1) with new devices like POCT (point of care technology) device using BioMEMS technology. Micro-fluidic chips are also playing key role to deliver new devices for better health care. The sensitivity and specificity of the POCT device would give earliest possible detection. Several promising directions for detection of bonemarker for OP have been interrogated (Arnaud, 1996; Singh, 2006, Singh, 2007, Singh, 2008, Singh, 2009).

Various researchers have studied OP disease for biological, chemically, physiological and engineering aspects in the past, by using different types of measurement techniques and methodologies (Arnaud, 1996; Korkia, 2002; Raiz, 1997; Singh, 2006). However, newer and newer techniques with new advances in technology, like micro/ nano technology, are being developed.

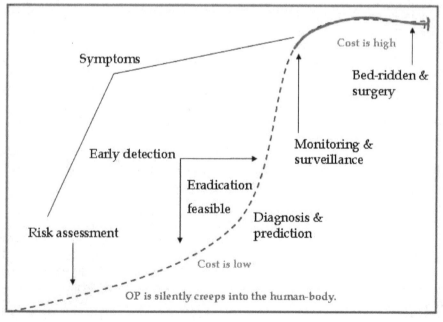

Fig. 1. Early Detection of OP (EDO)

S.No	Specification	Consequences
1	Early detection	Screening for large number of population
2	Minimal invasive	Uses only micro amounts of biofluids
3	Site-specific	Bone turnover specific bonemarkers
4	Diagnostics levels	OP-specific
5	User-friendly	Self testing is possible, easy to use
6	Simple, low cost	Portable, home care

Table 1. Importance of EDO(Singh, 2006)

3. Technical terminologies

3.1 Osteoproteogerin
Osteoprotegerin, also known as osteoclastogenesis inhibitory factor (OCIF), is a cytokine and a member of the tumor necrosis factor (TNF) receptor superfamily. It is a basic glycoprotein comprising 401 amino acid residues arranged into 7 structural domains. It is found as either a 60 kDa monomer or 120 kDa dimer linked by disulfide bonds.

3.2 Biological MEMS (BioMEMS)
It is a combination of a Micro-electromechanical system (MEMS) with the biological systems, like protein, DNA or cell. It includes micro- and nanosystems for genomics, proteomics, and drug delivery analysis; molecular assembly, tissue engineering, biosensor development, and nanoscale imaging (Singh et al., 2007, 2009, Vijayendran et al., 2003).

3.3 Microfluidics
Microfluidics is a multidisciplinary field comprising physics, chemistry, engineering and biotechnology that studies the behavior of fluids at the microscale and mesoscale, that is, fluids at volumes thousands of times smaller than a common droplet. It also concerns the design of systems in which such small volumes of fluids are used (Singh, 2007; Vijayendran et al., 2003).

3.4 Electrochemical sensor
The biosensor in which a biological process is harnessed to an electrical sensor system, such as an enzyme electrode. Other types couple a biological event to an electrical one via a range of mechanisms, such as those based on oxygen and pH (Heineman, 2001, Singh et al, 2008, 2009).

3.5 Immunosensor
Immunosensor uses the immuno-compounds (antibodies or antigens) as biological receptors configures the so-called immunosensors, which are usually the result of the integration in one device of an immunoassay and a directly associated transducer. The antigen-antibody complex formation can be detected either directly (without using any labeled compound) by certain physical (potential, capacitance, conductivity compound) measurements or indirect approaches in which one immuno-compound is conjugated with an indicator molecule (Bakker and Quin, 2006).

3.6 Spectroscopy
It is a non-invasive analytical technique with an infinitely broad range of applications, especially in medical field. This gives a non-destructive analysis. It helps in identification of

the elements and the elucidation of atomic and molecular structure by measurement of the radiant energy absorbed or emitted by a substance in any of the wavelengths of the electromagnetic spectrum in response to excitation by an external energy source (Chittur, 1998; Clark and Hester. 1996).

3.7 Lab-on-a-chip (LOC)

LOC is to integrate multiple functions on a single chip of only millimeters to a square centimeters in size and that are capable of handling extremely small fluid volumes down less than pico liters, LOC device is a sub-set of MEMS device (Chittur, 1998; Clark and Hester, 1996). The term "Lab-on-a-Chip" was introduced later on when it turned out that µTAS (Micro Total Analysis System) technologies were more widely applicable than only for analysis purposes.
(http://en.wikipedia.org/wiki/Lab-on-a-chip).

4. Classification of OP detection techniques

There are several methods for detection of OP as shown in Fig. 2 (Singh, 2006).

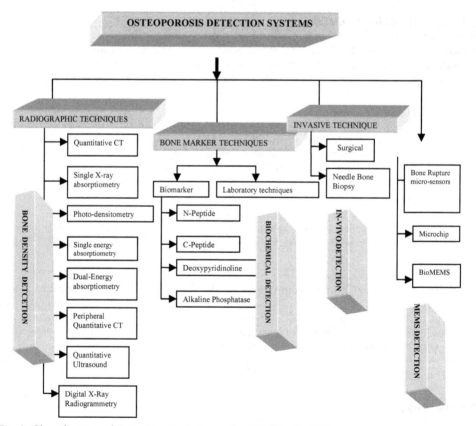

Fig. 2. Classification of Detection Techniques for OP (Singh, 2006)

4.1 Radiographic diagnosis

Radiogrammetry, a technique that has been in use for more than 30 years, relies on the measurement of the cortical thickness of bones in the hand (metacarpals) to estimate bone mass. This technique suffers from relatively poor accuracy and reliability and has largely been supplanted with new techniques(Bianchi, 2000)

The following diagnostic techniques are generally used for the detection of osteoporosis (Arnaud, 1996; Sartoris, 1996, Bianchi, 2005)

Bone Mineral Density Technique (BMD) is an effective approach for detection of osteoporosis. A decrease in the amount of bone, resulting in thin, weakened bones that are susceptible to fractures. Several techniques are available for BMD testing. For example; dual-energy X-RAY absorptiometry (DXA) remains the standard for testing the BMD. Dual energy absorptiometry measures the bone density within a given area of bone (g/cm^2). This technique offers the advantages of higher precision, minimal ionizing radiation exposure, rapid scanning time and the ability to access cortical and trabecular bone mass at appendicular and axial sites. Limitation, include equipment expense, the need for certified X-Ray technician and non-portability. In addition, DXA scans of the spine may show a false increase in spinal BMD in patients with osteophyes, aortic calcifications and degenerative arthritic changes.

The conception of osteoporosis relates bone health to bone strength, rather than mass. A bone's health implies that it should have enough strength to keep voluntary loads from causing spontaneous fractures. Thus, the diagnosis of osteoporosis would be a biomechanical matter concerning both bone strength and muscle strength (Martin et al., 1998). This supposes two kinds of problems, namely: (a) to properly assess bone material properties, structural design and strength; and (b) to correlate the respective indicators with suitable indicators of muscle strength. As a standard densitometry is unsuitable to assess muscle strength or bone strength, it should use of other, preferably cross-sectional analyses of bone structure as those provided by quantitative computed tomography (QCT), peripheral quantitative computed tomography (pQCT), MRI, or similar procedures. The value of pQCT lies in the ability of the software to account for all the `mass', material and architectural factors in whose-bone strength and to provide data on muscle cross-sections (Burr, 1997, Boyle et al, 2003, Singh et al, 2006).

4.2 Quantitative CT

This provides the evaluation of trabecular bone density of the lumbar spine based on bone volume. Quantitative computed tomography (QCT) may be less practical than DXA because of the lower precision, higher cost and increased radiation exposure (Singh et al, 2006).

4.3 Peripheral bone densitometry

These devices used for many devices single-energy X-ray absorptiometry, peripheral DXA and peripheral CT. these device have the advantages of less expense, portable equipment, reasonable precision, and low radiation exposure. The use of quantitative ultrasonography for screening of osteoporosis and assessing fracture risk has increased. Using the speed of sound and broadband ultrasonic attenuation measurements, ultrasonic densitometry provides on bone elasticity and structure in peripheral sites. Advantages of this method, is low cost and lack of ionization radiation (Singh et al, 1997, 1998, 1999, 2006).

4.4 Single-energy absorptiometry

Single-energy absorptiometry measures bone mineral at peripheral sites such as the wrist and heel. Single photon absorptiometry (SPA) used a radioactive energy source, usually iodine125 to estimate the amount of bone mineral at peripheral measurement sites. In recent years, Single-energy X-ray absorptiometry (SXA) has supplanted SPA for measurements of the peripheral skeleton (heel and wrist) because of its better reproducibility and ease of use. SXA avoids the necessity of obtaining and disposing of radioactive energy sources. It requires immersion of the part in water bath and hence can measure bone mass in peripheral bones like bones of forearm and legs (Singh et al, 2006, Blair et al, 2003).

4.5 Dual-energy absorptiometry

Bone density tests are painless, non-invasive and safe. Dual-energy absorptiometry was developed to measure bone in parts of the skeleton (lumbar spine, hip, and total body) that could not be measured with single-energy devices. Currently dual-energy X-ray absorptiometry (DXA) is the most widely used technique for measuring bone at these sites. DXA devices also are capable of measuring bone at the heel and wrist with high accuracy and precision, with very low exposure to radiation (Singh et al, 2006).

4.6 Peripheral quantitative CT (pQCT)

Quantitative computed tomography (QCT) measures the density of vertebral trabecular bone, the spongy bone in the center of the vertebra. pQCT devices are QCT instruments that have been adapted for measurements at peripheral sites such as the wrist (Singh et al, 2006).

4.7 Quantitative ultrasound (QUS)

Quantitative ultrasound devices measure bone at several skeletal sites, including the heel, hand, finger, and lower leg. The heel measurement it is composed of primarily trabecular bone, similar to the composition of the spine. Ultrasound devices based on the changes in the speed of sound (SOS), as well as specific changes in sound waves (broadband attenuation or BUA) as they pass through bone. QUS measurements provide information on fracture risk by providing an indication of bone density and possibly also information on the quality of the bone. Ultrasound devices do not expose the patient to ionizing radiation. Ultrasound devices do not expose the patient to ionizing radiation (Singh, 2006, Sartris, 1996)

4.8 Digital X-ray radiogrammetry (DXR)

Recently, the computer technology has renewed interest in this old technique. The Pronosco X-posure system estimates forearm bone mass from measurements of the cortical width of bones in the hand using computerized digital x-ray radiogrammetry from a single plain radiograph of the hand and wrist. The BMD estimate, referred to as DXR-BMD, is corrected for cortical porosity and striation. The results indicate that this technique is highly reproducible and appears to be at least as good as other peripheral bone assessment techniques in its ability to discriminate among patients with low bone mass at the spine and/or hip and osteoporotic fractures (Sartoris, 1996).

4.9 Photodensitometry

Previously, radiographic absorptiometry (RA) uses standard X-ray images of the hand and distal forearm are taken with a graduated aluminum reference. The radiographic image of the hand and wrist is captured by a video camera and the levels of grey seen on the hand image are quantified and compared with the grey levels of the reference standard, resulting in an estimate of bone mineral density (BMD). The cortical thickness of the bones can also be measured. Radiographic photo densitometry comprises of comparing the optical density of bone X-ray with standard calibrative, aluminium-step-wedge. Although inexpensive and easily accessible, this method had poor reproducibility. Computer-assisted methods have reduced these errors and several commercial systems have been developed in recent years. Although RA is generally less precise than DEXA, radiographic absorptiometry holds promise as a cost-effective method to screen cases of osteoporosis. Further research is needed to evaluate its effectiveness in predicting fracture and monitoring therapy (Sartoris, 1996, Singh et al, 2006, Blair et al, 2006, Bouxsien and Mary, 2005).

4.10 Double photon absorptiometry
The principle of dual photon absorptiometry (DPA) is the use of a photon beam that has two distinct energy peaks. One energy peak will be more absorbed by soft tissue and the other by bone. The soft tissue component then can be mathematically subtracted and the BMD thus determined (Sartoris, 1996).

4.11 Neutron activation analysis
A limb is bombarded by slow neutron from a generator. This is taken up by the soft tissue to convert it into thermal neutron. This thermal neutron is captured by the nucleus of calcium ion. The nucleus becomes radioactive. Decay of the nuclei emits photon which can be measured by a Geiger counter, giving an idea of bone mass. This is reduced in osteoporosis.
(source: www.iupac.org/publications/pac/1995/pdf/6711x1929.pdf).

4.12 Biochemical techniques
Biomarkers are substances found in an increased amount in the blood, other body fluids, or tissues and which can be used to indicate the presence the presence of osteoporosis. Biomarkers of bone remodeling (formation and breakdown), such as alkaline phosphatase and osteocalcin (serum markers) and pyridinolines and deoxypyridinolines (urinary markers), help in evaluating risk for osteoporosis. The research studies show that biomarkers correlate with changes in indices of bone remodeling and may provide insights into the mechanisms of bone loss which may give a basic detection method. The method may not be precise or accurate but it is quick, early, cheap and non-invasive way of detection. This method gives an indication of the onset of the disease (Sia, 2003).

4.13 Bone markers
There is a need for the development a non-invasive and repeated measurement of bone turnover which demands precision, accuracy and specificity. These kind of independent measurements of bone formation and resorption are done at organ or tissue level. The validated biochemical markers are urine and serum (see Table 2).
The two main biochemical markers for bone formation are serum alkaline phosphatase and serum osteocalcin. Markers for bone resorbtion include urinary calcium and urinary hydroxyproline: Alkaline phosphatase, which reflects osteoclast activity in bone, is measured in serum, but it lacks sensitivity and specificity for osteoporosis, because it can be

elevated or decreased with many diseases. It is increased with aging (see Table 2). Urinary calcium can give some estimate of resorbtion (loss of) bone, but there are many variables that affect this measurement. Urinary hydroxyproline is derived from degradation of collagen, which forms extracellular bone matrix. However, hydroxyproline measurement is not specific for bone, because half of the body's collagen is outside the bony skeleton. It is also influenced by many diseases, as well as diet. Several ELISA kits are developed by Osteomark Company for detection of Osteoporosis (www.osteomark.org).

S.No	Osteoblastic Activity	Osteoclastic Activity
1	S-alkaline phosphatase - Total alkaline phosphatase (S-tAP) - Bone alkaline phosphotase (S-bAP)	U-Hydroxyproline(U-OHPr)
2	S-osteocalcin(S-BGP)	U-collagen crosslinks - Pyridinoline(U-Pyr) - Deoxypryridine(U-D-Pyr)
3	S-carboxyterminal propeptide of human type I collagen(S-PICP)	S-C Terminal pyridine crosslinked telopeptide domain of type I collagen (S-ICTP) S-Tartrate-resistant acid phosphatase(S-TRAP)

Table 2. Urine and serum markers (Sartoris, 1996)

4.14 Laboratory methods
There are several preliminary tests to identify the loss of bone mass. A number of laboratory tests may be performed on blood and urine samples (Singh et al, 2006).
The most common blood tests evaluate:
- blood calcium levels
- blood vitamin D levels
- thyroid function
- parathyroid hormone levels
- estradiol levels to measure estrogen (in women)
- follicle stimulating hormone (FSH) test to establish menopause status
- testosterone levels (in men)
- osteocalcin levels to measure bone formation.

4.15 Needle bone biopsy
Needle bone biopsy is not a very common assessment technique of bone density. This test has limited availability, and is best utilized as a research technique for analysis of treatment regimens for bone diseases. The best clinical use of bone biopsy combines double tetracycline labeling to determine appositional bone growth and rule out osteomalacia. Doses of tetracycline are given weeks apart, and the bone biopsy is embedded in a plastic compound, sliced thinly, and examined under fluorescent light, where the lines of tetracycline (which auto fluoresce) will appear and appositional growth assessed (Singh et al, 2006).

5. Recent novel techniques

Osteoporosis is the disease which creeps into one's body silently without showing a significant symptom. The nature of the disease asymptotic until a gross deformity occurs in one's body. This is can be very serious and deadly for the patient. The time the patient realizes structural support of the body has totally deteriorated. The diagnosis and treatment is sometimes unaffordable for a common man. The patient has the control over prevention of this disease or is reliable, easy and cheap way is available for such deadly disease than proper care can be taken. There are several researches going on in order to achieve some cheap, easy early detection of osteoporosis (Singh et al, 2006). The latest trend is in miniaturizing the device which make it portable, useful for homecare, user-friendly, cheap, Non-invasive and provides a kind early indication for OP. This technique is based on MEMS based technique.

5.1 Bone fracture detection micro-sensor

The method for detection or investigation of osteoporosis is with the help of a micropump (Yung et al, 2004). The micropump has been designed using the electromagnetic principle to actuate the piston in two directions. A closed loop system is used for circulating the fluid with the pumping device. This is kind of pump is useful for blood sampling or drug delivery. Here the oscillating micropump is used to study the mechanosensitivity of bone cell for better investigation of osteoporosis. There is another research which has proposed an implantable, telemetry-based MEMS bone sensor (Singh et al, 2003, 2009) with the capability of determination of bone stress via wireless RF interface. The bone stress is detected using the embedded piezoresistive strain gauges with polysilicon layer and a CMOS chip (Singh, 1997).

Another design of micro-fabricated strain gauge array is used to monitor bone deformation *in vitro* and *in vivo* for detection of osteoporosis. These kinds of microsensor provide a map of distributed strain data over the area of interest on the surfaces of bone to monitor the structural integrity of bone. This type of strain membranes are wireless and implantable embedded in flexible membrane. A simulation experiment was conducted to develop such micro-strain gauge for study of osteoporotic bone (Yang et al, 2004).

A bone sensor has been used for the piezoelectric BioMEMS. An attempt has been made to develop bone-based piezoelectric sensors to detect the stress in bone (Singh, 2003). Another micro-scale sensor for bone surface strain measurement is discussed. This kind of sensor is used for studying the structural effects of osteoporosis. Designs and simulation using ANSYS finite element modeling tool of thin-film metal strain gauge. Metal films for electrical interconnection encapsulated in PDMS have been studied. The PDMS membrane was characterized to facilitate encapsulation designs. The basic fabrication steps like silanization, PDMS preparation, photolithography, PDMS metallization, wire bonding and finally device separation. With experiments were performed for optimizing and characterizing the device like mechanical testing, electrochemical testing and adhesion testing (Yang et al, 2004), and there is a new design which has been discussed here.

Another latest technology is detecting osteoporosis with the study of the brittleness of the bone. The bone mass and bone density play an important role in bone strength. It is important to measure the brittleness or fragility or the bone mechanics. Certain walking studies are done and it is found that as the heel strikes the ground it creates force pulse, energy that passes up through the body and it is absorbed by bone. The osteoporosis reduces the quality of the bone so by attaching the skin-mounted sensors for measuring the electrical pulses of the muscles which is an active part of the skeletal system. If the person has osteoporosis the energy which passes up to the body is disrupted due to porous nature of the bone (http://www.uc.edu/news/NR.asp?id=3280).

5.2 Microfluidic channels – Detection by biomarkers

The total Alkaline phosphatase (AP) is the mostly widely used bone marker in the clinics and hospitals. AP have physiological substrates which splits the inorganic phosphatase with organic phosphatase, increasing the calcium-phosphatase product and enabling mineralization. AP is essential for normal mineralization of the bone. Bone AP (bAP) constitutes approximately 50% serum AP and the serum has the half-life of 24-48hrs. Though the half-life is relatively large but it may differ on cardiac rhythm, with peak levels in afternoon and night. The exact metabolic pathway is unknown. AP is measured with the help of spectrophotometer using p-nitrophenylphosphate as substrate. The bone and liver AP may be separated by electrophoresis but this method is time consuming and gives semi-quatitaive results. The concentration of bAP concentration may be measured using two antibodies with small differences in affinity toward the isoforms (Singh et al, 2006).

MEMS based detection with alkaline phosphatase has been attempted by Kang and Park (2005). A microfluidic device has been used for enzyme assay. The measurement of enzyme-substrate reaction will to do the substrate consumed. A lab-on-a-chip (LOC) device is developed for controlling the flow containing small volumes of liquids in microchannel which can speeed up and simplifies sample preparation steps in LOC which offers high throughput, low version of traditional research. The microfluidic device is fabricated by the casting process with PDMS. It consists of three parts part I is the injection system, part II is the reaction chamber and part III is the microchannel. This particular microchannel measures the ALP activity using a micro-plate reader. Microfluidic mixing for single enzyme assay was applied and with mathematical prediction the enzymatic (Singh et al, 2006).

5.3 Biochemical based BioMEMS chip

A novel BioMEMS chip, based on gold nanoparticles, for the detection of osteoproteogerin (OPG). This biochip is used to evaluate the bone conditioning which is directly related to the diagnosis and prognosis of the osteoporosis, in an effective manner. The flow visualization of the mixing capabilities are characterized using micro-scale laser-induced fluorescence (LIF). The BioMEMS chip detection is based on competitive immunoassay. The monoclonal OPG antibody (anti-OPG) is immobilized onto the AuNPs deposited conducting polymer, using covalent bonding with a carboxylic acid group. The catalytic reduction is monitored amperometrically at - 0.4 V versus Ag/AgCl. The linear dynamic range is between 2 to 24 ng/ml with the detection limit of 2 ng/ml (Singh et al., 2007). Fig. 3 depicts schematic of the microfluidic chip.

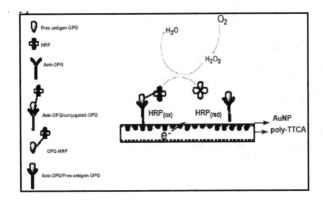

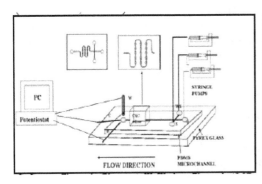
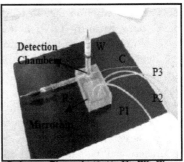

Fig. 3. Microfluidic technique for early detection of OP(Singh et al., 2007 & 2009)

Bone Formation	Bone Resorption
• Osteocalcin (OC) • Bone-specific alkaline phosphatase (BAP) • Amino terminal propeptide of type I collagen (PINP) • Carboxy terminal propeptide of type I collagen (PICP)	• Pyridinoline (Pyr) • Deoxypyridinoline (dPyr) • Amino terminal telopeptide of type I collagen (NTx) • Carboxy terminal telopeptide of type I collagen (CTx)

Table 3. Biochemical Indices (Singh et al., 2006)
(http://www.scielo.br/img/revistas/abem/v50n4/31869t2.gif)

5.4 BioMEMS-based sensors

BioMEMS using electrochemical immunoassay with microfluidic system (Heineman et al, 2001) help in blood sample analysis using the heterogeneous immunoassay. Two concepts of immunoassay are studied in this research. First is based on analogous microcapillary immunoreactor and other combines the reaction and detection chamber within the area of electromagnet. Both are MEMS based system for alkaline phosphatase study.

Another MEMS microvalve with PDMS diaphragm and two chambers with thermo-pneumatic actuator for integrated blood test system with silicon have been suggested for point of care device. The blood test system can be reduced to reasonable cost with MEMS technology (Singh, 2006). The microvalve with long stroke has been fabricated with two chamber thermo-pneumatic actuator.

5.5 Spectroscopic techniques for early detection of OP

Optical techniques such as Fourier Transform Infrared Spectroscopy (FTIR) and Ultra Violet Visible Spectroscopy (UV-Vis) are employed to find the bone markers with an emphasis on the noninvasive modalities for early detection of osteoporosis. Blood plasma samples procured from two groups, patients and healthy persons were tested. Both of the optical techniques revealed obvious differences in the spectra; between two groups, for example, increase in intensity for OP persons. New peaks were found at 1588, 1456 and 1033 cm⁻¹ in FTIR spectra, as shown in Fig. 4. On the other hand, in UV-Visible spectroscopy results, a new peak appeared in the OP patients' spectra at the wavelength of 420 nm, as shown in Fig. 5. These differences in the spectra of the two types of samples, allow rapid and cost-effective discrimination of the potential patients with the optical techniques which were verified by the bone densitometer in the hospitals. The new technique used here is quick, reliable and effective.

A hierarchical algorithm is used to investigate and quantify the mutual relevance between successive clusters in terms of heterogeneity values as shown in the Fig.6.

Fig. 6 represents the classification with the spectra at 1539-1542 cm⁻¹. This gives clear distinction between the patients and healthy groups for the amide II group.

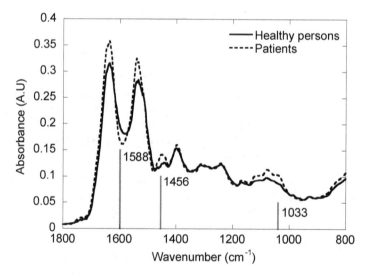

Fig. 4. FTIR results for EDO (Singh et al., 2010)

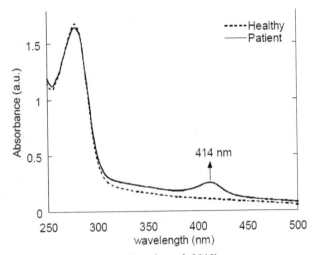

Fig. 5. UV-visible spectroscopy for EDO (Singh et al.,2010)

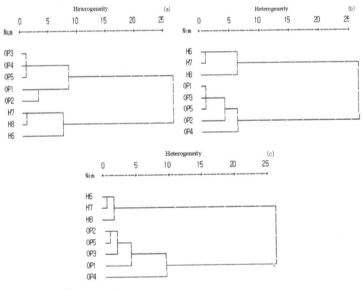

Fig. 6. Cluster analysis(Singh, 2010)

6. Discussions

6.1 Bone density testing

There is several bone density measurement testing techniques which have been discussed with their working principles. The recent developments in the instruments for BMD measurement have also been discussed. But there are several limitations in these devices. The testing with these devices is very expensive, early detection is not easy, these are invasive measurement, errors in magnification may occur, accuracy is not achievable, scan time is high, harmful radiation may cause problems in the body, home care is not possible and the instruments are not portable. Specially trained persons are required to operate such sophisticated equipments. Though BMD measurement is the most accurate method for detection of Osteoporosis but it is unable to help in early detection and is very expensive. Early detection of such a silent and deadly disease is important for the mankind. Hence there is a need for new, novel, portable, cheap detection systems to be developed for point of care testing.

6.2 Invasive technique
The invasive technique has several risks involved like skin is punctured. There is a slight chance that the needle may cause fracture the bone being sampled or injure one of the nerves, blood vessels, or organs near the biopsy site. If complications occur, another surgery may be needed to treat the problem. After a bone biopsy, there is a slight chance that the bone may become infected, osteomyelitis or not heal properly. In rare instances, the bone from which the biopsy sample was taken may become weak and break, fracture at a later time. This type detection is only good for extreme severe cases.

6.3 Biochemical measurement
There are several bone markers or the biomarkers available for the early detection of the osteoporosis which control the osteoblastic and osteoclastic activity. The biochemical detection is not accurate detection but it gives the indication for onset of osteoporosis detection.

6.4 MEMS-based techniques
The MEMS-based techniques are portable, handheld, easy to use, can be used for home care and point-of-care testing. But the accuracy of the detection may be achieved by using bone mineral density testing (BMD) (Singh et al., 2009, 2010).

7. Conclusions

The radiographic techniques are needed for the accurate detection of osteoporosis as they give precise data for detection of the deadly disease. Generally, the patients are just unaware of the disease as osteoporosis creeps silently within a human body. Osteoporosis is a silent killer and is a very progressive disease. The time the person realizes the detection and treatment becomes unaffordable for patient. This research paper focuses on the urgent need for the development on early, non-invasive, cheap, and handheld POCT device for such a dangerous disease. These characteristics can be achieved by using a micro-size (MEMS/ Nano based techniques). There have been several attempts in this direction as mentioned in the paper above. But this area needs more of research and deep studies.

8. References

Ahn C.H; Choi JW, Beaucage G, Nevin JH, Lee JB, Puntambaker A, Lee J., (2004). Disposable smart lab on a chip for point-of-care clinical diagnostics. *Proc. IEEE* 92: pp.154-173.

Arnaud, C.D.; (1996). Osteoporosis: using bone markers for diagnosis and monitoring. *Geriatrics,* Vol. 51, 24-30.

Atkinson, P.J.; (1964). Age-related structural changes in trabecular and cortical bone: Cellular mechanisms and biomechanical consequences *Nature,* Vol. 201, 373 – 375.

Auroux, P.A., Iossifidis, D., Reyes, D.R and Manz, A.,(2002). Micro total analysis systems. 2. Analytical standard operations and applications. *Anal. Chem.,*Vol. 74, 2637-52.

Bagur, A.,(2001). Epidemiology of osteoporosis in Argentina, *Bone* 29 (3), 298.

Bakker, E., Quin Y., 2006. Anal. Chem. Vol.78, 3965-3982.

Bal, S.K., McCloskey, E.V., (2002). Menopause and bones. *Current Obst & Gynaec.* Vol.12, 354-357.

Ban, C., Chung, S., Park, D-S., Shim, Y-B, (2004). Nucleic Acids Res.32(13), e110.

Becerra-Rojas, F. and Jupari, M., (2001). Epidemiology of osteoporosis in Peru, *Bone* , Vol.29 (3), 297.

Berthonnaud L, F., Chotel , J., Dimnet, I., (2002).The anatomic patterns of the lower limb from three-dimensional radiographic reconstruction of bones (3drrb). *ITBM-RBM,* Vol. 23, 290-302.

Bianchi, M.L, (2005). How to manage osteoporosis in children? *Bone Prac. & Res Clinical Rheumatology,* Vol. 19, Issue no.6, 991-1005.

Bianchi, M..L., Cimaz, R., Bardare, M., et al, (2000). Efficacy and safety of alendronate for the treatment of osteoporosis in diffuse connective tissue diseases in children: a prospective study. *Arthritis & Rheum,* Vol.43, 1960.

Blair, J.M, Zhou, H., Seibel, M.J., Dunstan, C.R., (2006). *Nat. Clin. Pract. Oncol.* Vol.3, 41 – 49.

Bouxsien, Mary L, (2005). Determinants of skeletal fragility: best practice and research. *Clinical Rheumatology,* Vol.19 (6), 897-911.

Boyle, W.J., Simonet, W.S., Lacey, D.L., (2003). Osteoclast differentiation and activation. *Nature,*Vol.423, 337-342.

Burr, D.B., Forwood, M.R., Fyhrie, D.P., Martin, R.B., Schaffler, M.B., Turner, C.H., (1997). Bone microdamage and skeletal fragility in osteoporotic and stress fractures. *J Bone Miner Res,* Vol.12, 6 – 9.

Clark, R.J.H., Hester, R.E., (1996). Biomedical applications of spectroscopy. New York: 1st ed., Wiley & Sons, New York.

Heineman, W.R, Thomas, J.H, Wijayawardhana, A, Brian Halsall et.al, (2001). BioMEMS: Electrochemical immunoassay with microfluidic systems, Analytic Sciences 17, i281-i284.

Korkia, P., (2002). Osteoporosis: process, prevention and treatment. J. Bodywork and Movement Therapies. 6, 156-169.

Raisz, L.G., (1997) The osteoporosis revolution. Ann Intern Med. 126,458-462.

Sia, K.S. and Whitesides, G.M., (2003). Microfluidic devices fabricated in polydimethylsiloxane) for biological studies. *Electrophoresis,* Vol.24, 3563-3576.

Sartoris, David, J.,Osteoporosis Diagnosis and treatment. 28/06/1996. Publisher Marcel Dekker Inc. ISBN 9780824795078

Singh, K.,(2007) Study of Biomechanical, Optical Spectroscopy & Electrochemical techniques for Early detection of Osteoporosis: Design and development of a new BioMEMS chip for the point of care testing (POCT) device. Ph.D dissertation, Pusan National University, South Korea. Supervisor: Prof.K.C.Kim

Singh, K., (2000). Development of MEMs using ASE, *National Symposium on Instrumentation (NSI),* Goa, India, Feb 2-4.

Singh, K., (1997). Electronic bone fracture detector, *Proc IEEE- EMBS Int Conf, Chicago (USA),* Oct 29 to Nov 3.

Singh, K., (1998). Portable battery operated bone fracture evaluator *Proc IEEE- EMBS Int. conf,* Hong Kong, Oct 28 to Nov 3, 2257-2259.

Singh, K., (1999). Development of a dynamic bone micro-sensor for biomedical Applications, *Proc. IEEE-EMBS Int. Conf.,* Atlanta, USA, Oct 29-Nov. 1.

Singh K., Singh V.R., (1999).A piezo-electric bone dynamic sensor for bio-medical applications *Proc First Joint BMES-EMBS Conf Sewing Humanity, Advancing Technology,* Atlanta.GA. USA, 831.

Singh, K., (2000). Biomedical MEMs using ASE technique. *Proc.11th Asia-Pacific Conf. on Biomedical Engineering,* Hangzhou, China, Sept 26-28.

Singh, K., (2003). Piezoelectric BioMEMs", *10th Congress World federation for Ultrasound in Medicine &Biology (WFUMB)* hosted by American Institute of Ultrasound in Medicine(AIUM), June 1-4, 2003, Montreal, Canada.

Singh, K, Kim, K.C, (2005). Biomechanics of Bone, *Proc. 7th Cross Straits Symp on Materials, energy and Environmental Sciences,* CSS7, 35-36.

Singh, K, (2004). A bone- based sensor. *Proc 26th Annual IEEE-EMBS Int Conf., San Francisco, USA,* 1-5th Sept.

Singh, K., Lee, S.H., Kim, K.C., (2006). Osteoporosis: new biomedical engineering aspects. *J. Mech. Eng. Sci. Technol.* 20, 2265-2283.

Singh, K., Kim, K.C., (2007). BioMEMS-early disease detection. Korean Society of Mechanical Engineers, *KSME Int. conference,* 30th April, Bexco, Busan, Korea..

Singh, K, Lee, S. G., Kim, S.G., Lee, D., Kim, K.C., (2007). Optical techniques for investigation of biofluid for early disease detection, *8rth Cross Straits Symposium on Material,* Busan, Korea.

Singh, K., (2003). Piezoelectric BioMEMs. *Proc.10th Congress World Fed for Ultrasound in Med &Biology (WFUMB) Am Institute of Ultr in Medicine(AIUM),* June 1-4, , Montreal, Canada.

Singh, K., (2003). Study of BioMEMS. *SICON: Int Conf. on Sensors,* Nov, 2003,USA.

Singh, K, Lee, S.G, Kim, S.G., Lee, D., Kim, K. C., (2006). Osteoporosis detection for normal and abnormal biofluids by FTIR. *The Korean Society of Visualization,* Workshop at Dongnae University, Busan, 1st Dec.

Singh, K, Lee, S.H., Kim, K.C., (2006). Osteoporosis: new biomedical engineering aspects. *J Mech Eng Sci Technol,* Vol.20, Issue no.12, 2265-2283.

Singh, K., Kim, H. H. and Kim K.C., (2007). Biomems for osteoproteogerin detection with gold nanoparticles. *Proc. MicroTAS,* 7 - 11 October 2007, Paris, France.

Singh, K., Kim, K.C., (2007). POCT for Diseases. *Cambridge Healthtech Institute, Inaugural Enabling Point-of-Care Diagnostics Conf,* August 14-15, 2007, Washington, D.C.

Singh K, Rahman Md.A, Son J-I, Kim K.C and Shim Y-B, An amperometric immunosensor for osteoproteogerin based on gold nanoparticles deposited conducting polymer, *Biosensors and Bioelectronics,* Vol 23, Issue 11, 15 June Pages 1595-1601, 2008

Singh. K. & Kim, K.C., (2009). BioMEMS for Early detection of bone diseases" *The 5th International Conference on Microtechnologies in Medicine and Biology, MMB 2009* Conference, Quebec City, Canada, April 1-9

Singh, K, Kim, K.C., (2009). Multiprong approaches to monitor the Biomechanical aspects of osteoporosis, Int. J. of biomedical engineering and technology, IJBET. *Int. J. Biomedical Engineering & technology,* Vol. 2, Number 3, 279-291.

Singh, K., Kim, K.C., (2009). Technology and Applications of Clinical BioMEMS, *Sensor Letters,* Vol 7, No.6, 1013-1024.

Singh K, Lee K-S, Lee D-G, Kim Y-K and Kim K.C (2010) Spectroscopic as a diagnostic tool for early detection of OP, *Journal of Mechanical Science and Technology* Vol.24 ,Issue no.8, 1661~1668

Vijayendran, R.A., Motsegood, K.M., Beebe, D.J and Leckband, D.E., (2003). Langmuir 19, 1824-1828.

Yang, G.Y, Vasudev, J.B., et al., (2004) Design of microfabricated strain gauge array to monitor bone deformation, in vitro and in vivo. Proc. 4th IEEE Symp on Bioinformatics and Bioengineering (BIBE'04).

9

Approach to the Screening and Diagnosis of Osteoporosis

H.J. Choi
Department of Family Medicine,
Eulji University School of Medicine
South Korea

1. Introduction

The goal of treatment of osteoporosis is to decrease the risk of fractures in patients with high risk for a first or subsequent fracture. The efficacy of treatment will depend on the efficacy and level of accomplishment of case finding to select patients at risk, the results of additional investigations, the efficacy, tolerance, and safety of medical intervention, and the adherence to treatment during follow-up. Each of these steps is critical in treatment in daily clinical practice. Failure to consider one or other step can result in suboptimal fracture prevention or overtreatment (Geusens, 2009).

On the other hand, measurement of bone mineral density (BMD), assessment of the fracture risk, and making decisions regarding to appropriate therapeutic intervention are the ultimate goal when evaluating patients for osteoporosis (NIH Consensus Development Panel on Osteoporosis Prevention, Diagnosis, and Therapy, 2001). Since many fractures among postmenopausal women occur in those with T-scores better than in the osteoporotic range (Siris et al, 2004; Schuit et al, 2004; Cranney et al, 2007), screening of the patients at high risk of fracture and early diagnosis are important.

2. Screening of osteoporosis

The aim of screening is obviously to direct interventions to those most in need, and to avoid treatment of healthy individuals who will never fracture. Bone mass is used conventionally as a proxy of overall bone strength and low bone mass is a major risk factor for osteoporotic fractures. Although BMD measurement is the standard test for the diagnosis of osteoporosis before fracture, ongoing research indicates that BMD measurement alone may not be adequate for detection of individuals at high risk of fracture (Kanis, 1994). Epidemiological studies have shown that a substantial proportion of osteoporotic fractures occur in postmenopausal women who do not meet BMD criteria for osteoporosis defined according to the WHO definition as a T-score of -2.5 or below (Siris et al, 2004; Schuit et al, 2004; Cranney et al, 2007). This suggests that factors other than BMD contribute to a patient's risk of fracture. Central dual-energy x-ray absorptiometry (DXA) is not available everywhere. Furthermore, although BMD measurement is specific, it lacks sensitivity when used alone, so that a number of high-risk patients escape identification (Kanis, 1994). Thus, the potential impact of extensive population-based screening with BMD in women at the time of menopause on the burden of fractures is less than optimal; screening the general population with BMD would not be cost-effective and is considered inadvisable in many countries (World Health Organization [WHO], 2004). In practice, most guidelines recommend using risk factor assessment tools such as Fracture Risk Assessment Tool FRAX® to help select patients for BMD measurement and/or treatment.

The National Osteoporosis Foundation (NOF), US Preventive Services Task Force (USPSTF), and the American Association of Clinical Endocrinologists (AACE) recommend that BMD testing should be performed to guide treatment decisions, based on the patient's risk profile (National Osteoporosis Foundation [NOF], 2003; US Preventive Services Task Force [USPSTF], 2002; Hodgson et al, 2001). Also, the NOF recommends that all postmenopausal women and men age 50 and older should be evaluated clinically for osteoporosis risk in order to determine the need for BMD measurement and considered the possibility of osteoporosis and fracture risk in men and women, based on the presence of the risk factors and conditions (NOF, 2010).

The National Osteoporosis Guideline Group (NOGG) recommends that patients are identified opportunistically using a case-finding strategy on the finding of a previous fragility fracture or the presence of significant clinical risk factors because, at present, there is no universally accepted policy for population screening in the UK to identify individuals with osteoporosis or those at high risk of fracture (Compston et al, 2009).

3. Diagnosis of osteoporosis

Osteoporosis is diagnosed on the basis of either a low-impact or fragility fracture or a low BMD. A low-impact fracture is one that occurs after a fall from standing height or less; a fragility fracture occurs spontaneously or with no trauma (cough, sneezing, sudden movement) (Mauck & Clarke, 2006).

Until recent years, diagnosis of non-fractured patients was based on the quantitative assessment of BMD, usually by central DXA. In 1994, the World Health Organization (WHO) developed a definition of osteoporosis on the basis of studies of women of various ages (Table 1) (Kanis et al, 1994). The BMD, measured with DXA, results are reported as a density measurement in gm/cm^2, in addition to T- and Z-scores.

Category	Fracture Risk	Action
Normal T-score at -1.0 or above	Below average	Be watchful for clinical triggers
Osteopenia T-score between -1.0 and -2.5	Above average	Consider prevention in peri- or post-MPW Be watchful for clinical triggers Possibly repeat investigations in 2-3 years
Osteoporosis T-score at -2.5 or below	High	Exclude secondary causes Therapeutic intervention indicated in most patients
Severe Osteoporosis T-score at -2.5 or below and already experienced one or more fractures	Established osteoporosis	Exclude secondary causes Therapeutic intervention indicated in most patients

Table 1. Definition of osteoporosis by the WHO

The T-score represent the number of SDs from the mean bone density values in normal gender-matched young adults. T-score is used to make a diagnosis of normal bone density, osteoporosis or osteopenia in postmenopausal women and in men age 50 years and older (Leib et al, 2004). Z-scores represent the number of SDs from the normal mean value for age- and gender-matched control subjects. A Z-score of -2.0 or lower may suggest the presence of a secondary cause of osteoporosis, although no definitive data support this hypothesis. Z-scores are used preferentially to assess bone loss in premenopausal women and men younger than age 50 years. A Z-score of -2.0 or lower is defined as "below the expected range for age"; a Z-score above -2.0 is "within the expected range for age." (Leib et al, 2004). Originally, the definition of osteoporosis was developed for the estimation of the prevalence of osteoporosis across populations. It was not for the assessment of osteoporosis in individual patient. In other words, diagnostic thresholds differ from intervention thresholds. The fracture risk varies at different ages, even with the same T-score. Other factors that determine intervention thresholds include the presence of clinical risk factors (CRFs), costs and and benefits of treatment.

4. Determination of fracture risk

In the past decade, a great deal of research has taken place to identify factors other than BMD that contribute to fracture risk. The consideration of well-validated CRFs, with or without BMD, is likely to improve fracture risk prediction and the selection of individuals at high risk for treatment. Some of these risk factors act independently of BMD to increase fracture risk whereas others increase fracture risk through their association with reduced BMD (e.g., some of the secondary causes of osteoporosis) (Table 2) (Compston et al, 2009).
Several models have been proposed to stratify osteoporotic fracture risk. These include strategies to identify patients with a high risk of low BMD (e.g., the OST index (Gensens et al, 2002), and the FRAX algorithm (Kanis, et al, 2008a, 2008b)) or with a high absolute risk of fractures based on CRFs, with or without BMD (e.g., FRAX algorithm (Kanis, et al, 2008a, 2008b)), Fracture Risk in Glucocorticoid Users (FIGS) (van Staa et al, 2005), the Garvan algorithm (Nguyen et al, 2008)), and simplified questionnaires.
Among these models, FRAX®, developed by WHO is an algorithm for individualized fracture risk prediction which is depend on population-based cohort from Europe, North America, Asia, and Australia.

4.1 Use of WHO Fracture Risk Assessment Tool (FRAX®)
FRAX® is a clinical tool for case finding for identifying patients at high risk for fractures, for selecting patients to measure BMD, and for treatment decisions. FRAX® should not be considered a gold standard but rather provides an aid to enhance patient assessment. The aim of FRAX® is to provide an assessment tool for the fracture prediction with use of CRFs with or without femoral neck BMD (Kanis et al, 2008a). These CRFs include age, sex, race, height, weight, body mass index (BMI), a history of fragility fracture, a parental history of hip fracture, use of oral glucocorticoid, rheumatoid arthritis, and other secondary causes of osteoporosis, current smoking, and alcohol intake of three or more units daily. These risk factors were identified and validated based on an analysis of 12 prospective studies, yielding a total of 250,000 person-years in 60,000 men and women with more than 5,000 osteoporotic fractures (Kanis, 1994). Because fracture probability also varies markedly among different regions of the

world, FRAX® allows fracture risk to be calculated for countries where the incidences of both fractures and mortality are known (Unnanuntana et al, 2010).

FRAX® has been developed for calculating the 10-year absolute fracture risk in individual patients in primary care settings for a major osteoporotic fracture (in the proximal humerus, the wrist, or the hip or a clinical vertebral fracture) and for a hip fracture calibrated to the fracture and death hazards. The relative risks are difficult to apply in clinical practice since their clinical significance depends on the prevalence of fractures in the general population. As a result, the concept of the absolute risk of fractures has emerged and refers to the individual's risk for fracture over a certain time period, e.g., over the next 5 or 10 years which is the usual duration of the effects of osteoporosis medications during and after use (van Geel et al, 2010).

The FRAX® algorithm is available at www.nof.org and at www.shef.ac.uk/FRAX. FRAX® is intended for postmenopausal women and men age 50 and older who have not been treated for osteoporosis; it is not intended for use in younger adults or children.

NOF starts case finding with age as a criterion (NOF, 2011). Below 65 years, NOF advocates clinical attention for the presence of CRFs (those included in FRAX, with the addition of other risks), and a DXA in the presence of CRFs. In all women older than 65 years, NOF advocates BMD. Treatment is advocated in women with osteoporosis or osteoporotic fracture and in women with osteopenia if FRAX® calculation with BMD indicates a high risk of fracture or when specific high risks (total immobilization and glucocorticoid use) are present.

Age
Sex
Low body mass index (≤ 19 kg/m^2)
Previous fragility fracture, particularly of the hip, wrist, and vertebrae including morphometric vertebral fracture
Parental history of hip fracture
Current glucocorticoid treatment (any dose, per oral for ≥ 3 months)
Current smoking
Alcohol intake of 3 or more units daily
Secondary causes of osteoporosis including:
Rheumatoid arthritis
Untreated hypogonadism in men and women
Prolonged immobility
Organ transplantation
Type 1 diabetes
Hyperthyroidism
Gastrointestinal disease
Chronic liver disease
Chronic obstructive pulmonary disease
Falls*

* Not presently accommodated in the FRAX® algorithm

Table 2. Clinical risk factors used for the assessment of fracture probability

The National Osteoporosis Society (NOS) starts case finding with CRFs of FRAX® in all postmenopausal women (Compston et al, 2009). Treatment is advocated in high-risk patients based on CRFs of FRAX® without DXA and in patients with intermediate risk when BMD results integrated in FRAX® indicate a high risk.

It should also be acknowledged that there are many other risk factors for fracture that are not incorporated into assessment algorithms. FRAX® does not include fall-related risk factors and other risk factors for fractures: dose and duration of some risk factors like glucocorticoid use; characteristics of previous fractures (location, number, and severity); vitamin D deficiency; and levels of biochemical markers of bone turnover (van Geel et al, 2010). Moreover, no randomized clinical trials focusing on prevention of fractures in patients who are included based on FRAX® are available (van Geel et al, 2010). Further studies will be needed on the ability to treatment to reduce fracture risk in subjects at high risk for fractures based on FRAX®. Another drawback is that FRAX® is only applicable in treatment naïve patients (Saag, 2009).

5. Clinical investigations

Comprehensive approach to the clinical evaluation of osteoporosis is recommended. A detailed history and physical examination together with BMD assessment and the 10-year estimated fracture probability are utilized to establish the individual patient's risk. The range of tests will depend on the severity of the disease, age at presentation, and the presence or absence of fractures. The aims of patient evaluation are to exclude diseases that mimic osteoporosis (e.g. osteomalacia, myeloma), identify the cause of osteoporosis and contributory factors, assess the risk of subsequent fractures and select the most appropriate form of treatment (Compston et al, 2009).

5.1 History and physical examination

Many metabolic bone diseases are associated with low BMD, therefore a complete and thorough history taking and physical examination are essential to establishing a correct diagnosis of osteoporosis. A complete history should be obtained, with specific attention given to the risk factors, including lifestyle, medical, family, and medication histories (Table 3) (NOF, 2010). Physical examination should include height and weight for BMI and determining any loss of height (historical height loss >4 cm). A thorough physical examination may detect kyphosis, a protruding abdomen, rib-iliac crest distance of less than 2 cm, height loss (prospective height loss >2 cm), acute or chronic back pain and/or tenderness, reduced gait speed or grip strength, and poor visual acuity. Certain other findings, such as nodular thyroid, hepatic enlargement, jaundice, or cushingoid features may reveal secondary causes of osteoporosis (Lane, 2006).

Since the majority of osteoporosis-related fractures result from falls, it is also important to evaluate risk factors for falling. The most important of these seem to be a personal history of falling, along with muscle weakness and gait, balance and visual deficits (Anonymous, 2001). All elderly should be asked annually about the occurrence of falls. Any patient who reports a single fall should undergo basic evaluation of gait/balance (e.g., "Get Up and Go test")(Anonymous, 2001). Items that should be included as a part of a fall risk assessment are summarized in Table 4 (NOF, 2010).

Lifestyle factors		
Low calcium intake	Vitamin D insufficiency	Excessive vitamin A
High caffeine intake	High salt intake	Aluminum (in antacid)
Alcohol (≥3 units/day)	Inadequate physical activity	Immobilization
Smoking	Falling	Thinness
Genetic factors		
Cystic fibrosis	Homocysteinuria	Osteogenesis imperfecta
Ehlers-Danlos	Hypophosphatasia	Parental history of hip fracture
Gaucher's disease	Idiopathic hypercalciuria	Porphyria
Glycogen storage disease	Marfan syndrome	Riley-Day syndrome
Hemochromatosis	Menkes steely hair syndrome	
Hypogonadal states		
Androgen insensitivity	Hyperprolactinemia	Turner's & Klinefelter's syndromes
Anorexia nervosa, bulimia	Panhypopituitarism	Athletic amenorrhea
Premature ovarian failure		
Endocrine disorders		
Adrenal insufficiency	Diabetes mellitus	Thyrotoxicosis
Cushing's syndrome	Hyperparathyroidism	
Gastrointestinal disorders		
Celiac disease	Inflammatory bowel disease	Primary biliary cirrhosis
Gastric bypass	Malabsorption	GI surgery
Pancreatic disease		
Hematologic disorders		
Hemophilia	Multiple myeloma	Systemic mastocytosis
Leukemia, lymphoma	Sickle cell disease	Thalassemia
Rheumatic and autoimmune diseases		
Ankylosing spondylitis	Lupus	Rheumatoid arthritis
Miscellaneous conditions and diseases		
Alcoholism	Emphysema	Muscular dystrophy
Amyloidosis	End stage renal disease	Parenteral nutrition
Chronic metabolic acidosis	Epilepsy	Post-transplant bone loss
Congestive heart failure	Idiopathic scoliosis	Prior fracture as an adult
Depression	Multiple sclerosis	Sarcoidosis
Medications		
Anticoagulants (heparin)	Chemotherapeutic drugs	GnRH agonists
Anticonvulsants	Cyclosporin A, tacolimus	Lithium
Aromatase inhibitors	Depo-medroxyprogesterone	Barbiturates
Glucocorticoid	Selective serotonin reuptake inhibitors	Thiazolidinediones
Proton pump inhibitors		

Table 3. Conditions, diseases, and medications that cause or contribute to osteoporosis and fractures

Environmental risk factors
Lack of assistive devices in bathrooms Loose throw rugs Low level lighting Obstacles in the walking path Slippery outdoor conditions
Medical risk factors
Age Anxiety and agitation Arrhythmia Dehydration Depression Female gender Impaired transfer and mobility Malnutrition Medications causing oversedation (narcotic analgesics, anticonvulsants, psychotropics) Orthostatic hypotension Poor vision and use of bifocals Previous fall Reduced problem solving or mental acuity and diminished cognitive skills Urgent urinary incontinence Vitamin D insufficiency (25(OH)D <30 ng/mL (75 nmol/L)
Neuro and musculoskeletal risk factors
Kyphosis Poor balance Reduced proprioception Weak muscles
Other risk factors
Fear of falling

Table 4. Risk factors for falls

5.2 Bone mineral density measurement

Although central DXA of the hip (femoral neck or total hip) is the gold standard for diagnosing osteoporosis, many experts including the International Society for Clinical Densitometry (ISCD), recommend using the lowest central DXA T-score of posteroanterior lumbar spine (L1-L4), femoral neck, or total hip (or the 33% distal radius of the non-dominant forearm, if measured) to make the diagnosis (Leib et al, 2004). DXA measurement of BMD at other sites (including the trochanter, Ward triangle, lateral lumbar spine, other forearm regions, heel, or total body) or with other technologies (calcaneal ultrasonography, peripheral DXA, quantitative computed tomography, single- or dual-photon radionuclide absorptiometry, or magnetic resonance imaging) are not recommended for use in diagnosing osteoporosis (Leib et al, 2004; Marshall et al, 1996).

As a spine region of interest, posteroanterior L1-L4 for spine BMD measurement and only exclude vertebrae that are affected by local structural change (e.g., degenerative change or compression fracture) or artifact should be used (Baim et al, 2008). However, BMD based diagnostic classification should not be made using a single vertebra. If only one evaluable vertebra remains after excluding other vertebrae, diagnosis should be based on different valid skeletal site.

As a hip region of interest, femoral neck or total proximal femur, whichever is lowest should be used (Baim et al, 2008). Forearm BMD should be measured under the following circumstances: hip and/or spine cannot be measured or interpreted; hyperparathyroidism; and very obese patients (over the weight limit for DXA table) (Baim et al, 2008).

Peripheral DXA (pDXA), quantitative computed tomography (QCT), and quantitative ultrasound densitometry (QUS) are also capable of predicting both site-specific and overall fracture risk (NOF, 2010). When performed according to accepted standards, these densitometry techniques are accurate and highly reproducible (USPSTF, 2002). However, T-scores from these technologies cannot be used according to the WHO diagnostic classification because they are not equivalent to T-scores derived from DXA (NOF, 2010). Moreover, these measurements are less useful in predicting the risk of fractures of the spine and proximal femur than central DXA (Lane, 2006).

The accuracy of QCT of the spine in predicting spinal fracture is comparable to that of DXA but has the advantage of measuring true volumetric or 3-demential BMD, in contrast to the areal BMD obtained from DXA (Miller, 1999). QCT can distinguish between cortical and trabecular bone and thus is more sensitive to changes in BMD caused by the higher bone turnover rate of trabecular bone (Brunader & Shelton, 2002). It is also precise enough to detect BMD changes over time, and it can be used to follow the disease state or to monitor the response of osteoporosis therapy (Brunader & Shelton, 2002). For this reason, QCT are not the gold standard at the moment, but are also recommended (if applicable) to evaluate osteoporosis.

5.3 Vertebral fracture assessment

Morphometric vertebral fractures are the most frequent fractures in women and men older than 50 years (Sambrook & Cooper, 2006). Independent of BMD, age, and other CRFs, radiographically confirmed vertebral fracture is a strong predictor of future vertebral, non-vertebral, and hip fracture risk (Lems, 2007). The presence of a vertebral fracture increases the relative risk of future vertebral fractures by 4.4-fold and increases the risk of fragility fractures at other skeletal sites as well (Klotzbuecher et al, 2000). The higher the grade (severity) of the existing vertebral fracture, or the more vertebral fractures present (one, two, or three), the greater the risk for future fractures (Gallagher et al, 2005; Black et al, 1999).

Clinical vertebral fractures represent one out of three to four morphometric vertebral fractures (van Helden et al, 2008). Because most morphometric vertebral fractures are not diagnosed until clinically suspected and imaging by x-ray is performed, vertebral fractures are often missed.

Imaging techniques to detect and evaluate vertebral fractures in clinical practice include plain radiography (x-ray), computed tomography (CT), magnetic resonance imaging (MRI) nuclear bone scanning, and vertebral fracture assessment (VFA). There are differences in each of these in terms of imaging resolution, radiation exposure, availability, cost, and patient convenience.

Vertebral Fracture Assessment (VFA) is a new method to evaluate the presence of morphometric vertebral fractures and deformities using central DXA. VFA reliably and accurately identified patients with vertebral fractures that have not been recognized, with greater patient convenience, lower cost, and less radiation than standard x-ray. VFA is indicated when there is a probability that a prevalent vertebral fracture will influence clinical management of the patient (Lewiecki & Laster, 2006). The use of VFA contributes to better define the fracture risk in women with osteopenia and contributes to treatment decisions identifies patients at high risk of fractures in the absence of BMD-based osteoporosis. Indications for VFA according to the ISCD are presented in Table 5 (Baim et al, 2008).

Postmenopausal women with low bone mass (osteopenia) by BMD criteria, plus any one of the following:
Age ≥70 years Historical height loss >4 cm (1.6 inch) Prospective height loss >2 cm (0.8 inch) Self-reported vertebral fracture (not previously documented) Two or more of the following: 　　Age 60-69 years 　　Self-reported prior non-vertebral fracture 　　Historical height loss of 2 to 4 cm 　　Chronic systemic diseases associated with increased risk of vertebral fractures (for example, moderate to severe chronic obstructive pulmonary disorder (COPD) or chronic obstructive airway disease (COAD), seropositive rheumatoid arthritis, Crohn's disease)
Men with low bone mass (osteopenia) by BMD criteria, plus any one of the following:
Age ≥80 years Historical height loss >6 cm (2.4 inch) Prospective height loss >3 cm (1.2 inch) Self-reported vertebral fracture (not previously documented) Two or more of the following: 　　Age 70-79 years 　　Self-reported prior non-vertebral fracture 　　Historical height loss of 3 to 6 cm 　　On pharmacologic androgen deprivation therapy or following orchiectomy 　　Chronic systemic diseases associated with increased risk of vertebral fractures (for example, moderate to severe COPD or COAD, seropositive rheumatoid arthritis, Crohn's disease)
Women or men on chronic glucocorticoid therapy (equivalent to 5 mg or more of prednisone daily for 3 months or longer)
Postmenopausal women or men with osteoporosis by BMD criteria, if documentation of one or more vertebral fractures will alter clinical management

Table 5. Indications for vertebral fracture assessment using x-ray absorptiometry

5.4 Biochemical markers of bone turnover

Bone turnover is the principal factor that controls both the quality and the quantity of bone in adult skeleton and it can be assessed by measuring biochemical markers in blood and urine samples. Bone turnover markers (BTMs) represent the products of bone formation and resorption that are released into the circulation (Table 6).

Resorption markers
Urine 　　N-telopeptide cross-links of type 1 collagen (uNTx) 　　C-telopeptide cross-links of type 1 collagen (uCTx) 　　Pyridinolines, free and total (Pyr) 　　Deoxypyridinolines, free and total (Dpd)
Serum 　　N-telopeptide cross-links of type 1 collagen (sNTx) 　　C-telopeptide cross-links of type 1 collagen (sCTx) 　　Cross-linked C-telopeptide of type 1 collagen (ICTP) 　　Tartrate-resistant acid phosphatase (TRAP)
Formation markers
Serum 　　Bone specific alkaline phosphatase (BSAP) 　　Osteocalcin (OC) 　　Amino-terminal propetide of type 1 collagen (P1NP) 　　Carboxy-terminal propetide of type 1 collagen (P1CP)

Table 6. Markers of bone turnover

Quantitative changes in BTMs reflect the dynamic process of bone metabolism. BTMs have been associated with increased osteoporotic fractures independently of BMD in large prospective studies. They also may predict bone loss and, when repeated after 3 to 6 months of treatment with FDA approved antiresorptive drugs, may be predictive of fracture risk reduction. However, BTMs are not a substitute for DXA in women at risk. The value of BTMs in the assessment of fracture risk is likely to be in combination with risk factors, including BMD (Delmas et al, 2000). Generally, their use in the diagnosis of osteoporosis is not recommended (Lash et al, 2009).

There are multiple factors that may cause variations in the levels of BTMs (Table 7). Therefore it is necessary to review certain factors that affect bone marker levels. The main source of variability is pre-analytical; mostly sample conservation and biological variability (Unnanuntana et al, 2010). Pyridinoline crosslinks are light sensitive and degraded under the influence of intense UV irradiation (Body et al, 2009). Osteocalcin concentrations are decreased by freeze-thaw cycles and hemolysis. Assays detecting only intact osteocalcin are particularly affected by in vitro degradation, so it may be advantageous to use assays recognizing both the intact molecule and the large N-terminal fragment (N-MID, 1–43 amino acid), which appear to be more stable, sensitive and reproducible. (Delmas et al, 1985) Some osteocalcin fragments are also released during bone resorption (Delmas et al, 1990). In adults, the main source of undesirable biological variability is the circadian rhythm, with higher values in the early morning hours (peak in 4:00 A.M. and 8:00 A.M.), then a steep decrease in the morning, to attain a nadir at the end of the afternoon (through in 1:00 P.M. and 11:00 P.M.) (Seibel et al, 2005). Most BTMs follow the same pattern, with the exception of alkaline phosphatase because of its longer half-life. Practically, it implies that the measurement of BTMs must be performed in the same lab using standard procedures; samples should be taken while fasting and always at the same time of day. For the urinary BTMs, it is best to obtain either a 24-hour urine collection or morning second voided urine sample. Creatinine excretion also contributes to the overall variability in the levels of urinary BTMs (Unnanuntana et al, 2010).

Biological factors	Analytical factors
Uncontrollable	Technical variability
Age	Sample conservation and processing
Sex	
Growth	
Menopausal status	
Immobilization	
Recent fracture	
Compromised renal and/or hepatic function	
Medical conditions (diabetes, thyroid disease, etc.)	
Medications (anticonvulsants, GnRH agonists, glucocorticoids, etc.)	
Controllable	
Circadian rhythm	
Menstrual cycle	
Exercise	
Food intake	
Seasonal variation	
Sample handling	

Table 7. Factors affecting levels of bone turnover markers

5.5 Laboratory tests

Among men, 30% to 60% of osteoporosis cases are associated with secondary cause. Among perimenopausal women, more than 50% of cases are associated with secondary causes (NIH Consensus Development Panel on Osteoporosis Prevention, Diagnosis, and Therapy, 2001). In patients referred for DXA in the clinical context of an osteoporosis clinic, contributors to secondary osteoporosis were already documented in one out of three postmenopausal women, previously undiagnosed contributors were found in an additional 30% of women (Tannenbaum et al, 2002).

General consensus exists among experts that a minimum screening laboratory tests should be considered for all patients who are diagnosed as having osteoporosis prior to treatment. Many experts have also suggested that patients who have osteoporosis and a Z-score of less than -2.0 should have more extensive laboratory tests for secondary cause of osteoporosis. A diagnosis of osteoporosis in men should also prompt a through work-up for secondary causes regardless of their Z-score (Mauck & Clarke, 2006).

The range of laboratory tests will depend on the severity of the disease, age at presentation, and the presence or absence of fractures. In patients with BMD-based osteoporosis or presenting with a clinical fracture or both, diagnostic evaluation is necessary and should include blood cell count, sedimentation rate or C-reactive protein, serum calcium, phosphate, alkaline phosphatase, liver transaminase, albumin, creatinine, thyroid stimulating hormone (TSH) and $25(OH)D_3$. According to the clinical features and suspicion, other measurements such as parathyroid hormone (PTH), protein immunolelectrophoresis and urinary Bence-Jones proteins, serum testosterone, sex-hormone binding globulin (SHBG), follicle stimulating hormone (FSH), and luteinizing hormone (LH) in men, serum prolactin, 24-hour urinary cortisol/dexamethasone suppression test, endomysial and/or tissue transglutaminase antibodies, 24-hour urinary calcium and creatinine looking for secondary causes are indicated (Compston et al, 2009). If a specific secondary cause of osteoporosis is suspected on the basis of the history and physical examination findings, further direct testing is indicated.

6. Conclusion

Many factors are associated with osteoporosis and fracture, including low peak bone mass, hormonal factors, the use of certain medications, cigarette smoking, low physical activity, low calcium and vitamin D intake, race, small body size, and a personal or family history of fracture. All these factors should be taken into account when assessing the risk of fracture to determine which patients require further assessment and/or treatment. Clinical guidelines help guide practice but should not replace clinical judgment and patient preferences. The final decision about screening, assessment, and/or treatment is ultimately at the discretion of the physician and the patient.

7. References

Anonymous. (2001). Guideline for the prevention of falls in older persons. *Journal of American Geriatric Society*, Vol.49, No.5, pp. 664-672, ISSN 0002-8614

Baim, S ; Binkley, N. Bilezikian, J.P. Kendler, D.L. Hans, D.B. Lewiecki, E.M. & Silverman, S. (2008). Official Positions of the International Society for Clinical Densitometry and executive summary of the 2007 ISCD Position Development Conference. *Journal of Clinical Densitometry*, Vol.11, No.1, pp. 75-91, ISSN 1094-6950

Black, D.M.; Arden, N.K. Palermo, L. Pearson, J. & Cummings, S.R. (1999). Prevalent vertebral deformities predict hip fractures and new vertebral deformities but not wrist fractures. Study of Osteoporotic Fractures Research Group. *Journal of Bone and Mineral Research*, Vo.14, No.5, pp. 821-828, ISSN 0884-0431

Body, J.J.; Bergmann, P. Boonen, S. Boutsen, Y. Devogelaer, J.P. Goemaere, S. Kaufman, J.M. Rozenberg, S. & Reginster, J.Y. (2010). Evidence-based guidelines for the pharmacological treatment of postmenopausal osteoporosis: a consensus document by the Belgian Bone Club. *Osteoporosis International*, Vol.21, No.10, pp. 1657-1680, ISSN 0937-941X

Brunader, R. & Shelton, D.K. (2002). Radiologic bone assessment in the evaluation of osteoprosis. *American Family Physician*, Vol.65, No.7, pp. 1357-64, ISSN 0002-838X

Compston, J.; Cooper, A. Cooper, C. Francis, R. Kanis, J.A. Marsh, D. McCloskey, E.V. Reid, D.M. Selby, P. Wilkins, M. & National Osteoporosis Guideline Group (NOGG). (2009). Guidelines for the diagnosis and management of osteoporosis in postmenopausal women and men from the age of 50 years in the UK. *Maturitas*, Vol.62, No.2, pp. 105-108, ISSN 0378-5122

Cranney, A.; Jamal, S.A. Tsang, J.F. Josse, R.G. & Leslie, W.D. (2007). Low bone mineral density and fracture burden in postmenopausal women. *Canadian Medical Association Journal*, Vol.177, No.6, pp. 575-580, ISSN 0820-3946

Delmas, P.D.; Christiansen, C. Mann, K.G. & Price, P.A. (1990). Bone Gla protein (osteocalcin) assay standardization report. *Journal of Bone and Mineral Research*, Vol.5, No.1, pp. 5-11, ISSN 0884-0431

Delmas, P.D.; Eastell, R. Garnero, P. Seibel, M.J. Stepan, J. & Committee of Scientific Advisors of the International Osteoporosis Foundation. (2000). The use of biochemical markers of bone turnover in osteoporosis. Committee of Scientific Advisors of the International Osteoporosis Foundation. *Osteoporosis International*, Vol.11, Suppl 6, pp. S2-17, ISSN 0937-941X

Delmas, P.D.; Malaval, L. Arlot, M.E. & Meunier, P.J. (1985). Serum bone Gla-protein compared to bone histomorphometry in endocrine diseases. *Bone*, Vol.6, No.5, pp. 339-341, ISSN 8756-3282

Gallagher, J.C.; Genant, H.K. Crans, G.G. Vargas, S.J. & Krege, J.H. (2005). Teriparatide reduces the fracture risk associated with increasing number and severity of osteoporotic fractures. *The Journal of Clinical Endocrinology and Metabolism*, Vo.90, No.3, pp. 1583-1587, ISSN 0021-972X

Geusens, P.; Hochberg, M.C. van der Voort, D.J. Pols, H. van der Klift, M. Siris, E. Melton, M.E. Turpin, J. Byrnes, C. & Ross, P. (2002). Performance of risk indices for identifying low bone density in postmenopausal women. *Mayo Clinic Proceedings*, Vol.77, No.7, pp. 629-637, ISSN 0025-6196

Geusens, P. (2009). Strategies for treatment to prevent fragility fractures in postmenopausal women. *Best Practice & Research. Clinical Rheumatology*, Vol.23, No.6, pp. 727-740, 1521-6942, ISSN 1521-6942

Hodgson, S.F.; Watt,s N.B. Bilezikian, J.P. Clarke, B.L. Gray, T.K. Harris, D.W. Johnston, C.C. Jr. Kleerekoper, M. Lindsay, R. Luckey, M.M. McClung, M.R. Nankin, H.R. Petak, S.M. Recker, R.R. & AACE Osteoporosis Task Force. (2003). American Association of Clinical Endocrinologists medical guidelines for clinical practice for the prevention and treatment of postmenopausal osteoporosis: 2001 edition, with selected updates for 2003. *Endocrine Practice*, Vol.9, No.6, pp. 544-564, ISSN 1530-891X

Kanis, J.A.; Burlet, N. Cooper, C. Delmas, P.D. Reginster, J.Y. Borgstrom, F. Rizzoli, R. & European Society for Clinical and Economic Aspects of Osteoporosis and Osteoarthritis (ESCEO). (2008). European guidance for the diagnosis and management of osteoporosis in postmenopausal women. *Osteoporosis International,* Vol.19, No.4, pp. 399-428, ISSN 0937-941X

Kanis, J.A.; McCloskey, E.V. Johansson, H. Strom, O. Borgstrom, F. Oden, A. & National Osteoporosis Guideline Group. (2008). Case finding for the management of osteoporosis with FRAX--assessment and intervention thresholds for the UK. *Osteoporosis International,* Vol.19, No.10, pp. 1395-1408, ISSN 0937-941X

Kanis, J.A.; Melton, L.J. 3rd. Christiansen, C. Johnston, C.C. & Khaltaev, N. (1994). The diagnosis of osteoporosis. *Journal of Bone and Mineral Research,* Vol.9, No.8, pp. 1137-1141, ISSN 0884-0431

Kanis, J.A.; Oden, A. Johansson, H. Borgström, F. Ström, O. & McCloskey, E. (2009). FRAX and its applications to clinical practice. *Bone,* Vol.44, No.5, pp. 734-743, ISSN 8756-3282

Kanis, J.A. (1994). Assessment of fracture risk and its application to screening for postmenopausal osteoporosis: synopsis of a WHO report. WHO Study Group. *Osteoporosis International,* Vol.4, No.6, pp. 368-381. ISSN 0937-941X

Klotzbuecher, C.M.; Ross, P.D. Landsman, P.B. Abbott III, T.A. & Berger, M. (2000). Patients with prior fractures have an increased risk of future fractures: a summary of the literature and statistical synthesis. *Journal of Bone and Mineral Research,* Vol.15, No.4, pp. 721-739, ISSN 8756-3282

Lane, N.E. (2006). Epidemiology, etiology, and diagnosis of osteoporosis. *American Journal of Obstetrics and Gynecology,* Vol.194, Suppl 2, pp. S3-11, ISSN 0002-9378

Lash, R.W.; Nicholson, J.M. Velez, L. van Harrison, R. & McCort, J. (2009). Diagnosis and management of osteoporosis. *Primary Care,* Vol.36, No.1 , pp. 181-198, ISSN 0095-4543

Leib, E.S.; Lewiecki, E.M. Binkley, N. Hamdy, C. & International Society for Clinical Densitometry. (2004). Official positions of the International Society for Clinical Densitometry *Journal of Clinical Densitometry,* Vol.7, No.1, pp. 1-6, ISSN 1094-6950

Lems, W.F. (2007). Clinical relevance of vertebral fractures. Annals of the rheumatic diseases, Vol.66, No.1, pp. 2-4, ISSN 0003-4967

Lewiecki, E.M. & Laster, A.J. (2006). Clinical applications of vertebral fracture assessment by dual-energy x-ray absorptiometry. *The Journal of Clinical Endocrinology and Metabolism,* Vol.91,No.11, pp. 4215-4222, ISSN 0021-972X

Marshall, D.; Johnell, O. & Wedel, H. (1996). Meta-analysis of how well measures of bone mineral density predict occurrence of osteoporotic fractures. *British Medical Journal,* Vol.312,No.7041, pp. 1254-1259, ISSN 0959-8138

Mauck, K.F. & Clarke, B.L. (2006). Diagnosis, screening, prevention, and treatment of osteoporosis. *Mayo Clinic Proceedings,* Vol.81, No.5, pp. 662-672, ISSN 0025-6196

Miller PD. (1999). Management of osteoporosis. *Disease-a-month,* Vol.45, No.2, pp. 21-54, ISSN 0011-5029

National Osteoporosis Foundation. (2010). *Clinician's Guide to Prevention and Treatment of Osteoporosis.* National Osteoporosis Foundation, ISBN 978-0-9798989-9-0, Washington (DC)

National Osteoporosis Foundation. (2003). *Physician's guide to prevention and treatment of osteoporosis.* National Osteoporosis Foundation, Washington (DC)

Nguyen, N.D.; Frost, S.A. Center, J.R. Eisman, J.A. & Nguyen, T.V. (2008). Development of prognostic nomograms for individualizing 5-year and 10-year fracture risks. *Osteoporosis International,* Vol.19, No.10, pp. 1431-1444, ISSN 0937-941X

NIH Consensus Development Panel on Osteoporosis Prevention, Diagnosis, and Therapy. (2001). Osteoporosis prevention, diagnosis, and therapy. *The Journal of the American Medical Association*, Vol.285, No.6, pp. 785-795, ISSN 0098-7484

Pluijm, S.M.; Koes, B. de Laet, C. Van Schoor, N.M. Kuchuk, N.O. Rivadeneira, F. Mackenbach, J.P. Lips, P. Pols, H.A. & Steyerberg, E.W. (2009). A simple risk score for the assessment of absolute fracture risk in general practice based on two longitudinal studies. *Journal of Bone and Mineral Research*, Vol.24, No.5, pp. 768-774 ISSN 8756-3282

Saag, K.G & Genusens P. (2009). Progress in osteoporosis and fracture prevention: focus on postmenopausal women. *Arthrotis Research & Therapy*, Vol.11, No.5, pp.251, ISSN 1478-6354

Sambrook, P. & Cooper, C. (2006). Osteoporosis. *Lancet*, Vol. 367, No.9527, pp. 2010-2018, ISSN 0140-6736

Schousboe, J.T.; Vokes, T. Broy, S.B. Ferrar, L. McKiernan, F. Roux, C. & Binkley. N. (2008). Vertebral Fracture Assessment: the 2007 ISCD Official Positions. *Journal of Clinical Densitomery*, Vol.11, No.1, pp. 92-108, ISSN 1094-6950

Schuit, S.C.; van der Klift, M. Weel, A.E. de Laet, C.E. Burger, H. Seeman, E. Hofman, A. Uitterlinden, A.G. van Leeuwen, J.P. & Pols, H.A. (2004). Fracture incidence and association with bone mineral density in elderly men and women: the Rotterdam Study. *Bone*, Vol.34, No.1, pp. 195-202, ISSN 8756-3282

Seibel, M.J. (2005). Biochemical markers of bone turnover: part I: biochemistry and variability. *The Clinical biochemist. Reviews*, Vol.26, No.4, pp. 97-122, ISSN 0159-8090

Siris, E.S.; Chen, Y.T. Abbott, T.A. Barrett-Connor, E. Miller, P.D. Wehren, L.E. & Berger, M.L. (2004). Bone mineral density thresholds for pharmacological interventions to prevent fractures. *Archives of internal medicine*, Vol.164, No.10, pp. 1108-1112, ISSN 0003-9926

Tannenbaum, C.; Clark, J. Schwartzman, K. Wallenstein, S. Lapinski, R. Meier, D. & Luckey, M. (2002). Yield of laboratory testing to identify secondary contributors to osteoporosis in otherwise healthy women. *The Journal of Clinical Endocrinology and Metabolism*, Vol.87, No.10, pp.4431-4437, ISSN 0021-972X

Unnanuntana A, Glandnick BP, Donnelly E, Lane JM. The assessment of fracture risk. J Bone Joint Surg Am 2010;92:743-53.

US Preventive Services Task Force. (2002). Screening for osteoporosis in postmenopausal women: recommendations and rationale. Annals of Internal Medicine, Vol.137, No.6, pp. 526-528, ISSN 0003-4819

van Geel, T.A.; van den Bergh, J.P. Dinant, G.J. & Geusens, P.P. (2010). Individualizing fracture risk prediction. *Maturitas*, Vol.65, No.2, pp.143-148, ISSN 0378-5122

van Helden, S.; van Geel, A.C. Geusens, P.P. Kessels, A. Nieuwenhuijzen Kruseman, A.C. & Brink, P.R. (2008). Bone and fall-related fracture risks in women and men with a recent clinical fracture. *The Journal of bone and joint surgery. American volume.* Vol.90, No.2, pp. 241-248, ISSN 0021-9355

van Staa, T.P.; Geusens, P. Pols, H.A. de Laet, C. Leufkens, H.G. & Cooper, C. (2005). A simple score for estimating the long–term risk of fracture in patients using oral glucocorticoids. *Monthly journal of the Association of Physicians.* Vol.98, No.3, pp.191-198, ISSN 1460-2725

WHO Scientific group on the assessment of osteoporosis at primary health care level. (2004). Summary meeting report, July,2011, Available from: www.who.int/chp/topics/Osteoporosis.pdf

10

Sophisticated Imaging Technology in the Assessment of Osteoporosis Risk

Huayue Chen[1], Tatsuro Hayashi[2], Xiangrong Zhou[2],
Hiroshi Fujita[2], Minoru Onozuka[3] and Kin-ya Kubo[4]
[1]Department of Anatomy, Gifu University Graduate School of Medicine
[2]Department of Intelligent Image Information,
Gifu University Graduate School of Medicine
[3]Department of Physiology and Neuroscience, Kanagawa Dental College
[4]Seijoh University Graduate School of Health Care Studies,
Japan

1. Introduction

Osteoporosis is a common disease characterized by low bone mass and microstructural deterioration of bone tissue, with an increased fracture risk. With an aging population, osteoporosis and its related fractures have become an increasingly important health and socioeconomic issue. The aim of osteoporosis screening and treatment is to prevent bone fracture. A fracture occurs when the external force applied to a bone exceeds its strength. The ability of a bone to resist fracture depends on its amount, spatial distribution, and intrinsic properties. Sophisticated bone imaging techniques, as new modalities, improve the potential for non-invasive study of bone anatomy, physiology and pathophysiology. The objective of bone imaging in osteoporosis is to minimize fracture occurrence by identifying the osteoporotic process at an early stage, differentiate distinctive patterns of bone loss, predict fracture risk accurately and monitor treatment response precisely. Non-invasive imaging techniques, such as computed tomography (CT) and magnetic resonance imaging (MRI), provide structural information, beyond bone mineral density (BMD). Non-invasive or non-destructive imaging techniques can provide important structural information about the local and systemic skeletal status and about the propensity to fracture. These advanced imaging techniques provide information about bone beyond standard bone mineral densitometry. In this chapter, we will discuss recent progress in bone imaging in a range from the macro- to micro-structures in order to investigate the structural basis of the skeletal fragility underlying osteoporosis.

2. Bone mineral density measurement

In bone fragility assessment, BMD is the main parameter to quantify because of its relationship to bone strength and prediction fracture risk. In the past two decades bone densitometry has been performed with direct methods such as dual X-ray absorptiometry (DXA) and quantitative computed tomography (QCT), which also evaluates bone structural characteristics. The most commonly used quantitative imaging measure in osteoporosis is the areal BMD assessed by DXA. The assessment of bone macro- and micro-architecture by using more sensitive three-dimensional (3D) methods is important to determine certain aspects of bone structure and quality. Research has especially focused on the assessment of compartmental BMD and bone microstructure, since it has become technologically possible to obtain relatively high resolution volumetric images of bone in vivo.

2.1 Dual X-ray absorptiometry

Bone mineral density (BMD) measurement by dual X-ray absorptiometry (DXA) has been available for clinical use since 1987. It provides a quantitative assessment of mineralized bone mass at the axial and appendicular skeleton in vivo. This technique is currently the most readily available surrogate marker of bone strength and fracture risk. DXA measures the attenuation of photons of two different energies during radiation transmission. Bone mineral content (BMC, g) and areal BMD (g/cm^2) of a region of interest are obtained. As low areal BMD is a strong risk factor for fractures, this technique provides the basis for the World Health Organization (WHO)'s guidelines for diagnosis of osteoporosis. DXA is limited in that it measures only areal BMD two-dimensionally. DXA is also limited in that it does not distinguish cortical and trabecular bone. Furthermore, measurements are subject to artefacts due to degenerative changes such as osteophytes and aortic calcification. Recommendations from the International Society for Clinical Densitometry regarding DXA examination for all ages have been updated. Although DXA is the gold standard for clinical assessment of fracture risk, its shortcomings are increasingly being recognized. Individual fracture risk has recently been standardized using the WHO Fracture Risk Assessment tool (FRAX), which was released in 2009 (Kanis et al., 2009). FRAX combines BMD from DXA with other well-known major risk factors for osteoporosis, such as age, sex and a parental history of hip fracture, to provide a 10-year risk of hip and other major fractures. Although it is not an ideal system, FRAX represents an important initiative in allowing clinicians to individualize fracture risk based on DXA examination and other factors.

2.2 Quantitative computed tomography (QCT)

In quantitative computed tomography (QCT), the X-ray source and detector rotate in synchronised fashion around the subject. Algorithms are used to reconstruct the attenuation data into 3D images. Use of a bone mineral or hydroxyapatite phantom allows calibration of the data, providing a measurement of bone density that is independent of bone size. Compared with DXA, one advantage of QCT is the capacity for separate analysis of the cortical and trabecular BMD. QCT also provides real bone density per bone volume (mg/cm^3). Recently, 3D volume data from the scanning of an entire bone, such as a vertebral body or proximal femur, can be reconstructed to adjust the exact selected region for several serial images in a longitudinal study, which enables monitoring of successive changes with very good precision. QCT-based bone measurements have been used to evaluate age-, sex- and ethnic-related differences in vertebral and femoral geometry and density, providing insights into the development of skeletal fragility.

2.2.1 Volumetric BMD assessment by QCT

CT image is a two step process of initial scan acquisition and then tomographic image reconstruction by a mathematical process of calculating from acquired raw data. All clinical

CT scanners are calibrated to the X-ray attenuation to the water, resulting in CT numbers, measured in Hounsfield Units (HU). To transform HU into bone mineral equivalents (mg/cm^3) an appropriate bone mineral phantom is included in the scan field. QCT is the unique modality that measures the real bone density in a determinate volume (mg/cm^3) without the overlapping of others tissues. QCT differs from DXA as it can allow a selective assessment of both trabecular and cortical bone. Trabecular BMD obtained by QCT shows a more rapid age dependent decrement than that measured by DXA. Single Energy QCT is normally used for clinical setting, though BMD estimation can be altered by quantity of fat tissue, which substitutes the red marrow in elderly people. This effect produces an increasing error of evaluation with the increase of elderly patients. Even if Dual Energy QCT improves the accuracy, nevertheless it uses higher radiation dose and longer scanning times without increasing QCT sensibility in discriminating between healthy and osteoporotic subjects. Over the last decade, technical developments in CT, including multi-detector CT (MDCT) have resulted in images of volumes of tissue being acquired very rapidly, and this has had an impact on QCT in that 3D volume images can be acquired rapidly. Such 3D volumetric QCT enables analysis of the hip, the important site of osteoporotic fracture, which was not feasible with 2D single slices.

2.2.2 Vertebral trabecular QCT assessment

The trabecular BMD, particularly in the vertebra, is metabolically more active and may therefore serve as an early indicator of osteoporosis treatment effect. Vertebral trabecular BMD was demonstrated to have a significant correlation with vertebral fracture. Worldwide, the number of subjects in thoracic and abdominal CT examinations has increased dramatically over the last two decades (McCollough et al., 2009). Several recent studies have shown how it is possible to obtain meaningful QCT BMD values from subjects undergoing thoraco-abdominal CT examinations without the use of a calibration phantom. Such BMD values have a high correlation with BMD values obtained from QCT. These studies demonstrate that it is technically feasible to obtain reasonably accurate BMD values in subjects undergoing thoracic or abdominal CT examinations for other reasons. It is very useful for subjects as it will allow predictions of vertebral fractures without additional radiation exposure (Lenchik et al., 2004). The analysis of BMD at different vertebral levels is necessary because most osteoporotic vertebral fractures are located in the thoracolumbar spine between T4 and L1, with the segments between T7 and L1 most affected (Wasnich, 1996). Osteoporotic fractures of the cervical spine are considered uncommon. The etiology of the striking segmental differences for osteoporotic vertebral fractures is not well explained. Recently we measured the trabecular BMD of thoracic and lumbar vertebrae from 1,031 subjects who had undergone MDCT examination (Hayashi et al., 2011). The vertebral trabecular BMD of both men and women tended to gradually decrease from Th1 to L3 in all age categories (Fig. 1). In relation to vertebral level, L3 had the lowest trabecular BMD among the thoracic and lumbar vertebrae. The correlation of the trabecular BMD among thoracic and lumbar vertebrae was also studied. On the whole, we found that the further the vertebrae were from each other, the weaker were their correlations of the trabecular BMD, and vice versa. This finding indicates that estimating the BMD of distant vertebrae existing beyond the scope of CT images is difficult. For example, if the BMDs of T7 and T12 are estimated using L3 BMD in CT images from abdominal organ examinations, the estimated accuracy of T12 (r=0.92) would be better than that of T7 (r=0.79) because T12 is nearer to L3 than T7 (Hayashi et al., 2011). That is to say, it may be appropriate to use an arbitrary vertebra as a first approximation for assessing vertebrae which are in the area of predilection for the fracture. If the BMD of one vertebra is known, the BMD of other vertebrae may be estimated using our knowledge of BMD correlations.

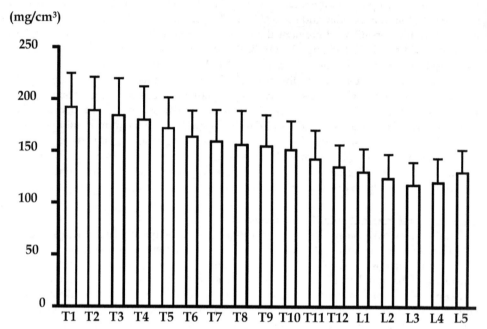

Fig. 1. The trabecular BMD of the thoracic and lumbar vertebrae. The BMD tends to decrease from the first thoracic to third lumbar vertebra (Hayashi et al., 2011)

3. Bone quality assessment

As BMD explains only part of the variation seen in bone strength and only some of the observed reduction in fracture risk that occurs with treatment, recent developments have focused more on measuring bone structure and quality of both cortical and trabecular bone rather than bone mass alone. This is done with the knowledge that a measure encompassing bone quality and structure along with bone mass will provide a better prediction of fracture risk than bone mass alone.

3.1 Conventional X-rays

Conventional radiography is a low-cost, readily available technique with high spatial resolution capable of providing fine bone detail, especially for appendicular skeleton such as the distal forearm and phalanges. It is widely available method, provides a good tissue contrast and has the potential to reflect bone microstructure. Conventional radiography is the first and most important method to identify fractures. The distal radius fractures are almost always identified by standard radiographs, while hip and especially spine fractures may have a difficult detection with important significance in their management, prognosis and therapy.

A more accurate evaluation of lateral chest radiographs routinely executed could lead to the detection of a major number of vertebral fractures and earlier diagnosis of osteoporosis. Although it is ideally suited for use in large population studies, the limitation of radiography is that as a projection imaging technique, it cannot consistently visualize individual trabecula and it depends heavily on the depth of tissues under investigation. Despite these limitations, the trabecular bone properties could be described by texture analysis. Good correlations were found between direct, 3D measures of trabecular architecture and a multiple parameter model, based on 2D texture parameters, such as fractal, statistical and anisotropy measures (Guggenbuhl et al., 2006). With increasing sophistication of structural analysis techniques and an improving ability to acquire high-resolution radiographic detail, interest remains in developing radiography to more precisely evaluate trabecular bone microstructure.

3.2 Multi-detector computed tomography (MDCT)

Computed tomography (CT) is a 3D X-ray imaging technique, which provides positive contrast of mineralized tissues. The image formation process begins with the acquisition of serial radiographic projections over a range of angular positions around the object of interest. The cross-sectional field of view is then reconstructed using established computational techniques. Similar to simple radiography, the reconstructed image intensity values represent the local X-ray attenuation. A material property related to the electron density. Several classes of CT devices are presently used for high-resolution imaging of trabecular and cortical bone microstructure. The multi-detector CT (MDCT) is a clinical CT technique, which is available in most diagnostic imaging departments and thus a dedicated scanner is not required. Since its inception, the number of detector rows on clinical CT units has increased from 4 to the current clinical standard of 64 rows, although 320-row MDCT systems are also commercially available. As expected, MDCT fared less well with trabecular thickness and number because the spatial resolution of all MDCT systems (250–300μm) remains larger than the trabecular thickness of 50 to 200μm (Issever et al., 2010). Nevertheless, structural parameters by MDCT provide a better discriminator of change than DXA. It has been shown that trabecular bone parameters obtained with MDCT correlate with those determined in contact radiographs from histological bone sections and micro-CT (Link et al., 2003). The advantage of MDCT technique is that more central regions of the skeleton such as the spine and proximal femur can be visualized. However, in order to achieve adequate spatial resolution and image quality the required radiation exposure is substantial, which offsets the technique's applicability in clinical routine and scientific studies. High-resolution CT scanning is associated with considerably higher radiation dose compared with standard techniques for measuring BMD. Using clinical imaging in more central regions of the skeleton such as spine and femur, it is still noted that the trabecular bone architecture visualized with MDCT is more a texture of the trabecular bone than a true visualization of the individual trabecular structure.

3.3 Peripheral quantitative CT and high-resolution peripheral quantitative CT

The peripheral QCT (pQCT) with a resolution comparable to that of MDCT has been available since 1990 to examine the peripheral skeleton. pQCT confers a smaller effective radiation dose and is particularly useful for studying cortical bone changes in metabolic bone disorders because the distal radius contains more cortical bone than the vertebral body. As pQCT units use low-power X-ray tubes, these examinations are slow, with a tendency toward motion artifact. With this limitation in mind, the feasibility of using clinical CT scanners with a dedicated forearm phantom as an alternative to pQCT has been investigated. The cortical and trabecular BMD, and bone geometrical parameters, such as marrow and cortical cross-sectional area, cortical thickness, periosteal and endosteal circumference, biomechanical parameters can be obtained, like cross-sectional moment of inertia, which is a measure of bending strength, polar moment of inertia, indicating bone strength in torsion and stress strain index (SSI). A non-invasive bone strength marker as SSI measured by pQCT, could be significantly correlated with a biomechanical bone strength index, as maximum load at bone failure, assessed by three-point bending test. pQCT can non-invasively determine bone mechanical properties by assessing parameters with accepted prognostic value on bone strength (Kokoroghiannis, et al., 2009). Bridging the clinical need for an imaging modality with lower radiation dose and better spatial resolution is the high-resolution pQCT (HR-pQCT). This can measure trabecular and cortical bone density and bone microstructure with an isotropic voxel of about 80μm. This technique has excellent precision for both density and structure measurements (Dalzell et al., 2009). In 2005, the first published clinical study assessing HR-pQCT found that postmenopausal women had lower BMD, trabecular number and cortical thickness compared with premenopausal women at the distal radius and tibia, although spine and hip BMD was similar. HR-pQCT is a useful modality for assessing changes in cortical and trabecular bone, with a precision of about 2% to 5% (Boutroy et al., 2005). The main limitation of HR-pQCT is that it requires a dedicated scanner, is confined to examination of distal forearm and leg, has some difficultly with registration in the Z plane and should take into consideration the expected difference among individuals of short or long radial or tibial length.

3.4 Micro-CT (μCT)

The earlier conventional tool for assessing trabecular bone architecture was histomorphometry from bone biopsies, which produces a two-dimensional representation of tissue structure, while bone structure is three-dimensional. In recent years, it has progressively been imposed the direct 3D analysis of biopsy specimens imaged by micro-CT (μCT). The most common application of this technology has been the in vitro quantitation of osteoporotic change in trabecular bone architecture. The μCT system has been demonstrated to be the first device able to non-destructively reveal the "real" trabecular architecture and is an X-ray-based technique that provides 3D images of very high spatial resolution below 8 μm. Since μCT allows the depiction of individual trabecula and enables the full characterization of the trabecular network, many investigators have used it to study the trabecular network at different skeletal sites, in direct relation to biomechanical properties or as a "gold standard" for evaluating other techniques, although most of the μCT are limited to ex vivo investigations. Microarchitectural 3D data elaborated by specific software consents to evaluate many metric and non-metric bone structural parameters, such as the bone volume (BV), tissue volume (TV), bone volume fraction (BV/TV), trabecular thickness (Tb.Th), trabecular number (Tb.N), trabecular separation (Tb.Sp), structure model index (SMI), connectivity degree (Conn.D) and degree of anisotropy (DA).

3.4.1 Hamster bone μCT assessment

Age-related bone loss, which is poorly characterized, is a major underlying cause of osteoporotic fractures in the elderly. In order to identify the morphological feature of age-related bone loss, we investigated sex and site (tibia, femur and vertebra) dependence of bone microstructure in aging hamsters from 3 to 24 months of age using µCT (Chen et al., 2008a). In the proximal tibia and distal femur, the trabecular BV/TV, Tb.N, Tb.Th and BMD increased to a maximum at 6 or 12 months and then declined progressively from 12 to 24 months of age (Fig. 2). Tb.Sp, trabecular bone pattern factor (TBPf) and SMI increased with age. As compared with male hamsters, BV/TV and Tb.N were significantly lower in females at 18 and 24 months of age. Age-related decrease of BV/TV in the vertebral body was less than that of the femoral and tibial metaphyses. In the mid-femoral diaphysis, cortical bone area remained constant from 3 to 24 months of age. Cortical thickness decreased from 12 to 24 months and cortical BMD declined significantly from 18 to 24 months of age. These findings indicate that skeletal site and sex differences exist in hamster bone structure. Age-related bone changes in hamsters resemble those in humans. Hamsters may be a useful animal model to study at least some aspects of bone loss during human aging.

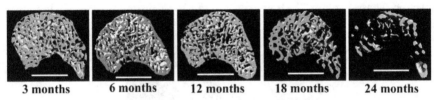

| 3 months | 6 months | 12 months | 18 months | 24 months |

Fig. 2. Three-dimensional images of the proximal tibial metaphysic in female hamsters at 3, 6, 12, 18 and 24 months of age. Trabecular bone volume is highest at 6 and 12 months of age, and declined at 18 and 24 months of age. Scale bar=1.0mm (Chen et al., 2008a)

3.4.2 Osteoporosis model mouse (SAMP6) bone µCT assessment

The senescence-accelerated mouse P6 (SAMP6) is a model of senile osteoporosis, which possesses many features of senile osteoporosis in humans. So far, little is known about the systemic bone microstructural changes that occur at multiple skeletal sites. Recently, we investigated site dependence of bone microstructure and BMD in SAMP6 and the normal control mouse (SAMR1) using quantitative µCT and imaging analysis software (Chen et al., 2009). As compared with SAMR1, the most prominent change in SAMP6 was the reduction of vertebral trabecular BV/TV (Fig. 3) and BMD. Moderate decrease of trabecular bone loss was observed in the proximal tibia and distal femur. Increased bone marrow area and periosteal perimeter were investigated, although the cortical area and cortical thickness had no marked changes in the mid-tibial and mid-femoral cortical bones. These results indicate that bone microstructural properties in SAMP6 are remarkably heterogeneous throughout the skeleton, which is analogous to changes that occur in human bones. These findings further validate the relevance of SAMP6 as a model of senile osteoporosis.

3.4.3 Human vertebral trabecular bone µCT assessment

The vertebral trabecular bone has a complex 3D microstructure, with inhomogeneous morphology. A thorough understanding of regional variations in the microstructural properties is crucial for evaluating age- and gender-related bone loss of the vertebra, and may help to gain more insight into the mechanism of the vertebral osteoporosis and the related fracture risks. Fifty-six fourth lumbar vertebral bodies from 28 women and men (57-98 years of age) cadaver donors were studied. Both women and men were divided into 3 age groups, middle-aged, old age and elderly groups. Five cubic specimens were prepared from anterosuperior, anteroinferior, central, posterosuperior and posteroinferior regions at sagittal section (Chen et al., 2008b). Bone specimens were examined by µCT and scanning electron microscope. The results showed that BV/TV, Tb.N and Conn.D decreased, while SMI increased significantly between middle-aged and old age groups, and between old age and elderly groups. As compared with women, men had higher Tb.N in the old age group, and higher Conn.D in the middle-aged and old age groups. The central and anterosuperior regions had lower BV/TV and Conn.D than their corresponding posteroinferior region (Fig. 4). Increased resorbing surfaces, perforated or disconnected trabeculae and microcallus formations were found with aging. Vertebral trabeculae are microstructurally heterogeneous. Decreases in BV/TV and Conn.D with age are similar in women and men. Significant differences between women and men are observed at some microstructural paramenters. Age-related vertebral trabecular bone loss may be caused by increased activity of resorption. These findings illustrate potential mechanisms underlying vertebral fractures.

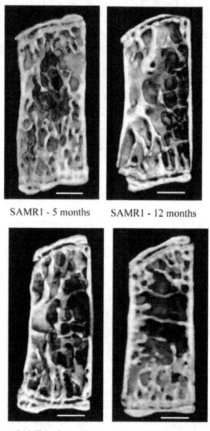

SAMR1 - 5 months   SAMR1 - 12 months

SAMP6 - 5 months   SAMP6 - 12 months

Fig. 3. Micro-CT images representative the fourth lumbar vertebral body in SAMP6 and SAMR1 mice at 5 and 12 months of age. Compared with SAMR1, the trabecular bone is reduced in SAMP6 both at 5 and 12 months of age. Scale bar=0.5mm (Chen et al., 2009)

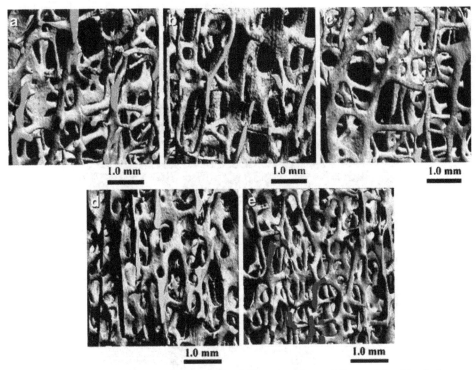

Fig. 4. Three-dimensional micro-CT image in different regions of the vertebral body from a woman aged 78 years: anterosuperior (a), anteroinferior (b), central (c), posterosuperior (d) and posteroinferior (e) regions. The trabecular bone is higher in the posterosuperior and posteroinferior regions than that of the central and anterosuperior regions (Chen et al., 2008b)

3.4.4 Human femoral neck μCT assessment

Femoral neck fracture, which is one of the most common outcomes of age-related and postmenopausal osteoporosis, is a significant cause of morbidity and mortality worldwide. Femoral neck fracture is attributed to both cortical and trabecular bone loss. The relative contribution of femoral neck cortical and trabecular bone to whole bone strength is unclear. We identified 3D microstructural changes of both cortical and trabecular bone simultaneously in human femoral neck from 57 to 98 years of age (Chen et al., 2010). The findings demonstrate that cortical thickness (Ct.Th) decreased by 10-15%, cortical porosity (Ca.V/TV) almost doubled between the middle-aged and elderly groups (Fig. 5).

The trabecular BV/TV declined by around 20% between the middle-aged and elderly groups. The most obvious age-related change in the femoral neck is the increase of Ca.V/TV. The decrease of BV/TV with age is more noticeable than that of Ct.Th. There was a significant inverse correlation between Ca.V/TV and BV/TV for both women and men. As compared with women, men had higher Ct.Th and BV/TV and lower Ca.V/TV. These findings may serve as reference for ethnic comparison with age and gender and may help to gain more insight into femoral neck fracture risk.

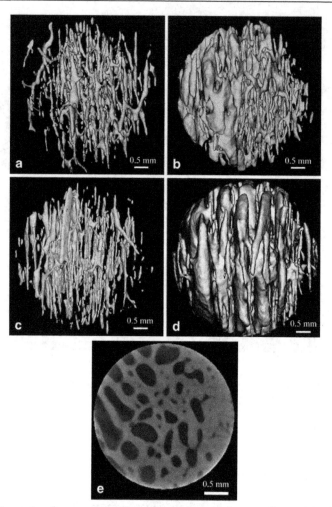

Fig. 5. Three-dimensional reconstructed images of the canal networks in the inferior femoral neck cortex from a man aged 62 years (a), a man aged 92 years (b), a woman aged 62 years (c) and a woman aged 92 years (d). There are more enlarged canals in the 92-year-old woman than that of the 62-year-old man. Representative two-dimensional micro-CT image of the femoral neck cortex from a woman aged 92 years (e) is shown. Periosteal surface faces right for all specimens (Chen et al., 2010)

3.4.5 Human proximal tibia μCT assessment

The analyses of local trabecular microstructure have been mainly performed in regions most susceptible to fractures, such as spine, proximal femur and radius. Studies of the proximal tibia also have an important clinical significance, as it is fractured in aging patients, specifically those suffering from osteoporosis. The proximal tibia, with its rich trabecular network, can be used as a donor site for bone grafting and it is the most easily accessible site for quantification of BMD and bone microstructure. The trabecular bone specimens from the medial compartment of the proximal tibial metaphyses were examined with μCT and scanning electron microscopy (Chen et al., 2011). It was shown that from 57 to 98 years of age, the trabecular BV/TV decreased by 6-7% and the trabecular BMD declined around 4% per decade at the proximal tibia. Figure 6 shows the typical 3D reconstructions of trabecular bone of the middle-aged and elderly groups for both women and men. The trabecular Tb.Th decreased between the middle-aged and elderly groups similarly in women and men. However, Tb.N decreased by 13% between the middle-aged and elderly groups in women and nearly doubled that in men. As compared with women, men had higher BV/TV and lower Tb.Sp in the old age and elderly groups, and higher Tb.N and Conn.D in the elderly group. Increased trabecular resorbing surfaces, perforated or disconnected trabeculae and microcallus formations were observed with age. These findings indicate that both BMD and BV/TV decreased at the proximal tibia with age similarly for women and men, but significant differences between women and men were observed for some microstructural parameters.

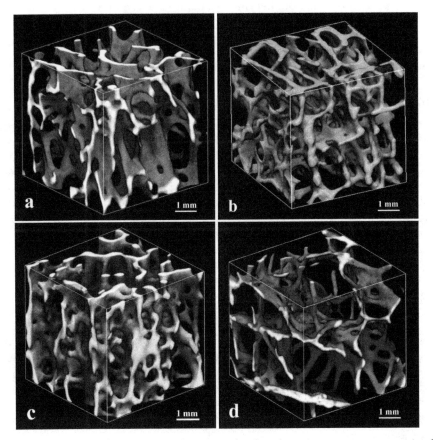

Fig. 6. Three-dimensional reconstructed images of trabecular microstructure at proximal tibia from a man aged 62 years (a), a man aged 92 years (b), a woman aged 62 years (c) and a woman aged 92 years (d). The trabecular bone volume fraction is highest in man aged 62 years and lowest in woman aged 92 years (Chen et al., 2011)

3.5 Magnetic resonance imaging (MRI)

Magnetic resonance imaging (MRI) is a non-ionizing method that uses a strong magnetic field in combination with specialized sequences of radio-frequency pulses to generate high-resolution 3D images of cortical and trabecular bone in vivo. Therefore, it is well suitable for assessing bone structure clinically (Link, 2010). With technical advances in MRI, such as optimized coil design, fast gradients, high gradients and high field strength, MRI scanners provide an in vivo spatial resolution close to the diameter of a single trabecula. MRI signal of trabecular bone itself is not visualized and trabeculae appear as a signal void, surrounded by high-intensity fatty bone marrows. As a result, the bone structure is assessed indirectly via measurements of the surrounding marrow and other soft tissues. Advances in the past decade have focused on image acquisition and analysis techniques to overcome inherent obstacles in MR imaging of bone. With the advent of parallel imaging, motion correlation techniques and new sequences, the limits of spatial resolution and scan time can be further overcome. This non-ionizing, 3D imaging technique is a very attractive tool to analyze trabecular bone structure, investigating bone structure and metabolism in osteoporosis or osteoarthritis. Various studies have been undertaken to optimize image acquisition and post processing, and to calibrate and validate measurements of the trabecular architecture. However, methods can be technically challenging to achieve and optimize.

4. Conclusion

Bone fragility, composite description of bone's biomechanical properties, is directly related to bone's susceptibility to fracture and is inversely related to bone's fracture resistance. As fractures compromise the quality of life and shorten life expectancy, the sophisticated bone imaging modalities play an important role in clearly and accurately identifying the presence and features of fragility fractures. The analysis of bone mass and bone microstructure is an exciting field in the assessment of osteoporotic risk. With the recent advances in MRI and CT, including the introduction of clinical μCT, imaging of true bone structure is becoming more feasible. These non-invasive sophisticated imaging techniques help us to gain more insight into the potential mechanism of metabolic bone diseases, particularly osteoporosis. However, further research is required for improvements in reproducibility, standardization and clinical application of these methods. New technological advances may further refine the imaging of osteoporotic bone and assessment of fracture risk. Recently various computer-aided diagnosis systems were developed for assessment of osteoporosis risks. The dental clinics took numerous panoramic radiographs for examining dental diseases worldwide. Several investigators demonstrated significant associations between mandibular cortical indices on panoramic radiographs and BMD of the skeleton generally, such as the spine and femur, biochemical markers of bone turnover and risk of osteoporotic fractures (Taguchi, 2010). So the computer-aided diagnosis system, based on digital panoramic radiography, may offer a new triage screening for osteoporosis risk in the near future.

5. Acknowledgment

The authors thank Dr. Ken-ichi Tezuka, Department of Tissue and Organ Development, Gifu University Graduate School of Medicine, for providing the micro-CT system used in this study.

6. References

Boutroy, S.; Bouxsein, ML.; Munoz, F. & Delmas, PD. (2005) In vivo assessment of trabecular bone microarchitecture by highresolution peripheral quantitative computed tomography. *Journal of Clinical Endocrinology & Metaboliam*, Vol.90, No.12, (December 2005), pp. 6508–6515, ISSN 0021-972X (Print); 1945-7197 (Electronic)

Chen, H.; Zhou, X.; Washimi, Y. & Shoumura, S. (2008a) Three-dimensional microstructure of the bone in a hamster model of senile osteoporosis. *Bone*, Vol.43, No.3, (September 2008), pp. 494-500, ISSN 8756-3282

Chen, H.; Shoumura, S.; Emura, S. & Bunai, Y. (2008b) Regional variations of vertebral trabecular bone microstructure with age and gender. *Osteoporosis International*, Vol.19, No.10, (October 2008), pp. 1473-1483, ISSN 1433-2965 (Print); 0937-941X (Electronic)

Chen, H.; Zhou, X.; Emura, S. & Shoumura, S. (2009). Site-specific bone loss in senescence-accelerated mouse (SAMP6): a murine model for senile osteoporosis. *Experimental Gerontology*, Vol.44, No.12, (December 2009), pp. 792-798, ISSN 0531-5565

Chen, H.; Zhou, X.; Shoumura, S.; Emura, S. & Bunai, Y. (2010) Age- and gender-dependent changes in three-dimensional microstructure of cortical and trabecular bone at the human femoral neck. *Osteoporosis International*, Vol.21, No.4, (April 2010), pp. 627-636, ISSN 1433-2965 (Print); 0937-941X (Electronic)

Chen, H.; Washimi, Y.; Kubo, K. & Onozuka, M. (2011) Gender-related changes in three-dimensional microstructure of trabecular bone at the human proximal tibia with aging. *Histology and Histopathology*, Vol.26, No.5, (April 2011), pp. 563-570, ISSN 0213-3911 (Print); 1699-5848 (Electronic)

Dalzell, N.; Kaptoge, S.; Morris, N.; Berthier, A.; Koller, B.; Braak, L.; van Rietbergen, B. & Reeve, J. (2009) Bone micro-architecture and determinants of strength in the radius and tibia: age-related changes in a population-based study of normal adults measured with high-resolution pQCT. *Osteoporosis International*, Vol.20, No.10, (October 2009), pp. 1683-1694, ISSN 1433-2965 (Print); 0937-941X (Electronic)

Guggenbuhl, P.; Bodic, F.; Hamel, L.; Basle, MF. & Chappard, D. (2006) Texture analysis of X-ray radiographs of iliac bone is correlated with bone micro-CT. *Osteoporosis International*, Vol.17, No.3, (January 2006), pp. 447–454, ISSN 1433-2965 (Print); 0937-941X (Electronic)

Hayashi, T.; Chen, H.; Miyamoto, K.; Zhou, X.; Hara, T.; Yokoyama, R.; Kanematsu, M.; Hoshi, H. & Fujita, H. (2011) Analysis of bone mineral density distribution at trabecular bones in thoracic and lumbar vertebrae using X-ray CT images *Journal of Bone and Mineral Metabolism*, Vol.29, No.2, (March 2011), pp. 174-185, ISSN 0914-8779

Issever, AS.; Link, TM.; Kentenich, M.; Rogalla, P.; Burghardt, AJ.; Kazakia, GJ.; Majumdar, S. & Diederichs, G. (2010) Assessment of trabecular bone structure using MDCT: comparison of 64- and 320-slice CT using HR-pQCT as the reference standard. *European Radiology*, Vol.20, No.2, (February 2010), pp. 458–468, ISSN 0938-7994 (Print); 1432-1084 (Electronic)

Kanis, JA.; Johansso,n H.; Oden, A. & McCloskey, EV. (2009) Assessment of fracture risk. *European Journal of Radiology*, Vol.71, No.3, (September 2009), pp. 392–397, ISSN 0720-048X

Kokoroghiannis, C.; Charopoulos, I.; Lyritis, G.; Raptou, P.; Karachalios, T. & Papaioannou, N. (2009) Correlation of pQCT bone strength index with mechanical testing in distraction osteogenesis. *Bone*, Vol.45, No.3, (Semptember 2009), pp. 512-516, ISSN 8756-3282

Lenchik, L.; Shi, R.; Register, TC.; Beck, SR.; Langefeld, CD. & Carr, JJ. (2004) Measurement of trabecular bone mineral density in the thoracic spine using cardiac gated quantitative computed tomography. *Journal of Computer Assisted Tomograpgy*, Vol.28, No.1, (January 2004), pp. 134-139, ISSN 0363-8715

Link, TM. (2010) The Founder's Lecture 2009: advances in imaging of osteoporosis and osteoarthritis. *Skeletal Radiology*, Vol.39, No.10, (October 2010), pp. 943–955, ISSN 0364-2348 (Print); 1432-2161 (Electronic)

Link, T.; Vieth, V.; Stehling, C.; Lotter, A.; Beer, A.; Newitt, D. & Majumdar, S. (2003) High resolution MRI versus Multislice spiral CT - Which technique depicts the trabecular bone structure best? *European Radiology*, Vol.13, No.4, (April 2003), pp. 663-671, ISSN 0938-7994 (Print); 1432-1084 (Electronic)

McCollough, CH.; Guimarães, L. & Fletcher, JG. (2009) In defense of body CT. *American Journal of Roentgenology*, Vol.193, No.1, (July 2009), pp. 28–39, ISSN 0361-803X (Print); 1546-3141 (Electronic)

Taguchi, A. (2010) Triage screening for osteoporosis in dental clinics using panoramic radiographs. *Oral Diseases*, Vol.16, No.4, (May 2010), pp. 316-327, ISSN 1354-523X (Print); 1601-0825 (Electronic)

Wasnich, RD. (1996) Vertebral fracture epidemiology. *Bone*, Vol.18, No.3 Suppl., (May 1996), pp. 179S-183S, ISSN 8756-3282

11

What We Learn from Bone Complications in Congenital Diseases? Thalassemia, an Example

Zohreh Hamidi
Endocrinology and Metabolism Research Institute of
Tehran University of Medical Sciences (EMRI-TUMS)
Islamic Republic of Iran

1. Introduction

The thalassemias, a group of inherited disorders of hemoglobin synthesis, are the most common monogenetic diseases worldwide and are curable by bone marrow transplantation (BMT). Many patients achieve a lifelong disease-free period after BMT. This has focused attentions on disease and treatment complications, for example bone complications. Some of bone disorders occur before and after transplantation and some of them (osteoporosis) and their complications are life threatening. For a better understanding of the bone complications in thalassemia, a brief review of normal bone is required. However, because thalassemia is a curable congenital disease and with an ethical background, the investigation of bone disorders in thalassemic patients (before and after transplantation), can provide a model of calcium and bone metabolism. This model, based on clinical and research findings before and after transplantation, can enlighten factors affecting bone and mineral metabolism throughout the life (disease period and cure period can be considered as periods of bone loss and bone gain through-out the normal life). This model can help in the understanding and management of bone disorders in other bone diseases and in primary osteoporosis. As a resident of a country with a large population of thalassemic patients (Iran), it is author's special interest that such studies help these patients achieve a better quality of life and decrease the burden of this disease not only in Iran but also in other countries worldwide.

2. What is thalassemia

2.1 Disease name and synonyms

The term thalassemia, has two components thalassa (sea) and haima (blood), both from Greek. Beta-thalassemia includes three main forms: thalassemia major ("Cooley's Anemia" or "Mediterranean Anemia"), Thalassemia Intermedia and Thalassemia Minor ("beta-thalassemia carrier", "beta-thalassemia trait" or "heterozygous beta-thalassemia") (Galanello & Origa, 2010). In this review the author's focus is on β-thalassemia major and its bone complications.

2.2 Definition

The thalassemias, hereditary hematologic disorders, are caused by defective synthesis of one or more of the hemoglobin (Hb) chains (Muncie & Campbell, 2009). Hb molecule is a tetramer composed of 4 -globin polypeptide (2 alpha-globin and 2 beta-globin) plus a heme prosthetic group, to form the complete molecule. In the α-thalassemias, defective production of α-globin chains results in an unstable Hb causes and mild to moderate hemolytic and hypochromic anemia (Sankaran & Nathan, 2010). Beta thalassemia is caused by reduced or absent synthesis of beta globin chains. Hemolysis and impaired erythropoiesis is the result of this imbalance of globin chains. Fatal hydrops fetalis, is seen in cases of Alpha thalassemia major with hemoglobin Bart's (Muncie & Campbell, 2009).

Beta-thalassemia minor (carrier state) patients , are clinically asymptomatic (they are diagnosed, generally accidental by specific hematological features). Thalassemia major patients are severely transfusion-dependent. Thalassemia intermedia patients, ranging in severity from the asymptomatic carrier patients to the severe transfusion-dependent patients (Cao & Galanello, 2010).

Galanello and Origa, in their article (Galanello & Origa, 2010) suggested the following classification:

- Beta-thalassemia
  • Thalassemia major
  • Thalassemia intermedia
  • Thalassemia minor
- Beta-thalassemia with associated Hb anomalies
  • HbC/Beta-thalassemia
  • HbE/Beta-thalassemia
  • HbS/Beta-thalassemia (clinical condition more similar to sickle cell disease than to thalassemia major or intermedia)
- Hereditary persistence of fetal Hb and beta-thalassemia
- Autosomal dominant forms
- Beta-thalassemia associated with other manifestations
  • Beta-thalassemia-tricothiodystrophy
  • X-linked thrombocytopenia with thalassemia

2.3 Epidemiology of thalassemia

The total annual incidence of symptomatic individuals is estimated to be 1 in 100,000 worldwide and 1 in 10,000 in the European Union (Galanello & Origa, 2010). Approximately 5% of the world's population has a globin variant, and only 1.7% has the alpha or beta thalassemia trait. Thalassemia affects men and women equally and occurs in approximately 4.4 of every 10,000 live births. Alpha thalassemia is most common in persons of African and Southeast Asian descent, and beta thalassemia occurs most often in persons of Mediterranean, African, and Southeast Asian descent. The thalassemia trait affects 5-30% of persons in these ethnic groups (Muncie & Campbell, 2009).

2.4 Genetics of thalassemia

The extent of imbalance between the alpha and non-alpha globin chains, relates to the clinical severity of beta-thalassemia. Cao & Galanello suggest that the beta globin (HBB) gene maps in the short arm of chromosome 11, in a region also containing the delta globin gene, the embryonic epsilon gene, the fetal A-gamma and G-gamma genes, and a pseudogene (_B1). Single nucleotide substitutions, deletions, or insertions of oligonucleotides that leads to frame shift, are the majority of mutations. Beta-thalassemia rarely results from gross gene deletion. In addition to the variation in the phenotype resulting from allelic heterogeneity at the beta globin locus, the phenotype of beta-thalassemia can also be modified by the action of genetic factors mapping outside the globin gene cluster and not influencing fetal hemoglobin (Cao & Galanello, 2010).

2.5 Pathophysiology of thalassemia

Fessas (1963), as cited in Sankaran & Nathan, 2010, described unbalanced globin chain synthesis, as the cause of the b-thalassemia syndromes. Intraerythroblastic inclusions of unpaired a-globin molecules , results disease manifestations (Sankaran & Nathan, 2010). Galanello & Origa explain two mechanisms for increase the clinical and hematological severity in beta-thalassemia heterozygote patients. In first mechanism, an excess of unassembled alpha chains (resulting in premature destruction of red blood cell precursors) is caused by the coinheritance of both heterozygous beta-thalassemia and triple or quadruple alpha globin gene arrangement, that increases the magnitude of the imbalance of alpha/non-alpha globin chain synthesis. In the other mechanism, premature destruction of red blood depends on the presence of a mutation in the beta globin gene, which causes extreme instability of the beta globin chains and the synthesis of truncated beta chain products (Galanello & Origa, 2010).

2.6 Diagnosis of thalassemia

Most individuals with the thalassemia trait are found incidentally when their complete blood count shows mild microcytic anemia. Hemoglobin electrophoresis with the beta thalassemia trait usually has elevated levels of HbA2.

Individuals with beta halassemia major are diagnosed during infancy. Symptoms appear during the second six months of life. The most common symptoms are pallor, irritability, growth retardation, abdominal swelling, and jaundice. Beta thalassemia intermedia patients (with microcytic anemia, but milder symptoms) have start of disease later in their life (Muncie & Campbell, 2009). Genetic sideroblastic anemias, congenital dyserythropoietic anemias, and other conditions with high levels of HbF (such as juvenile myelomonocytic leukemia and aplastic anemia) are considered as differential diagnosis (Galanello & Origa, 2010).

2.7 Signs, symptoms and complications of thalassemia

Hemolytic anemia, poor growth, and skeletal abnormalities during infancy, are major sign and symptoms of beta thalassemia major (Muncie & Campbell, 2009). Growth retardation, pallor, jaundice, poor musculature, hepatosplenomegaly, leg ulcers, the development of masses from extramedullary hematopoiesis, and skeletal changes (results of the bone marrow expansion) are found in untreated or poorly transfused individuals with thalassemia major (Galanello & Origa, 2010). Thalassemia major patients are diagnosed within the first 2 years and require regular blood transfusions to survive (Sankaran & Nathan, 2010). Iron overload is the result of regular blood transfusions. Complications of iron over load includs endocrine complications (growth retardation, failure of sexual maturation, diabetes mellitus, and insufficiency of the parathyroid, thyroid, pituitary, and less commonly, adrenal glands), dilated myocardiopathy, liver fibrosis and cirrhosis. Patients with thalassemia intermedia present later in life with moderate anemia and do not require regular transfusions. Though the thalassemia intermedia patients, come to medical attention later, may show an extended list of complications like hypertrophy of erythroid marrow with medullary and extramedullary hematopoiesis and its complications (osteoporosis, masses of erythropoietic tissue that primarily affect the spleen, liver, lymph nodes, chest and spine, and bone deformities as well as typical facial changes), gallstones, painful leg ulcers and increased predisposition to thrombosis. Moderate anemia may be the only sign of thalassemia minor patients and they are in general, clinically asymptomatic (Galanello & Origa, 2010).

2.8 Genetic counseling and prenatal diagnosis in thalassemia

As there is big population of thalassemic patients in some countries and there is high carrier rate for thallassemic mutations in certain populations (explained before in part 2.3), population screening is ongoing in them. Availability of genetic counseling and prenatal diagnosis, makes such screening in these countries more usefull (Cao & Galanello, 2010) and use of prenatal diagnosis may be stressed in such countries (Galanello & Origa, 2010).

Analysis of DNA extracted from fetal cells obtained by amniocentesis (at 15–18 weeks gestation), in high-risk pregnancies in which both members are defined carriers of beta-thalassemia, is possible for prenatal diagnosis. Chorionic villus sampling is useful and is performed at approximately 10–12 weeks gestation (Cao & Galanello, 2010).

2.9 Treatment of thalassemia

Many patients with b-thalassemia, and some patients with severe forms of a-thalassemia, require regular transfusions to survive. In the case of b-thalassemia, this therapy has an important effect on reducing the massive ineffective erythropoiesis and organ infiltration and bone destruction that is seen in β-thalassemia patients that are untreated. (Sankaran & Nathan, 2010). With multiple transfusions, iron overload and organ failure (particularly cardiac iron overload and heart failure) are the leading causes of death (Au, 2011), Therefore, after 10–12 transfusions, chelation therapy (an effective but non-absorbable iron chelator, such as desferrioxamine B (DFO) with a short plasma half-life) is initiated 5–7 days a week by 12-hour continuous subcutaneous infusion via a portable pump (Cao & Galanello, 2010).

2.9.1 Splenectomy

Splenectomy is recommended if the annual red cell requirement exceeds 180-200 ml/kg of RBC (assuming that the Hct of the unit of red cells is about 75%). Symptoms of splenic enlargement, leukopenia and/or thrombocytopenia and increasing iron overload despite good chelation, are considered as other indication for splenectomy (Galanello & Origa, 2010).

2.9.2 Bone marrow transplantation (BMT) in thalassemia

It is explained extensively in part 5.

2.9.3 Therapies under investigation in thalassemia

The potential of new chelation strategies, including combination or alternate treatment with available chelators, induction of HbF synthesis that can reduce the severity of beta-thalassemia by improving the imbalance between alpha and non-alpha globin chains, several pharmacologic compounds including 5-azacytidine, decytabine, butyrate derivatives and gene therapy in the management of beta-thalassemia syndromes are described by Cao and Galanello, Sankaran and Nathan as under investigation therapies (Cao & Galanello, 2010; Sankaran & Nathan, 2010).

2.9.4 Treatment of thalassemia in developed versus underdeveloped countries

In United States and Europe (as developed countries), there are approximately 10,000 homozygous patients with thalassemia. In such countries, due to effective prevention methods, the number of new cases is progressively decreasing. The result of high-quality medical care is longer life expectancy and a relatively good quality of life. BMT and gene therapy, is performed in such countires. The need of Western cultures is to develop improved support for patients with thalassemia and their families (Rund & Rachmilewitz, 2005). In a recent study by Hamidi et al, in Iran, low bone mass was significantly less prevalent in thalassemic patients in comparison to previous studies (Hamidi et al, 2010). Good bone health in patients may also be due to better and developing health network services in Iran and in other countries with high populations of these patients, thus providing a good health service. In Iran there are more than 300 transplanted thalassemic patients (Abolghasemi et al., 2007; Ghavamzadeh, 2009).

The treatment situation of thalassemia patients is different in less developed countries. It is very important because big population of thalassemic patients live there. Safe transfusion and chelation are not universally available. Consequently, many patients with thalassemia in underdeveloped nations die in childhood or adolescence (Rund & Rachmilewitz, 2005).

2.10 Prognosis in thalassemia

Following recent medical advances in transfusion, iron chelation and BMT therapy, prognosis in these patients has improved substantially in the last 20 years. However, the main cause of death in patients with iron overload, remains cardiac disease (Galanello & Origa, 2010).

- As a congenital disease, bone disorders in thalassemic patients are mainly due to bone growth problems and begin in childhood, thus a brief insight into normal bone growth and related matters are discussed in the following section.

3. Normal bone growth

3.1 Normal bone development

Schonau, explains the first phase of bone development so: in development period of embryo, the axial skeleton and extremities are initially in the form of cartilage. The first spontaneous mineralization occurs in the diaphysis. As a result of the activities of osteoclasts and osteoblasts, this mentioned tissue will be replaced by the mature bone matrix. Bones' longitudinal growth take place in the specialized epiphyseal growth plates in which chondrocytes synthesize cartilage matrix, that will be changed to primary and secondary spongiosa in the metaphyseal junction. The growth of The axial skeleton thickness happens due to periostal and endosteal growth(Schonau, 1998). Turn-over of the bones is necessary for either normal mineralized bone matrix maintenance or bone's growth. In healthy adults, resorption and formation of bones take place together in the remodeling process. Though this process is important for maintaining normal skeletal integrity, it does not have any role in changes in bone shape. Diversely, growth of childhood skeletal takes place in bone modeling, a process in which increased bone mass and changes in bone shape, happens. If bone resorption exceeds bone formation a problem occurred named Osteopenia. Which can occur in 2 different ways. It happens when bone resorption exceeds bone formation or when bone formation diminishes, but resorption is normal. (von Scheven, 2007). When muscular strength and parallel biomechanical usage increase, an increase in cortical thickness and area must be happened. The ratio of cortical thickness to bone diameter (corticalis index) increases as child grows up (Schonau, 1998). The velocity of increase of bone density in children, mostly mimics height growth velocity. It means, a first gradual phase of bone acquisition happens in early childhood and a more accelerated phase of accumulation, approximately 8% per year, occurs during adolescence. (von Scheven, 2007). A decrease phase of bone density happens after 20 or 30 years old, before that, bones mass increases to peak bone mass (PBM). Schonau, suggests that the percentage of ash weight of the individual skeletal sections however does not change significantly with age. On the other hand, physiological content of mature bone tissue (matrix plus minerals) does not change essentially with age and represents a kind of "constant." Morogulis (1931) as cited in Schonau, 1998 , also showed that the calcium and phosphate contents of the of very different animal species's skeletal systems were nearly the same . In contrast the water content does change. Up to years 20 the water content in bone tissue decreases . It is because of the high vascularity of the bones during the elevated phase of remodeling and modeling processes in growth time. It decreases later. (Schonau, 1998).

3.2 How peak bone mass is gained

The increase of total skeletal calcium(from approximately 25 g at birth to 900 and 1200 g in adult females and males, respectively), is gotten through bone growth, modeling and remodeling, which proceed at different rates at various skeletal sites. (Rabinovich, 2004). During childhood and adolescence, changes in size and shape of the skeleton happens together. And also bone grow up in width and and cortical thickness. Genetic, hormonal and environmental factors influence all these processes. (Bianchi, 2007). Bone mass increase is faster in adolescence , 25% of the PBM acquired during the two-year period close to peak height velocity. Rabinovich suggests that maximal rates of bone mineral accrual lag behind peak height velocity by 6–12 months, resulting in relatively undermineralized bone and increased fracture risk in the peri-pubertal years. At peak height velocity, males and females have reached 90% of their adult stature but have acquired only 57% of their adult total body bone mineral content (BMC). Bone mineral accrual continues after linear growth is complete, but the timing of PBM remains debatable (Rabinovich, 2004). About 85% of human skeleton is cortical bone and 15% is trabecular. The bone gain and loss during growth or in later age affects these 2 parts, in different ways. Hormonal/metabolic factors influence strongly the trabecular bone density througout the sexual maturation. Cortical bone consolidates slower. Bianchi states that Although the timing of peak values has not been precisely determined, the PBM is probably reached at the end of the second decade in the axial skeleton (predominantly trabecular bone), but only later in the appendicular skeleton (predominantly cortical bone) (Bianchi, 2007). Rabinovich says that is suggested that, though at least 90% of PBM is achieved by age 18, 5–12% of bone mineral density is reached during the third decade (Rabinovich, 2004).   Heritable factors is supposed to attribute to approximately 60–80% of the variations in peak bone mass(Bachrach, 2001), Bianchi results that these changes are not only continuous, but also subject to great individual variation, mostly related to the variability of pubertal development, and this is essential for the correct evaluation of BMD in young subjects (Bianchi, 2007).

3.3 Gender differences

Rabinovich explains difference between girls and boys in growing bone: during puberty, estrogen in girls inhibits periosteal formation while stimulating endocortical bone formation, thus limiting the medullary space. In contrast, in boys, androgens stimulate periosteal formation, bone diameter, and cortical thickness (Rabinovich, 2004). Also, van Kuijk suggests that, both the starting age of the pubertal spurt and the growth process happens earlier in girls, but the duration of the growth spurt and the maximal peak of growth are greater in boys. Increase in bone density starts around the age of 10 in girls and around the age of 12 in boys. (Van Kuijk, 2010).

3.4 Genetics of low bone mass

As Marini and Brandi categorized in their 2010 article (Marini & Brandi, 2010), the main osteoporosis candidate genes are: Calciotrophic and sex hormones and their receptors ((i) Vitamin D receptor (VDR), (ii) Parathyroid hormone (PTH) and PTH receptor (PTHR), (iii) Estrogen Receptor Alpha and Beta (ERα and ERβ), (iv) Calcitonin (CT) and its receptor (CTR), (v) Aromatase (CYP19A1), (vi) Androgen receptor (AR), (vii) Calcium-sensing receptor (CaSR), (viii) Glucocorticoid receptor (GR)), cytokines, growth factors and local regulators ((i) Interleukin-6 (IL6), (ii) Insulin-like growth factor 1 (IGF-I), (iii) Transforming growth factor β1 (TGFβ-1), (iv) Bone morphogenetic protein 7 (BMP7, OP1), (v) Bone morphogenetic protein 4 (BMP4), (vi) Bone morphogenetic protein 2 (BMP2)), Bone matrix proteins ((i) Collagen type I alpha1 (COLIA1), (ii) Collagen type I alpha2 (COLI-A2), (iii) Osteopontin (OPN, SPP1), (iv) Osteocalcin (OCN, BGLAP), (v) Osteonectin (ON, SPARC)) and miscellaneous genes such as (i) Low-density lipoprotein receptor-related protein 5 (LRP5), (ii) Low-density lipoprotein receptor-related protein 6 (LRP6), (iii) Receptor activator of nuclear factor kappa B (RANK), (iv) RANK ligand (RANKL), (v) Osteoprotegerin (OPG), (vi) Sclerotin (SOST), (vii) Chloride channel 7(CLCN7) and (viii) Methylenetetrahydrofolate reductase (MTHFR) (Marini &Brandi, 2010).

3.5 Low bone mass in pediatrics

Congenital connective tissue disorders such as osteogenesis imperfecta and Ehler–Danlos syndrome are important causes of pediatric osteoporosis. Neuromuscular disorders (cerebral palsy and Duchenne muscular dystrophy), childhood cancer, endocrine disorders (Turner Syndrome and juvenile diabetes mellitus), and inborn errors of metabolism (Gaucher disease) and chronic diseases like thalassemia are secondary causes of pediatric osteoporosis include. Don't forget pharmacological treatment, that are used for treatment of common pediatric conditions (iatrogenic causes. Among these, Glucocorticoids and anticonvulsants are known causes. Some add various forms of chemotherapy to this list (Bogunovic et al., 2009). However idiopathic juvenile osteoporosis is an acknowledged cause of osteoporosis in children and may it is the cause of a higher than expected prevalence of inadequate BMD in the pediatric population.

3.6 Problems with DXA in pediatrics

Bone density measurement by dual energy X-ray absorptiometry (DEXA) the standard method for bone mineral Densitometry. It is also one of most non-invasive techniques for the assessment of bone mass (Hamidi et al., 2008). Not surprising, it is used for many pediatric studies that produced many papers in the field of bone densitometry and in body composition (Van Kuijk, 2010). The WHO based the diagnosis of postmenopausal osteoporosis on the presence of a BMD T-score of 2.5 or greater below the mean for young women (Hamidi et al., 2008). The term "low bone mineral density for age" was mentioned at the "2007 ISCD Pediatric Position Development Conference" as a criterion for low bone mass in children, and is described as a child with a Z-score below -2.0. The difference between adult and pediatric criterion for low bone mass is that children have not reached PBM, yet. Instead, a child's Z-score (comparison of BMD of patient to age and sex matched normal children in reference data of pediatric software) must be noticed. (Daniels et al., 2003). However, must not forget that DXA has challenging aspects in pediatrics densitometry. True bone density is defined as BMC (g) divided by volume (cm3). Bogunovic explains that as DXA is a 2-dimentional projectional technique. In DXA , a two-dimensional projection, measures a three-dimensional object, bone. As a result, the BMD measured by DXA is defined as BMC (g) divided by the projected area (cm2) not devided by the projected volume (cm3). As a consequence of this area measurement of density, smaller bones appear to have a lower BMD than larger bones (Bogunovic et al., 2009). Van Kuijk, reminds us that in adults, bone size does not change over time. In contrast, bone size changes in growing children in 3 dimensions. When measuring children using DXA and following them over time, growth is measured more than actual changes in bone density (Van Kuijk, 2010). Another challenge, as Bogunovic believes is that the assignment of DXA Z-scores is dependent on the comparison of the patient's BMD to normative childhood data for age and sex. The wide variation in height, and, therefore, of bone size in children complicates the interpretation of BMD results especially in short children. Longitudinal evaluation of a given patient over time is complicated by the ever-changing size of the growing skeleton. Furthermore, the rates of skeletal growth vary with each bony dimension (Bogunovic et al., 2009). All these problems, pose a question: To Do or Not to Do DXA for the measurement of bone density and fracture risk in children? In response we must remember some points related to DXA, 1) patients are exposed to less radiation when measuring BMD by DXA, which is very important in children, 2) it is less fearful for children (less noisy with no tunnel) 3) DEXA is used worldwide and many pediatric studies have been published in the field of bone densitometry and in body composition studies, by using this method and 4) Studies suggest that bone mass may contribute to fracture risk in childhood (Van Kuijk, 2010). Therefore, the answer may be that carrying out DXA for the measurement of bone density and fracture risk in children, is a helpful method, although, it must be remembered, as Bogunovic reminds us, that bone fragility in children extends beyond a single BMD measurement and is influenced by bone geometry and body size and the diagnosis of osteoporosis requires the presence of both a clinically significant fracture history and low bone mass (Bogunovic et al., 2009).

3.6.1 Special considerations in the comparison of normal children and children with chronic disease, some points on the BMD of chronically ill children

As explained above, the measurement of BMC (g/cm) and BMD (g/cm2) are not only dependent on the mineral density of cortical and spongious bone, but also on the geometric configuration. This situation is of great importance in pediatrics. Schonau concludes that if BMC or BMD measurement results in decreased values for children with short stature (e. g., with "smaller bones"), this does not necessarily describe a mineral deficiency or a mineralization disorder, as is often thought (Schonau, 1998). Wide variation in age at onset and progression of puberty is another problem. It means a wide variation in the age at attainment of PBM. Some diseases, like juvenile arthritis, is thought to delay pubertal onset and development. As it is believed that one-third to one-half of the total mineralization in the lumbar spine in adult women is accumulated during the 3 years around the onset of puberty. Therefore Rabinovich concludes that, comparing the BMD of a well-grown 13-year-old girl who is in mid-puberty with that of a small pre-pubertal 13-year-old with juvenile arthritis is fraught with problems. She suggests that a DXA scan is not needed to tell who has the lower BMD. The question then is, is the BMD finding in this small pre-pubertal girl normal? (Rabinovich, 2004). As van Kuijk suggested, children with chronic disorders or medication, should never be compared with age-matched reference (normal) values. They should be compared with children with the same maturation status (skeletal age) (Van Kuijk, 2010).

3.7 Fractures in pediatrics

Fragility fractures are raising in pediatric population. This may be due to growing number of chronic disease in this population. It caused the increase of use of DXA in children. Healthy children with frequent fragility fracture, have been the focus of research. This is changing, may be because escalating of children with chronic diseases and fragility fractures. When an atraumatic event, cause fracture, fragility fracture come true. The difficulty looms here because as Bogunovic et al state, in young children especially, distinction between traumatic and atraumatic fractures may prove to be a challenge (Bogunovic et al., 2009). Other side of this problem, appear there, when there are many papers on fractures in childhood, but very few of these focus to identify fragility fractures, and fewer focused on the concept of osteoporosis in the young in relation to fractures. Bianchi reminds us that fractures, especially in infants, and especially if multiple or repeated, may be the consequence of violence and child abuse. However, fractures are common events in children. Landin, 1997, as cited in Bianchi, 2007, estimated that 42% of boys and 27% of girls sustain a fracture between 0 and 16 years of age. The must fractures in them, occurs between 10 and 15 years and forearm is the most common site (Bianchi, 2007). Is low BMD a risk factor for fractures? Bone mass may contribute to fracture risk in childhood (Bogunovic et al., 2009). Adverse reactions to cow milk, low dietary calcium intake, early age at first fracture, asthma and overweight (Goulding et al., 2005), and low physical activity are suggested as risk factors for fractures in children. Others suggested that lower BMD for body size, lower milk intake and lower physical activity related with recurrent fractures (Manias et al., 2006). Carbonated beverages also had some relations to fragility fractures. In children with chronic diseases, no systematically collected data is available. Bianchi reviewed that and suggested that some studies found no significant differences in the fracture rate between patients and controls. In contrast, many studies found an increased fracture risk in children affected by various diseases such as acute lymphoblastic leukemia, cerebral palsy, celiac disease, organ transplantation and glucocorticoids users (Bianchi, 2007).

3.8 Treatment of low bone mass in children

Unfortunately, though general measures (optimizing the intake of calories, vitamin D and calcium; providing appropriate weight-bearing activity; replacing GH or sex steroids; and minimizing doses of glucocorticoids) are recommended for better acquisition and maintaining of bone mass in children, they may not be sufficient to prevent or restore deficits in bone mass. Anti-resorptive agents (eg. Bisphosphonates), found valuable in treating some disorders, such as steroid-induced osteoporosis.   In steroid-induced osteoporosis, increased bone loss also contributes to the deficit, so anti-resorptive agents, seem affective. The ideal is treatment children to improve the failure of bone mineral acquisition, but they are not recommended yet (Bachrach, 2001). However, the use of different anti-osteoporotic agents (anabolic or anti-resorptive) in pediatric patients is not very common or recommended, especially in young children, due to a lack of large and systematic studies and comprehensive data supporting their efficacy or addressing their adverse effects in pediatric patients.

4. Bone and thalassemia

Osteopenia and are observed in 40–50% of beta-thalassemia Major patients, and so osteoporosis can be considered prominent causes of co-morbidity in this population, which significantly increases fracture risk (Gaudio et al., 2010).
Before discussing bone disorders in thalassemia patients, it is necessary to understand normal bone function and remodeling.

4.1 Bone in normal individuals

Voskaridou & Terpos, explain the role of skeleton, bone properties and BMU as so: the skeleton provides mechanical support for the body and is a reservoir for normal mineral metabolism. Bone is an active tissue constantly being remodeled and changing metabolically through the balanced activity of osteoclasts and osteoblasts on trabecular surfaces. On a microscopic level, bone metabolism always occurs on the surface of the bone at focused sites, each of which is termed a bone metabolism unit (BMU) (Voskaridou & Terpos, 2004). Mundy suggests that the sequence is always the same, osteoclastic bone resorption followed by osteoblastic bone formation to repair the defect. The resorptive phase of the remodeling process has been estimated to last 10 days. This period is followed by repair of the defect by osteoblasts attracted to the site of the resorption defect which then presumably proceed to make new bone. This part of the process takes approximately 3 months (Mundy, 1999). After the lacunae are filled with osteoids, Voskaridou & Terpos state that this newly formed matrix is mineralized with hydroxyapatite, giving the BMU tensile strength (Voskaridou & Terpos, 2004).

4.1.1 Osteoclasts

Hodge et al, describe Osteoclasts as multinucleated cells which differentiate from early myelomonocytic progenitors rather than more differentiated monocyte/macrophage progenitors (Hodge et al., 2004). Roodman describes their function as they reabsorb bone by secreting proteases which dissolve the matrix and produce acid that releases bone mineral into the extracellular space under the ruffled border of the plasma membrane of osteoclasts (Roodman, 2004). Voskaridou & Terpos say osteoclastogenesis requires contact between osteoclast precursors and stromal cells or osteoblasts. They say the adherence of osteoclasts to the bone surface is critical for the bone resorptive process, since agents that interfere with osteoclast attachment, such as cathepsin K, block bone resorption (Voskaridou & Terpos, 2004).
Wittrant et al, state the role of colony-stimulating factor-1 (CSF-1), released by osteoblasts, as it stimulates the proliferation of osteoclast progenitors via the c-fms receptor (CSF-1R) and,

in combination with the receptor activator of nuclear factor-κB ligand (RANKL), leads to the formation of mature osteoclasts (Wittrant et al., 2009). These two molecules are expressed by bone marrow stromal cells, also (Voskaridou & Terpos, 2004). Wittrant et al names the cells of the mononuclear phagocytic lineage including osteoclast progenitors and mature osteoclasts as well as placental trophoblasts, uterine decidual cells, smooth muscle cells, microglia, renal mesangial cells and osteoblasts, as other sites that express CSF-1R (Wittrant et al., 2009). PTH administration in 7-14 first days, to enhances RANKL- and M-CSF–stimulated osteoclast formation and bone resorption was shown in vivo (Jacome-Galarza et al., 2011). Thyroxine, 1,25-dihydroxyvitamin D3, and cytokines that use gp130 as part of their receptor, such as interleukin-6 (IL-6) and oncostatin M, are named as other factors which enhance RANKL expression (Voskaridou & Terpos, 2004).
Rankle/OPG system has a characteristic position in osteoporosis and metabolic bone disease. Osteoprotegerin (OPG), a secreted member of the tumor necrosis factor receptor superfamily, has been identified as an osteoblast-derived regulator of bone resorption . OPG neutralizes RANK that is essential for osteoclast formation and activation (Morabito et al., 2004). Alteration in the Rank/Rankl/OPG system may favors osteoclasts and osteoporosis formation (Toumba & Skordis, 2010).

4.1.2 Osteoblasts

Marie & Kassem explain in detail that bone formation is dependent on the recruitment of a sufficient number of osteoblasts as well as the activity of individual osteoblasts. They suggest that osteoblastic cells are recruited to bone forming surfaces mainly from a group of skeletal stem cells with osteogenic differentiation potential (referred to as skeletal, mesenchymal stem cells (MSC), or stromal stem cells. Some believe that some of these cells are pericytes located on the outer surface of blood vessels and sinusoids in the bone marrow, though, the exact location of mesenchymal stem cells in vivo is still debatable (Marie & Kassem, 2011).
Wnt signaling pathway is named as a key pathway involved in the regulation of bone mass. Johnson et al in an article in 2004, explained that Wnt signaling is also required for a diverse number of developmental events including mesoderm induction, organogenesis, CNS organization and limb patterning. In addition, a number of Wnt's have been implicated in vertebrate skeletal development. For example, there is evidence that Wnt3a, Wnt4, Wnt5a, Wnt5b, and Wnt7a all have important roles in chondrogenesis. Another member of the Wnt family, Wnt9A (formerly Wnt14), can induce morphological and molecular signs of joint formation when inappropriately expressed, indicating that Wnt9A plays a crucial role in the initiation of synovial joint development. Wnt9A expression can also lead to the arrest and reversal of chondrogenic differentiation in vitro (Johnson et al., 2004). We explained before, the PTH role in resorption. PTH also have anabolic effects and Marie & Kassem explain that the anabolic effects of PTH on bone formation are mediated through PTH receptor-dependent mechanisms. PTH enhances osteoblastic cell proliferation and function, extends the lifespan of mature osteoblasts through antiapoptotic effects, enhances Wnt signaling through inhibition of the Wnt antagonist, sclerostin, and enhances the local production of bone anabolic growth factors such as insulin-like growth factor 1 (IGF1) (Marie & Kassem, 2011). Though the differentiation of osteoblasts is less well understood than the differentiation of osteoclasts (Voskaridou & Terpos, 2004), bone morphogenetic proteins (BMPs) are critical factors that stimulate the growth and differentiation of osteoblasts (Marie

& Kassem, 2011). Voskaridou & Terpos name several factors such as Basic fibroblast growth factor (bFGF), Insulin-like growth factors (IGF, type I and II), Transforming growth factors (TGF, beta 1 and beta 2) and platelet-derived growth factor (PDGF) and a number of hormones, such as PTH, thyroxine, oestrogen, cortisol, insulin, and calcitonin, as well as vitamin D, are involved in the regulation of bone metabolism, effecting both progenitors and mature osteoblastic cells and osteoclasts (Voskaridou & Terpos, 2004).

4.2 Bone complications in thalassemic patients

Peculiar mongoloid appearance, caused by enlargement of the cranial and facial bones, combined with skin discoloration, anemia, splenomegaly and some enlargement of the liver were included in the first description of thalassemia by Cooley & Lee (Wonke, 1998). Galanello & Origa explain Skeletal changes include typical craniofacial changes such as bossing of the skull, prominent malar eminence, depression of the bridge of the nose, tendency for a mongoloid slant of the eye, and hypertrophy of the maxillae, which tend to expose the upper teeth (Galanello & Origa, 2010).

Some experts suggest that, the thalassemic anemia and the need for transfusion, as earlier as appear in the disease course, the facial changes are more prominent, and all agree that the disease course changes are only seen or are more prominent in untreated patients or in those with no regular transfusion program (Cao & Galanello, 2010). Tyler et al suggest that the skeletal changes in untreated thalassemia are due to ineffective erythropoiesis and expansion of the bone marrow which affect every part of the skeleton. These changes include osteoporosis, growth retardation, platyspondyly and kyphosis (Tyler et al., 2006). Anemia, hemosiderosis, iron chelation therapy, and associated hormonal disorders, are described as main causes of spinal deformity (Haidar et al., 2011). Salehi et al. , suggest that expanded erythropoiesis occurs at extra-medullary sites, most commonly resulting in a para-spinal mass but occasionally affecting organs containing pluripotential stem cells (Salehi et al., 2004). Tyler et al., state that skeletal dysplasia, predominantly affects the rapidly growing long bones, in particular the distal ulna, causing irregularity and sclerosis of the physeal–metaphyseal junction and causing splaying of the metaphysis. They say , Deferoxamine (DFX) also exacerbates the observed growth retardation. DFX-induced skeletal dysplasia, may cause toxicity, which is associated with visual and auditory impairment (Tyler et al., 2006).

Among the spinal deformities observed, Papanastasiou et al suggest that an increased prevalence of frontal curves was reported of at least, 5° in 67% of patients with TM. However, scoliosis curvatures of more than 10° and less than 14° were observed in 21.7% of examined patients. It seemed that location, direction, and pattern of the curvatures, age of onset, gender, and rate of progression of this type of scoliosis associated with TM, differed those in patients with idiopathic scoliosis. They, in their greater than 10-year study reported that the prevalence of frontal curves of at least 5° in 43 TM patients was approximately 80%. Scoliosis of at least 10° and not more than 19° was revealed in 28% to 35% of patients. The most common scoliosis curve pattern was the S-shaped (right thoracic, left lumbar). The prevalence of scoliosis was not gender related, irrespective of age and curve magnitude. Progression of scoliosis in the 10-year period was only detected in four (12%) of 34 patients with scoliosis of 5° to 14°, a rate much lower than that reported in patients with idiopathic scoliosis. Only one patient (2.9%) developed scoliosis of 65° that progressed to 85°, and no other patient developed scoliosis curves that required bracing or operative treatment. No correlation was shown between scoliosis progression and (remaining) growth potential, curve pattern, gender, or curve magnitude (Papanastasiou et al., 2002). As Haidar et al., mention around 24% of curves showed spontaneous resolution, this was equally distributed among all but the right thoracic curve patterns. Left lumbar and thoraco-lumbar scoliosis improved at a rate of 22% and 33%, respectively. However, most of the curves showed a magnitude of less than 10°. This remarkable absence of progression and spontaneous resolution in small curves depicts the unique etiology of scoliosis in this hematologic condition. Of note, thoracic kyphosis increased with patient age, whereas lumbar lordosis decreased with age and followed the changes of thoracic kyphosis. The 'junction' thoracolumbar kyphosis increased with patient age, but independently from thoracic kyphosis and lumbar lordosis. However, neither scoliosis magnitude nor progression was correlated to thoracic kyphosis (Haidar et al., 2011).

4.2.1 Bone and joint pain

Bone or joint pain, reported in 34% of participants during the 30 days before enrollment, in one study in all thalasemic patients. Vogiatzi et al., state that 6 percent required prescription pain medication and an additional 12.2% used analgesics as over-the-counter. They report that age, sex, and thalassemia syndrome were all independent predictors of the presence and severity of bone and joint pain and the odds of more severe pain, increased 47% for each 5-yr age increase. 40% of females, but only twenty-eight percent of males complained of recent pain. Bone pain was reported more frequently among b TM participants (40%) compared with b TI and E-b participants (16% and 19%, respectively) (Vogiatzi et al., 2009). As Haidar et al suggested, though arthralgia has been mainly attributed to iron overload or use of iron chelators, back pain is mainly associated with osteoporosis, compression fractures, and intervertebral disc degeneration. They report that in one study by the Thalassemia Clinical Research Network (TCRN), young adults with thalassemia experienced pain comparable to the general population, whereas older adults (aged 35+) experienced greater pain. There was an association between pain and low vitamin D level. (Haidar et al., 2011). Vogiatzi et al report that GH-deficient patients were reported to have more severe bone pain, as did those with a history of medicated heart disease, cirrhosis, or hepatitis C (Vogiatzi et al., 2009).

4.2.2 Intervertebral disc changes

Haidar et al. In an extended report about bone disease and skeletal complications in patients with β thalassemia major, suggest that a significant difference in disc degeneration severity has been demonstrated between TM patients and controls on MRI and radiographs. The pattern of disc degeneration was different in TM patients as they exhibited multilevel disease with all levels of the lumbar spine involved. Although no clear mechanism has been suggested for the development of disc changes in TM patients, an underlying metabolic basis has been suggested. They say that the degeneration of intervertebral discs results, in part, from weakening of the annulus fibrosus. The chelating agent, deferoxamine, commonly used in patients with TM, is thought to deleteriously affect the integrity and strength of the annulus fibrosus fibers. Alternatively, the injurious effect of iron overload is also postulated as a factor (Haidar et al., 2011).

4.2.3 Osteoporosis

Several sensitive techniques are available for the quantitative assessment of the degree of total bone mass. Bone density measurement by dual energy X-ray absorptiometry (DEXA) of the lumbar spine and femoral neck is recommended as one of the most reliable non-invasive techniques for the assessment of bone mass (Kanis, 1994).

According to the World Health Organization (WHO, 1994), osteoporosis is a disease characterized by low bone mass and micro-architectural deterioration of bone tissue, leading to enhanced bone fragility and a consequential increase in fracture risk. The WHO based the diagnosis of postmenopausal osteoporosis on the presence of a BMD T-score of 2.5 SD or greater below the mean for young women (Hamidi et al., 2008). The term "low bone mineral density for age" was mentioned at the "2007 ISCD Pediatric Position Development Conference" as a criterion for low bone mass in children, and is described as a child with a Z-score below -2.0 (Daniels et al., 2003).

In spite of adequate transfusion and iron chelation, Thalassemia-induced osteoporosis (TIO) is seen in 30–50% of TM patients, that can cause substantially compromised quality of life in thalassemic patients (Mamtani & Kulkarni, 2010).

4.2.3.1 Genetics of bone density in thalassemic patients

Voskaridou and Terpos, reported that polymorphism at the Sp1 site of the collagen type Ia1 (COLIA 1) gene (collagen type I is the major bone matrix protein) was found in approximately 30% of TM patients who were heterozygotes (Ss) and in 4% who were homozygotes (SS) for the Sp1 polymorphism. They reported the female to male ratio was 2:1. This means that male patients with TM carrying the Sp1 mutation may develop severe osteoporosis of the spine and the hip more frequently than patients who do not carry this mutation. The COLIA 1 polymorphism has been also associated with reduced BMD in postmenopausal osteoporosis, and predisposes women to osteoporotic fractures (Voskaridou & Terpos, 2004). Marini & Brandi reported a similarity between this finding and genetic findings in non-thalassemic patients (Marini & Brandi, 2010).

A possible beneficial effect of BsmI on patient response to alendronate therapy should be emphasized (Gaudio et al., 2010). Haidar et al report the vitamin D receptor (VDR) BsmI and FokI polymorphisms to constitute risk factors for bone mineral damage, low BMD, and short stature in pre-pubertal and pubertal patients with TM, (Haidar et al., 2011).

As Gaudio et al say, it should be remembered that the pathogenesis of osteoporosis is multifactorial, and includes environmental (diet, lifestyle, and drugs) as well as acquired (bone marrow expansion, hemochromatosis, chelation therapy, hepatitis, deficiency of growth hormone or insulin growth factor I, and hypogonadism) and genetic factors (Gaudio et al., 2010).

4.2.3.2 Altered modeling/remodeling in thalassemic patients

Haidar et al, believe that most acquired factors act mainly through the inhibition of osteoblastic activity. They suggest that histomorphometry studies have revealed that increased osteoid thickness, increased osteoid maturation and mineralization lag time, and defective mineralization are common in TM pediatric patinets (Haidar et al., 2011). Mildly increased resorption found in adult patients with beta TM (Vogiatzi et al., 2010). Baldini et al explain an interesting hypothesis that the chronic request for blood cell production can play a role in the etiology of osteoporosis through overstimulation of the hematopoietic system, increasing the number of osteoclasts and osteoblasts resulting in accelerated bone turnover (Baldini et al., 2010). However, Domrongkitchaiporn et al., suggest that increased resorption may be a cause of hypogonadism in these patients (Domrongkitchaiporn et al., 2003).

4.2.3.3 Gender differences in bone density in thalassemic patients

Some studies support that gender of thalassemic poatients affects not only the prevalence, but also the severity of osteoporosis syndrome in TM. However the results are contradicted and some studies showed no gender differences in patients with TM, when they were hypogonadal (Toumba & Skordis, 2010).

4.2.3.4 Acquired factors contributing to reduced BMD in beta-thalassemia

4.2.3.4.1 Bone marrow expansion

Expansion of hematopoiesis and bone marrow expansion, caused severe bone deformities with marked facial and limb changes that were originally described by Cooley et al in 1927 in untreated thalassemia major patients (Jensen et al., 1998). As Wonke, also suggests, the bone marrow expansion due to ineffective erythropoiesis is a typical finding in patients with TM and is considered a major cause of bone destruction. The commonest sites for extramedullary hematopoiesis are the spleen, liver and chest; less common sites are para-vertebral masses and brain lesions. As the ribs contain hematopoietic marrow at all ages, overactive marrow results in, osteoporosis of the ribs, localized lucencies, cortical erosions, and 'rib within rib' deformities (Wonke, 1998). Mechanical interruption of bone formation, leading to cortical thinning, increased distortion and fragility of the bones, occurs due to Marrow expansion (Voskaridou & Terpos, 2004). Tyler et al. refer to ineffective hematopoiesis as a cause of severe anemia and increased erythropoietin production, resulting in expansion of the bone marrow by a factor of 15 to 30. They suggest that even with an optimal transfusion regimen, the bone marrow remains hyperactive. The appearance of "cob-webbing" in the pelvis is the reason of the expanded bone marrow that destroys the medullary trabeculae with initial cortical and trabecular thinning and subsequent trabecular coarsening (Tyler et al., 2006).

Salehi et al., even reported spinal cord compression that is seen in these patients, which can cause neurologic compromise and is, in part, due to extramedullary hematopoiesis (Salehi et al., 2004).

4.2.3.4.2 Endocrine complications

4.2.3.4.2.1 General

Idiopathic hemochromatosis (Iron overload), are commonly associated with hypogonadism and diabetes, while the other endocrinopathies seen in patients with β-thalassemia major and Iron overload, are less common in them. As Perera et al. suggest, a significant predictor of endocrine failure is the duration of transfusion therapy (Perera et al., 2010). In below, we explain endocrine disorders in thalassemic patients, more extensively, as these disorders are major and important causes of bone complication in thalassemic patients.

4.2.3.4.2.2 Growth failure

Homozygous b-thalassemias, have almost invariably growth retardation. Soliman et al . describe thes changes as significant size retardation that is observed in stature, sitting height, weight, biacromial (shoulder), and bicristal (iliac crest) breadths (Soliman et al., 2009). All studies do not show such results (Cao & Galanello, 2010). Soliman et al., state that after the age of 4 years, the longitudinal growth patterns, display rates consistently below those of normal controls and the bone age is frequently delayed after the age of 6-7 years. Growth retardation becomes markedly severe with failure of the pubertal growth spurt

(Soliman et al., 2009). Though hemosiderosis-induced damage of the endocrine glands is one of the main causes for their growth failure, Cao & Galanello, Muncie & Campbell, Toumba & Skordis and Soliman et al, state that other factors could considerably contribute to the etiology of this growth delay including (i) chronic anemic hypoxia secondary to low hemoglobin concentration (Muncie & Campbell, 2009) (ii) toxicity of desferrioxamine treatment (Cao & Galanello, 2010); (iii) increased energy expenditure due to high erythopoietic turnover and cardiac work; (iv) nutritional deficiencies including calories, folic-acid, zinc, and vitamin A (Soliman et al., 2009); (v) disturbed calcium homeostasis and bone disease (Toumba & Skordis, 2010) (vi) hepatic and pancreatic dysfunction (Soliman et al., 2009).

Perera et al., emphasize that normal stature is rarely attained, even in the well-managed patient. They report the administration of GH in some centers internationally at the judgment of individual clinicians, but the role or response to GH is not clearly understood in these patients and probably has no clear benefit unless GH deficiency is confirmed by formal testing (generally as a consequence of early childhood pituitary failure) (Perera et al., 2010).

4.2.3.4.2.3 Delayed puberty/hypogonadism in thalassemia

Both primary and secondary sexual development are usually delayed in both genders in b-thalassemia major (Vogiatzi et al., 2005). An association between hypogonadotrophic hypogonadism and osteoporosis in adult patients with TM has been reported in the past. Jensen et al (1998), found that hypogonadotrophic hypogonadism is a substantial contributor to the development of osteoporosis. Hypogonadotrophic hypogonadism is the commonest endocrinological complication in β-thalassaemia major and is present in 42% of patients (Jensen et al., 1998). Perera et al. describe the finding in thses patients as menarche is frequently delayed by an average of 1–2 years, breast development is poor and female patients frequently have oligomenorrhoea/amenorrhoea even if menarche occurs. Men frequently have poor or absent virilization, reduced libido and oligo/azospermia. They report both genders less fertile and commonly require reproductive assistance to achieve a successful pregnancy (Perera et al., 2010). Toumba & Skordis explains the complacation as disruption of gonadotrophin production (due to iron deposition in gonadotrophic cells) and delayed puberty and hypogonadotrophic hypogonadism. They say secondary amenorrhea will invariably develop with time, especially in patients poorly compliant with chelation therapy. Also primary is common. Men also develop hypogonadotrophic hypogonadism and secondary gonadal failure. So low testosterone secretion is common. They report also primary gonadal failure due to iron deposition in the testes and ovaries. (Toumba & Skordis, 2010).

Perera et al,, in an overview of endocrinopathies associated with b-thalassemia major, (2010), highlighted the high prevalence of hypogonadism with resultant growth failure and infertility, and suggested the following approach and managent protocol in these patients:

1. Formal surveillance from the age of 10–12 years to identify changes associated with puberty, including the development of primary or secondary sexual characteristics. Consideration of an endocrine consultation in cases of suspected delayed puberty.
2. In adults, in addition to regular clinical review, annual monitoring of gonadotropin levels and sex hormone levels for both men and women should be organized. If clinically indicated, use of appropriate hormone replacement therapy in cases of hypogonadism.
3. Regular monitoring (1–3 times/year) of zinc levels, especially if patient is on deferiprone. In cases of zinc deficiency, supplementation to normal levels would also be

reasonable until further clarification of the relationship between zinc deficiency and hypogonadism becomes available (Perera et al., 2010).

4.2.3.4.2.4 Fertility in thalassemia

Pregnancy reported generally safe if baseline cardiac function is good (Rund & Rachmilewitz, 2005). Psihogios et al., suggested that with optimal therapy, most young adults with homozygous β-thalassemia can achieve reproductive, sexual, and social experiences similar to those of their healthy peers (Psihogios et al., 2002).

4.2.3.4.2.5 Impaired glucose tolerance and diabetes mellitus in thalassemia

There are different reports on the prevalence of diabetes in thalassemia major, however, Holger Cario reported that the prevalence is about 5%, while impaired glucose tolerance is found in up to 27% of patients (Cario et al., 2003).

Immune system activation against pancreatic beta cells in beta-thalassemia patients, is reported and pancreatic iron deposition is considered as factors that triggers the autoimmune response (iron deposisions act as environmental factor) and immune response, in turn, contributes to selective beta-cell damage (Najafipour et al., 2008). Perera et la.,did not report family history as a risk factor in thalassemic patient (Perera et al., 2010). In the study by Najafipour et al., risk factors reported for impaired glucose metabolism were, age, amount of blood transfused and duration of blood transfusion. Because not all of the patients with thalassemia major could be correctly diagnosed by fasting glucose alone, the authors preferred to use the oral glucose tolerance test (OGTT) rather than fasting blood glucose levels (BGLs) for the diagnosis of abnormal glucose tolerance in thalassemic patients (Najafipour et al., 2008).

Duration of transfusion therapy, in some studies was the strongest predictor for the development of diabetes (every decade of transfusion exposure further increasing the odds of developing diabetes by 2.5 times). The fact that diabetes mellitus is generally seen in the 3rd or 4th decade, may be is explainable by these findings.. Perera et al state that it is prudent to begin screening for diabetes after the 1st decade of transfusions (regular 6th monthly or annual) by assessing fasting BGLs followed by a 75-g 2-h OGTT if fasting results are abnormal (Perera et al., 2010).

Glyburide treatment and antidiabetic compounds improve insulin sensitivity. Treatment with basal-bolus insulin therapy is also used in these patients. However must not forget that effective iron chelation may improve glucose tolerance (Perera et al., 2010; Cario et al., 2003). Some believe that HbA1c is not a good tool for measuring glycemic control because of reduced red cell lifespan, ineffective hematopoiesis and frequent blood transfusions (affect the validity of HbA1c results). They propose serum fructosamine as an alternative way of monitoring glycemic control, though there is some limitations in its use. Blood glucose self monitoring and regular pre-transfusion venous blood glucose measurements may be use for measuring glycemic control, as an alternative ways in these patinets (Perera et al., 2010).

4.2.3.4.2.6 Hypothyroidism in thalassemia

The severity of thyroid dysfunction is variable in thalasemic patients and the reports of prevalence are very different. Najafipour et al, reported the prevalence of hypothyroidism in their patients 16%, but found the prevalence of 13% to 60% in different studies of patients with thalassemia. However they believe that milder forms of thyroid dysfunction are much more common in thalassemic patients (Najafipour et al., 2008). Primary thyroid damage (from iron infiltration) or secondary problems (due to pituitary dysfunction due to hemosiderosis of thyrotroph cells) are reported in these patients. Duration of transfusion therapy, has been the strongest predictor for development of hypothyroidism (Perera et al., 2010).

4.2.3.4.2.7 Short stature in thalassemia

As an important complication of thalassemia major, we discuss short stature in an independent section, not attached to growth failure. Najafipour et al, reported that 49% of thalassemic patients had a height standard deviation score less than -2 and 83% of thalassemic patients had a height standard deviation score less than -1. Normal stature is rare even in optimally treated patients. (Najafipour et al., 2008).

Even in well treated patients, it is prevalent and this is may be due to endocrine disorders, lifestyle, iron overload and high doses of desferrioxamine (DFX) when tissue iron burden is not very high (Ferrara et al., 2002).

4.2.3.4.2.8 Hypopituitarism in thalassemia

Hypogonadotropic hypogonadism occures in a large proportion of patients, because pituitary gland is one of the most vulnerable target organs to the early toxic effects of iron overload(Cao et al., 2011). Pan-hypopituitarism is a rare (especial in patients with good chelation therapy). Perera et al, describe the usual sequence for onset of pituitary dysfunction as begins with FSH, LH, GH and followes by ACTH and TSH (Perera et al., 2010).

4.2.3.4.2.9 The Rankl/OPG system in thalassemia

The increase in RANKL, followed by unmodified OPG levels, with the consequent increase in the RANKL/OPG ratio may represent the cause of uncoupling in bone turnover observed in thalassemia patients (Toumba & Skordis, 2010). Haidar et la, report a negative correlation between 17-b estradiol in female and the RANKL and RANKL and free testosterone in male thalassemia patients. They reason that there is a role for the RANKL/OPG system on the action of sex steroids on bone (Haidar et al., 2011).

4.2.3.4.2.10 GH and IGF1 axis in thalassemia

According to the importance of the GH and IGF1 axis, we investigate this axis in detail in the following:

Despite normal response to provocation, some studies have shown that spontaneous GH secretion is defective in some short patients with TM,. Soliman et al, emphasize that these data means the GH–IGF-I–IGFBP-3 axis in thalassemic children is defective. Structural abnormalities of their pituitary glands is also reported in association with defective GH secretion in thalassemic children. Impaired liver functions (secondary to siderosis and/or chronic viral hepatitis) may cause low IGF-I synthesis. Interestingly, Soliman et al, suggest that increased caloric dietary intake significantly increased IGF-I levels in thalassemic pediatric patinets (Soliman et al., 2009).

4.2.3.4.2.11 Parathyroid gland dysfunction in thalassemia

Hypoparathyroidism is another factor contributes to osteopenia and subsequently osteoporosis. It is believed that this complication develops more in late adolescence A recent study reported a prevalence of up to 13.5% with no sex differences (Angelopoulos et al., 2006 (a)). Main causes of hypoparathyroidism, are iron deposition on parathyroid cells (Galanello & Origa, 2010). Typical biochemical picture of hypoparathyroidism with low calcium and high phosphate levels, is seen in these patinets. Low calcium and phosphorus are found in 24-hour urine collection. Bone X-rays are characteristic for osteoporosis. Abnormal cerebral CT findings are reported to be related to hypoparathyroidism in thalassemics (Karimi et al., 2009; Angelopoulos et al., 2006 (a)).

4.2.3.4.3 Nutrition, Vitamins, Calcium, minerals and calorie intake in thalassemia

Vitamin C deficiency in iron-overloaded patients, is seen with increases the risk of osteoporotic fractures at the level of ephysial lines (Wonke, 1998). Vitamin D deficiency (although it is not reported in all studies in thalassemic patients) is also implicated in the pathogenesis of osteoporosis in TM patients due to the regulatory effect of vitamin D in both osteoclasts and osteoblasts. Adequate calcium intake during skeletal development can increase bone mass in adolescents (Voskaridou & Terpos, 2004). It was shown that increased caloric dietary intake significantly increased IGF-I levels in thalassemic children. Soliman et al., emphasized that aggressive nutritional therapy and/or GH/IGF-I therapy with vitamin D supplementation and/or calcium may improve bone growth and mineralization and prevent the development of osteoporosis and consequent fractures in these patients. They report that many studies, have also shown that improving caloric intake and supplying micronutrients including vitamin D, zinc, and carnitine have a positive effect on linear growth that can be mediated through increasing IGF-I synthesis (Soliman et al., 2009).

4.2.3.4.4 Liver disease in thalassemia

Liver diseases is a known risk factor for osteoporosis (Toumba & Skordis, 2010). The effect of iron overload in the liver is so huge and prominent that determination of liver iron concentration in a liver biopsy specimen shows a high correlation with total body iron accumulation and is considered the gold standard for the evaluation of iron overload (Galanello & Origa, 2010). Complications of iron overload include involvement of the liver (chronic hepatitis, fibrosis, and cirrhosis) (Cao & Galanello, 2010). Several factors are implicated in the reduction of bone mass in TM as well as liver disease (La Rosa et al., 2005). Growth retardation and short stature in these patients and low vitamin D are described as complications of liver disease (Baldini et al., 2010).

4.2.3.4.5 Iron overload in thalassemia

As described, iron overload causes many complications in thalassemic disease which affect bone. However, there are some bone complications that are related to iron overload directly. Some authors suggest direct iron toxicity on osteoblasts (Origa et al., 2005; Galanello & Origa, 2010). Mahachoklertwattana et al, suggest that iron deposition in bone may impair osteoid maturation and inhibit mineralization locally, resulting in focal osteomalacia (Mahachoklertwattana et al., 2003). Although all studies do not agree with these findings (Domrongkitchaiporn et al., 2003), the mechanism by which iron interferes with osteoid maturation and mineralization is explained by Toumba & Skordis as the incorporation of iron into crystals of calcium hydroxyapatite, which consequently affects the growth of calcium hydroxyapatite crystals and increases osteoids in bone tissue (Toumba & Skordis, 2010). Mahachoklertwattana reported a study on the effect of iron overload on bone remodeling in animals showed decreased osteoblast recruitment and collagen synthesis, resulting in a decreased rate of bone formation. Iron deposits in bone and low circulating IGF-I levels may partly contribute to the above findings (Mahachoklertwattana et al., 2003). Domrongkitchaiporn et al., described extensive iron staining on trabecular surfaces and a marked reduction in trabecular bone volume without significant alteration in bone formation and bone resorption rates, as well as a significant reduction in BMD in 18 thalassemic patients (Domrongkitchaiporn et al., 2003). Thus, it seems that further studies are needed to address the effect of iron toxicity on bone metabolism in thalassemia.

4.2.3.4.6 Chelation therapy in thalassemia

Chelation therapy is a known risk factor for bone problem in thalassemia patients (Origa et al., 2005; Vogiatzi et al., 2010) Growth failure and bone abnormalities, and cartilage alterations are reported as chelating therapy complication (Toumba & Skordis, 2010). Wonke et al., described the role of desferrioxamine in osteoporosis of thalassemic patients as follows: Desferrioxamine inhibits DNA synthesis, fibroblast proliferation and collagen formation, and may also cause zinc deficiency. Growth arrest and a reduction in growth velocity, difficulty in walking, frequently complain of pain in the hips and lower back is seen in patients who receive inappropriately high doses of desferrioxamine, specially when the iron burden is low, (Wonke, 1998).

4.2.3.4.7 Physical activity in thalassemia

As Haidar et al. Suggest, the association between mechanical stress and bone mass was first recorded by Galileo in 1683, who noted the relationship between body weight and bone size. They say that the low bone mass in TM patients is associated with reduced physical activity due to complications of the disease and overprotective parents, who do not encourage muscle activity (Haidar et al., 2011). However, bone disease management in these patients now includes increased physical activity (Rund & Rachmilewitz, 2005; Haidar et al., 2011; Wonke, 1998; Toumba & Skordis, 2010). What must not forget is that there is some conditions requiring special attention in recommending physical activity like severe heart disease , splenomegaly, and osteoporosis (Galanello & Origa, 2010).

4.2.3.5 Fractures in thalassemia

From self-reporting and a review of medical records, fractures occur in 36% of thalassemic patients, with 8.9% reporting three or more lifetime fractures. Extremity fractures are most common at 33%, followed by back and hip fractures at 3.6% (in one study, 10% of all fractures were reported in the spine, hip and pelvis). Low bone mass, sex hormone replacement therapy, and at least one iron overload-related endocrinopathy, was related to the prevalence of fracture. Multiple fractures are also a problem in TM patients (Haidar et al., 2011). Vogiatzi et al found The cumulative risk of fractures increased almost linearly with age. Overally, they didn't find,sex difference ; though among participants <20 years of age, males were more likely to have a fracture compared with females. Whites participants had reports of fracture rates more than Asian. Other their findings was that spine and femur BMD Z-score and total body BMC were negatively associated with fracture rate. For a 1-SD decrease in spine or femur BMD Z-score, the mean fracture rate increased by 37% or 47%, respectively (p < 0.001 for both) (Vogiatzi et al., 2009).

The peak age of fracture was the mid to late 30s. Interestingly, the percentage of subjects who remained fracture-free by the age of 18 years was significantly higher than population estimates of healthy children without hemoglobinopathies. There did not appear to be an increase in fracture prevalence during the adolescent growth spurt or surrounding the initiation of menstruation, as is typically observed in healthy reference cohorts. This may be attributed to anemia which leads to decreased physical activity and fewer opportunities for recreational fractures. There is decreased time available for sports and physical activity as these patients spend a significant amount of their time at health care centers, or overprotected by parents and caregivers. In summary, these findings confirm that the epidemiology of fractures in TM remains unique, as it is not correlated with risk taking behavior but is mainly due to vitamin D deficiency or low BMD which become more severe with age in this cohort of patients. (Haidar et al., 2011).

4.2.3.6 Management of thalassemia-induced osteoporosis

Prevention is essential for the effective control of this potentially debilitating morbidity in TM. Annual follow-up of BMD, starting in adolescence, is considered crucial. Haidar et al., recommend that Physical activity must always be encouraged and smoking should be discouraged. Adequate iron chelation, adequate calcium and zinc intake in combination with the administration of vitamin D , may prevent bone loss and fractures later and in adulthood. Hypogonadism and its prevension and treatment in thalassemic patients is very important in management of bone complication in thalassemia (Haidar et al., 2011). Despite the aforementioned measures, patients with TM still continue to lose bone mass and require treatment. Hormonal replacement, Calcitonin, Hydroxyurea, Bisphosphonates (clodronate, alendronate, pamidronate, and zoledronic) are used in the management of osteoporosis in thalassemic patients. Calcitonin, may decrease bone pain. (Voskaridou & Terpos, 2004 and Haidar et al., 2011).

Of course, it must be remembered that the use of these agents in pediatric patients is not very common or recommended, especially in young children, due to a lack of large systematic studies and comprehensive data supporting their efficacy or address their adverse effects in pediatric patients.

4.2.3.7 Bone mineral density in adult thalassemic patients

The thalassemic patients live longer now. Therefore, it is necessary to assess the bone problems in adult thalassemic patients. The increased survival of these patients during the last decade is due to regular transfusion associated with adequate iron chelation. Specific bone deformities are more rare but osteopenia and osteoporosis are more common . Low bone mass occurs despite transfusions, effective chelation, calcium, and vitamin D supplementation and hormonal deficiency replacement (Baldini et al., 2010). Though hypogonadism is important in low bone mass in TM patients, it may not be overt. Even in eugonadal women, as a delay of menarche which is common, a subtle deficiency in ovarian function cannot be ruled out (Carmina et al, 2004). Napoli et al demonstrated, at least in women with thalassemia major, that hormone replacement therapy was unable to prevent bone loss. This suggests that several mechanisms potentially contribute to low bone mass. One of these mechanisms may be vitamin D deficiency. It should be noted that TM patients progressively develop iron overload, and it is possible that a deficiency in liver hydroxylation of vitamin D, or in vitamin D absorption, can appear in older thalassemic patients (Napoli et al., 2006). However, all studies are not agree with high prevalence of low Vit-D in thalassemic patinets. Another problem in these patients is GH-IGF1 axis. It was demonstrated that the GH–IGF-I–IGFBP-3 axis in thalassemic children is defective (Soliman et al., 2009) and it is shown that GH is important in adult life and that replacement therapy should not be ignored in adults with hypopituitarism (La Rosa et al., 2005).

Baldini et al., found that the femoral site is more influenced (by biochemical and clinical factors) than the spinal site. (Baldini et al., 2010). Christoforidis et al., suggested that optimal conventional treatment in β-thalassemia major can help to achieve normal bone mass acquisition. They stated major contributors to this, as the regression of marrow expansion due to regular transfusions, the prevention of endocrine complications following adequate chelation therapy, and the reduction in deferioxamine-induced bone toxicity with the additional administration of deferiprone. As patients with thalassemia are in greater danger of developing predisposing factors for osteoporosis, optimal bone acquisition, comparable to the normal population, is essential in order to reduce future risks of osteoporosis in adult life. They recommend close surveillance with regular screening, preventive intervention and early management of possible endocrine complications are important in order to secure normal bone health. Life prolongation for patients with thalassemia major also requires improvement in quality of life (Christoforidis et al., 2006). In addition, Baldini et al. suggested that transfusion and chelation treatment can prevent bone demineralization only when applied early in childhood (Baldini et al., 2010).

5. Bone and thalassemia after bone marrow transplantation

5.1 General
Osteoporosis is increased in recipients of heart, kidney, lung, and liver transplants (Petropoulou al., 2010). Patients undergone bone marrow transplantation have some difference with other transplant recipients. Their underlying disease, organ dysfunction, age, and the median interval between diagnosis and transplantation is different. That interval is usually shorter for BMT. Kerschan-Schindl et al., conclude that BMT recipients may receive less pre-treatment impairing bone metabolism, experience fewer restrictions in mobility, and have a more normal nutritional status. Additionally, BMT recipients generally receive less subsequent immunosuppressive therapy which may induce osteopenia (Kerschan-Schindl et al., 2004).

Thalassemic patients are in an increased risk of accelerated bone loss and thus osteoporosis, because BMT is a curative treatment for thalassemia, and many patients achieve a lifelong disease-free period after BMT. Several factors inhance bone loss in them, including gonadal failure, prolonged immobility, decreased osteoprogenitor cells, conditioning regimens, vitamin D deficiency, secondary hyperparathyroidism, cyclosporine and high-corticosteroid use for graft-versus-host disease (D'Souza et al., 2006). Though some of them are not uncommon before transplantation (Angelopoulos et al., 2006 (b)).

Many investigators such as D'Souza et al. (D'Souza et al., 2006) and Schulte et al. (Schulte & Beelen, 2004) reported the significant lowering effect of corticosteroids on BMD in transplanted patients. However, their studies were not specifically on pediatric thalassemic patients, and a study by Daneils et al. did not find a statistically significant correlation between glucocorticoid exposure and BMD in transplanted children.

Kerschan-Schindl et al., suggest the amount of bone loss and the pattern of loss are controversial. The amount of bone loss within 1 year after transplantation varied and was approximately 2% for the lumbar spine and 12% for the femoral neck. At 5 years after allogeneic BMT, the lumbar spine BMD was within normal limits, but the femoral neck BMD was decreased; osteopenia was present in 43% and osteoporosis in 7% of patients (Kerschan-Schindl et al., 2004). Schulte & Beelen, demonstrated data of rapid bone loss during the first 6 months after transplantation (5.7% at the lumbar spine and 6.9% to 8.7% at the femoral neck sites) with no further decline between months 6 and 12, and recovery of bone mass during further follow-up (Schulte & Beelen, 2004).

As stated by Klopfenstein et al. in the study by Petryk et al., the incidence of osteopenia was 18% and the incidence of osteoporosis was 16% prior to BMT, which increased to 33% and 18%, respectively, 1 year after transplantation (Klopfenstein et al., 1999). In the study by Schulte et al., the lowest BMD in the femoral neck was seen 24 months after transplantation (Schulte & Beelen, 2004). However, as BMT is the only curative treatment for thalassemia, some investigators showed that the changes in BMD after transplantation may change in a positive direction (Leung et al., 2005).

5.2 Special considerations
5.2.1 Special consideration in children (Short stature)
Short stature is present in a significant number of transplanted thalassemic children. A close correlation between age at transplant and subsequent growth rate has been demonstrated (subjects who received BMT after 7 years of age, failed to achieve their full genetic potential), however, growth impairment in these subjects is due to multifactorial deranged function of the hypothalamic-pituitary-gonadal axis, abnormal hepatic conversion of steroid hormones to their active metabolites and defective hepatic biosynthesis of insulin-like growth factor (IGF-I). It is possible that iron overload is primarily involved in this phenomenon. Chronically transfused, inadequately chelated patients develop hepatocellular injury and late growth failure within the first decade of life. This is followed in adolescence by pubertal failure and dysfunction of various endocrine organs (De Simone et al., 2001).

5.2.2 Special consideration in older recipients
It must be remembered that early experience suggested that the results of transplantation for thalassemia were particularly poor for patients older than 16 years. However, Lucarelli et al., found that when the revised regimen for class 3 pediatric patients was used for older class 3 patients, the results were much improved (Lucarelli et al., 1999). However, Kaste, et al., recommend routine screening of BMD for all alloBMT patients. They suggest that patients should be advised to evaluate all behaviors which adversely affect bone health eg. avoid smoking, limit intake of caffeine and carbonated beverages, establish a weight-bearing exercise regimen after orthopedic consultation, and ensure adequate dietary intake of calcium and vitamin D. Patients should also be treated for other conditions that affect BMD such as hypogonadism and hypothyroidism (Kaste, et al., 2004).
In Iran, there is a large population of thalassemic patients and after Italy, the largest population of transplanted thalassemic patients. Thus, special attention to bone diseases before and after transplantation is necessary in these patients, and such studies may be helpful in improving life quality in affected individuals.

6. What we have learned about bone and thalassemia

The thalassemias, a group of inherited disorders of hemoglobin synthesis, are the most common monogenetic diseases worldwide and these diseases are curable by BMT. Many patients achieve a lifelong disease-free period after BMT. Thus, special attention to bone diseases before and after transplantation in these patients is necessary, and such studies may be helpful in improving life quality in affected individuals. Coping with huge problems related to the main disease and during and after BMT, the provision of a normal and safe life for these patients is a humanitarian problem. Some special points on the prevention, diagnosis, management and monitoring of bone disease in thalassemic patients are listed below:

- Assessment of bone conditions in thalassemic patients before and after transplantation is ethical and many assessments are routine.
- As a multifactorial disease (ineffective erythropoiesis and bone marrow expansion, endocrine complications, iron overload and iron chelation therapy (deferoxamine), vitamin deficiencies, and decreased physical activity all affect bone in thalassemic patients), the assessment of any of these risk factors and factors effecting them, are grounds for research which can be used to provide a better life for these patients. This is true for bone diseases following BMT.
- As a congenital disease that affects bone from an early age and is completely curable, the assessment of patients in a cohort before and after transplantation, provides an opportunity to investigate factors which affect bone in a positive or negative way, when bone is being destroyed by the main disease and when the main disease is cured.
- Genetic studies provide a way of identifying the genes responsible for low bone mass in non-thalassemic and normal individuals, especially when there are similarities in genes which cause low bone mass in thalassemic patients and non-thalassemic osteoporotic patients.
- It is questionable whether the international criteria for defining osteopenia and osteoporosis are relevant to patients with TM; also the diagnostic methods used for osteoporosis in thalassemic patients are questionable as multiple factors and micro-structural characteristics are involved in the pathogenesis of osteoporosis.
- Progression from childhood to puberty and adulthood in these patients provides ground for extended and ethical research on cohort changes in bone density and bone metabolism between these periods. As screening for low bone mass is ethical and routine in pediatrics and adults, there is a unique opportunity to assess the correlation between the diagnostic criteria for low BMD in adult and children.
- Assessment of the effects of different preventive and treatment methods and drugs on bone and different risk factors that affect bone in these patients.
- With an ethical background for investigating bone problems in thalassemic patients, providing a model of calcium and bone metabolism, and factors affecting this metabolism, throughout the life (in periods of bone gain and bone loss), is possible. This is possible by using clinical and research findings in these patients. As thalassemia is a congenital disease which is also curable, finding ways for understanding and management of bone disease in other bone disorders and in primary osteoporosis is possible.

7. Conclusion

With the expanding number of thalassemia and transplanted thalassemic patients worldwide, a better understanding of bone diseases is necessary to provide a better and safer life for these patients. The findings from these studies can be used in a model to better understand human bone diseases and help in the management of these conditions.

8. Acknowledgements

The author thanks Dr. B. Larijani (the director of EMRI-TUMS), Dr. F. Mohseni, Dr. MR. Mohajeri Tehrani, Dr. AA. Hamidieh, Mrs. A. Oojaghi and the Special Medical Center of Charity Foundation for Special Disease of Iran for their valuable assistance in this study.

9. References

Abolghasemi, Hassan. Amid, Ali. Zeinali, Sirous. Radfar, Mohammad H. Eshghi, Peyman. Rahiminejad, Mohammad S. Ehsani, Mohammad A. Najmabadi, Hossein. Akbari, Mohammad T. Afrasiabi, Abdolreza. Akhavan-Niaki, Haleh. Hoorfar, Hamid. (2007). Thalassemia in Iran: epidemiology, prevention, and management. *Journal of Pediatric Hematology/Oncology. Vol. 29, No. 4, (Apr 2007), pp. 233-238,* 1077-4114 (Print)

Angelopoulos (a), Nicholas G. Goula, Anastasia. Ombopoulos, Grigorios. Kaltzidou, Victoria. Katounda, Eugenia. Kaltsas, Dimitrios. Tolis, George. (2006). Hypoparathyroidism in transfusion-dependent patients with beta-thalassemia. *Journal of Bone and Mineral Metabolism. Vol. 24, No. 2, (2006), pp. 138-145,* 0914-8779 *(Print)*

Angelopoulos (b), Nicholas G. Katounda, Eugenia. Rombopoulos, Grigorios. Goula, Anastasia. Kaltzidou, Victoria. Kaltsas, Dimitrios. Ioannis, Pappas, Tolis, George. (2006). Evaluation of bone mineral density of the lumbar spine in patients with beta-thalassemia major with dual-energy x-ray absorptiometry and quantitative computed tomography: a comparison study. *Journal of Pediatric Hematology/Oncology. Vol. 28, No. 2, (Feb 2006), pp.73-78,* 1077-4114 (Print)

Au, W Y. Lee, V. Lau, C W. Yau, J. Chan, D. Chan, E Y T. Cheung, W W W. Ha, S Y. Kho, B. Lee, C Y. Li, R C H. Li, C K. Lin, S Y. Ling, A S C. Mak, V. Sun, L. Wong, K H F. Wong, R. Yuen, H L. (2011), A synopsis of current care of thalassaemia major patients in Hong Kong. *Hong Kong Medical Journal. Vol. 17, No. 4, Aug 2011, pp. 261-6, 1024-2708 (Print)*

Bachrach, L K. (2001). Acquisition of optimal bone mass in childhood and adolescence. *Trends in Endocrinology and Metabolism: TEM, Vol. 12, No. 1, (Jan-Feb 2001), pp. 22-28, 1043-2760 (Print)*

Baldini, Marina. Forti, Stella. Marcon, Alessia. Ulivieri, Fabio Massimo. Orsatti, Alessandra. Tampieri, Benedetta. Airaghi, Lorena. Zanaboni, Laura. Cappellini, Maria Domenica. (2010). Endocrine and bone disease in appropriately treated adult patients with beta-thalassemia major. *Annals of Hematology, Vol. 89, No. 12, (Dec 2010), pp.* 1207-1213, 1432-0584 (Electronic)

Bianchi, Maria Luisa. (2007). Osteoporosis in children and adolescents. *Bone, Vol. 41, No. 4, (Oct 2007), pp. 486-495,* 8756-3282 *(Print)*

Bogunovic, Ljiljana. Doyle, Shevaun M. Vogiatzi, Maria G. (2009). Measurement of bone density in the pediatric population. *Current Opinion in Pediatrics, Vol. 21, No. 1, (Feb 2009), pp. 77-82, 1531-698X (Electronic)*

Cao, Antonio, Moi, Paolo. Galanello, Renzo. (2011). Recent advances in beta-thalassemias. *Pediatric Reports, Vol. 3, No. 2, (Jun 2011), p. e17, 2036-7503 (Electronic)*

Cao, Antonio. Galanello, Renzo. (2010). Beta-thalassemia. *Genetics in Medicine, Vol. 12, No. 2, (Feb 2010), pp. 61-76, 1530-0366 (Electronic)*

Cario, Holger. Holl, Reinhard W. Debatin, Klaus-Michael M. Kohne, Elisabeth. (2003). Insulin sensitivity and beta-cell secretion in thalassaemia major with secondary haemochromatosis: assessment by oral glucose tolerance test. *European Journal of Pediatrics, Vol. 162, No. 3, (Mar 2003), pp. 139-146, 0340-6199 (Print)*

Carmina, E. Di Fede, G. Napoli, N. Renda, G. Vitale, G. Lo Pinto, C. Bruno, D. Malizia, R. Rini, G B. (2004). Hypogonadism and hormone replacement therapy on bone mass of adult women with thalassemia major. *Calcified Tissue International, Vol. 74, No.1 (Jan 2004). pp. 68-71.* 0171-967X (Print)

Christoforidis, Athanasios. Hatzipantelis, Emmanouil. Tsatra, Ioanna. Kazantzidou, Eirini. Katzos George. Athanassiou-Metaxa, Miranda. (2006). Bone mineral density in children and young adults with beta-thalassemia major conventionally treated. *Pediatric Blood & Cancer, Vol 47, No. 1, (Jul 2006). pp.113-114, 1545-5009 (Print)*

Daniels, Mark W. Wilson, Darrell M. Paguntalan, Helen G. Hoffman, Andrew R. Bachrach, Laura K. (2003). Bone mineral density in pediatric transplant recipients. *Transplantation. Vol. 76, No. 4, (Aug 2003), pp. 673-678, 0041-1337 (Print)*

D'Souza, A B. Grigg, A P. Szer, J. Ebeling, P R. (2006). Zoledronic acid prevents bone loss after allogeneic haemopoietic stem cell Transplantation. *Internal Medicine Journal, Vol. 36, No. 9, (Sep 2006), pp. 600-603, 1445-5994 (Electronic)*

De Simone, M. Verrotti, A. Iughetti, L. Palumbo, M. Di Bartolomeo, P. Olioso, P. Rosato, T. (2001). Final height of thalassemic patients who underwent bone marrow transplantation during childhood. *Bone Marrow Transplantation. Vol. 28, No. 2, (Jul 2001), pp. 201-205, 0268-3369 (Print)*

Domrongkitchaiporn, Somnuek. Sirikulchayanonta, Vorachai. Angchaisuksiri, Pantep. Stitchantrakul, Wasana. Kanokkantapong, Chavasak. Rajatanavin, Rajata. (2003). Abnormalities in bone mineral density and bone histology in thalassemia. *Journal of Bone and Mineral Research, Vol. 18, No. 9, (Sep 2003), pp. 1682-1688, 0884-0431 (Print)*

Ferrara, Mara. Matarese, Sofia M R. Francese, Matteo. Borrelli, Barbara. Coppola, Antonietta. Coppola, Lina. Esposito, Luigi. (2002). Effect of VDR polymorphisms on growth and bone mineral density in homozygous beta tlassaemia. *British Journal of Haematology, Vol. 117, No. 2, (May 2002), pp. 436-340, 0007-1048 (Print)*

Galanello, R. Origa, R. (2010). Beta-thalassemia. *Orphanet Journal of Rare Disease , Vol. 5:11, May 2010, 1750-1172 (Electronic)*

Gaudio, Agostino. Morabito, Nancy. Xourafa, Anastasia, Curro, Monica. Caccamo, Daniela. Ferlazzo, Nadia. Macri, Ilaria. La Rosa, Maria Angela. Meo, Anna. Ientile, Riccardo. (2010). Role of genetic pattern on bone mineral density in thalassemic patients. *Clinical Biochemistry. Vol. 43, No. 10-11, (Jul 2010), pp. 805-807, 1873-2933 (Electronic)*

Ghavamzadeh, Ardeshir. Alimoghaddam, Kamran. Jahani, Mohammad. Mousavi, Seied Asadollah. Iravani, Masood. Bahar, Babak. Khodabandeh, Ali. Khatami, Farnaz. Gaffari, Fatemeh. Jalali, Arash. (2009). Stem cell transplantation; Iranian experience. *Archives of Iranian Medicine, Vol. 12, No. 1, (Jan 2009), pp. 69-72, 1029-2977 (Print)*

Goulding, Ailsa. Grant, Andrea M. Williams, Sheila M. (2005). Bone and body composition of children and adolescents with repeated forearm fractures. *Journal of Bone and Mineral Research. Vol. 20, No. 12, (Dec 2005), pp. 2090-2096, 0884-0431 (Print)*

Haidar, Rachid. Musallam, Khaled M. Taher, Ali T. (2011). Bone disease and skeletal complications in patients with beta thalassemia major. *Bone, Vol. 38, No. 3, (Mar 2011), pp. 425-32, 1873-2763 (Electronic)*

Hamidi, Zohreh. Sedaghat, Mojtaba. Hejri, Soroosh Mortaz. Larijani, Bagher. (2008). Defining cut-off values for the diagnosis of osteoporosis in postmenopausal women by quantitative ultrasonography of the phalanx. *Gynecological Endocrinology, Vol. 24, No. 10, (Oct 2008), pp. 546-8, 1473-0766 (Electronic)*

Hamidi, Zohreh. Hamidieh, Amir Ali. Mohajeri, Mohammad Reza. Nedaeifard, Leila. Heshmat, Ramin. Alimoghaddam, Kamran. Ghavamzadeh, Ardeshir. Larijani, Bagher. (2010). Affects Of allogenic hematopoietic stem cell transplantation on bone density of pediatric patients with beta thalassemia major. *Proceedings of ASBMR 2010 Annual Meeting*, ISBN: 1523-4681 (Electronic), Toronto, October 2010. DOI: 10.1002/jbmr.5650251305(p S363-S502)

Hodge, Jason M. Kirkland, Mark A. Aitken, Cathy J. Waugh, Caryll M. Myers, Damian E. Lopez, Carolina M. Adams, Brendan E. Nicholson, Geoffrey C. (2004), Osteoclastic potential of human CFU-GM: biphasic effect of GM-CSF. *Journal of Bone and Mineral Research. Vol. 19, No. 2, (Feb 2004), pp. 190-199*, 0884-0431 (Print)

Jacome-Galarza, Christian E, Lee, Sun-Kyeong. Lorenzo, Joseph A. Aguila, Hector Leonardo, (2011), Parathyroid hormone regulates the distribution and osteoclastogenic potential of hematopoietic progenitors in the bone marrow. *Journal of Bone and Mineral Research. Vol. 26, No. 6 ,(Jun 2011), pp. 207-16, 1523-4681 (Electronic)*

Jensen, C E. Tuck, S M. Agnew, J E. Koneru, S. Morris, R W. Yardumian, A. Prescott, E. Hoffbrand, A V. Wonke, B. (1998). High prevalence of low bone mass in thalassaemia major. *British Journal of Haematology, Vol. 103, No. 4, (Dec 1998), pp. 911-915, 0007-1048 (Print)*

Johnson, Mark L. Harnish, Kimberley. Nusse, Roel. Van Hul, Wim. (2004). LRP5 and Wnt signaling: a union made for bone. *Journal of Bone and Mineral Research. Vol. 19, No. 11, (Nov 2004), pp. 1749-1757, 0884-0431 (Print)*

Kanis, J A. (1994). Assessment of fracture risk and its application to screening for postmenopausal osteoporosis: synopsis of a WHO report. WHO Study Group. *Osteoporosis International. Vol. 4, No. 6, (Nov 1994), pp. 368-381, 0937-941X (Print)*

Karimi, M. Rasekhi, A R. Rasekh, M. Nabavizadeh, S A. Assadsangabi, R. Amirhakimi, G H. (2009). Hypoparathyroidism and intracerebral calcification in patients with beta-thalassemia major. *European Journal of Radiology. Vol. 70, No. 3, (Jun 2009), pp. 481-484, 1872-7727 (Electronic)*

Kaste, S C. Shidler, T J. Tong, X. Srivastava, D K. Rochester, R. Hudson, M M. Shearer, P D. Hale, G A(2004). Bone mineral density and osteonecrosis in survivors of childhood allogeneic bone marrow transplantation. *Bone Marrow Transplantation, Vol. 33, No. 4, (Feb 2004), pp. 435-441, 0268-3369 (Print)*

Kerschan-Schindl, K. Mitterbauer, M. Mitterbauer M. Fureder, W. Kudlacek, S. Grampp, S. Bieglmayer, C. Fialka-Moser, V, Pietschmann, P, Kalhs, P. (2004), Bone metabolism in patients more than five years after bone marrow transplantation. *Bone Marrow Transplantation. Vol. 34, No. 6, (Sep 2004), pp. 491-496, 0268-3369 (Print)*

Klopfenstein, Kathryn J. Clayton, Julie. Rosselet, Robin. Kerlin, Bryce. Termuhlen, Amanda, Gross, Thomas. (1999). Prevalence of abnormal bone density of pediatric patients prior to blood or marrow transplant. *Pediatric Blood & Cancer, Vol 53, No. 4, (Oct 2009), pp. 675-677. 1545-5017 (Electronic)*

La Rosa, Clementina. De Sanctis, Vincenzo.Mangiagli, Antonino. Mancuso, Michele. Guardabasso, Vincenzo. Galati, Maria Concetta. Caruso-Nicoletti, Manuela. (2005).

Growth hormone secretion in adult patients with thalassaemia. *Clinical Endocrinology. Vol. 62, No. 6, (Jun 2005), pp. 667-671, 0300-0664 (Print)*

Leung, T F. Hung, E C W. Lam, C W K. Li, C K. Chu, Y. Chik, K W. Shing, M M K. Lee, V. Yuen, P M P. (2005). *Bone Marrow Transplantation, Vol. 36, No. 4, (Aug 2005), pp. 331-336, 0268-3369 (Print)*

Lucarelli, G. Clift, R A. Galimberti, M. Angelucci, E. Giardini, C. Baronciani, D. Polchi, P. Andreani, M. Gaziev, D. Erer, B. Ciaroni, A. D'Adamo, F. Albertini, F. Muretto, P. (1999). Bone marrow transplantation in adult thalassemic patients. *Blood, Vol. 93, No. 4, (Feb 1999), 0006-4971 (Print)*

Mahachoklertwattana, Pat. Sirikulchayanonta, Vorachai. Chuansumrit, Ampaiwan. Karnsombat, Patcharee. Choubtum, Lulin. Sriphrapradang, Arporn. Domrongkitchaiporn, Somnuek. Sirisriro, Rojana. Rajatanavin, Rajata. (2003). Bone histomorphometry in children and adolescents with beta-thalassemia disease: iron-associated focal osteomalacia. *The Journal of Clinical Endocrinology and Metabolism. Vol. 88, No. 8, (Aug 2003). pp. 3966-3972, 0021-972X (Print)*

Mamtani, M. Kulkarni, H. (2010), Bone recovery after zoledronate therapy in thalassemia-induced osteoporosis: a meta-analysis and systematic review. *Osteoporosis International, Vol. 21, No. 1, (Jan 2010), pp. 183-7, 1433-2965 (Electronic)*

Manca, Laura. Masala, Bruno. (2008). Disorders of the synthesis of human fetal hemoglobin. *IUBMB Life. Vol. 60, No. 2, (Feb 2008), pp. 94-111, 1521-6543 (Print)*

Manias, Karen. McCabe, Debbie. Bishop, Nick. (2006). Fractures and recurrent fractures in children; varying effects of environmental factors as well as bone size and mass. *Bone. Vol. 39, No. 3, (Sep 2006), pp. 652-657, 8756-3282 (Print)*

Marie, Pierre J. Kassem, Moustapha. (2011). Osteoblasts in osteoporosis: past, emerging, and future anabolic targets. *European Journal of Endocrinology. Vol. 165, No. 1, (Jul 2011), pp. 1-10, 1479-683X (Electronic)*

Marini, Francesca. Brandi, Maria Luisa. (2010). Genetic determinants of osteoporosis: common bases to cardiovascular diseases? *International Journal of Hypertension, Vol. 2010, (2010), LID - 394579 [pii], 2090-0392 (Electronic)*

Morabito, Nunziata. Gaudio, Agostino. Lasco, Antonino. Atteritano, Marco. Pizzoleo, Maria Antonia. Cincotta, Maria. La Rosa, Mariangela. Guarino, Roberta. Meo, Anna. Frisina, Nicola. (2004). Osteoprotegerin and RANKL in the pathogenesis of thalassemia-induced osteoporosis: new pieces of the puzzle. *Journal of Bone and Mineral Research. Vol. 19. No. 5, (May 2004), pp. 722-727, 0884-0431 (Print)*

Muncie, HL Jr. Campbell, J. (2009). Alpha and Beta Thalassemia, *American Family Physician, Vol. 80, No. 4, Aug 2009, pp. 339-44, 0002-838X (Print)*

Mundy, G R. (1999). Cellular and molecular regulation of bone turnover. *Bone. Vol. 24, No. 5 supply, (May 1999), 8756-3282 (Print)*

Najafipour, Farzad. Aliasgarzadeh, Akbar. Aghamohamadzadeh, Naser. Bahrami, Amir. Mobasri, Majid. Niafar, Mitra. Khoshbaten, Manouchehr. A cross-sectional study of metabolic and endocrine complications in beta-thalassemia major. *Annals of Saudi Medicine, Vol. 28, No. 5, (Sep-Oct 2008), pp. 361-366, 0256-4947 (Print)*

Napoli, N. Carmina, Enrico. Bucchieri, Salvatore. Sferrazza, C. Rini, G B. Di Fede, G.(2006). Low serum levels of 25-hydroxy vitamin D in adults affected by thalassemia major or intermedia. *Bone, Vol. 38, No. 6, (Jun 2006). pp. 888-892, 8756-3282 (Print)*

Origa, R. Fiumana, E. Gamberini, M R. Armari, S. Mottes, M. Sangalli, A. Paglietti, E. Galanello, R. Borgna-Pignatti, C. (2005). Osteoporosis in beta-thalassemia: Clinical and genetic aspects. *Annals of the New York Academy of Sciences, Vol. 1054, (2005), pp. 451-456, 0077-8923 (Print)*

Papanastasiou, Dimitris A. Ellina, Aikaterini. Baikousis, Andreas. Pastromas, Basilis. Iliopoulos, Panos. Korovessis, Panagiotis. (2002). Natural History of Untreated Scoliosis in beta-Thalassemia. *Spine, Vol. 27, No. 11, (Jun 2002), pp. 1186-1890, 1528-1159 (Electronic)*

Perera, N J. Lau, N S. Mathews, S. Waite, C. Ho, P J. Caterson, I D. (2010). Overview of endocrinopathies associated with beta-thalassaemia major. *Internal Medicine Journal, Vol. 40, No. 10, (Oct 2010), pp. 689-696, 1445-5994 (Electronic)*

Petropoulou, Anna D. Porcher, Raphael. Herr, Andree-Laure. Devergie, Agnes. Brentano, Thomas Funck. Ribaud, Patricia. Pinto, Fernando O. Rocha, Vanderson. Peffault de Latour, Regis. Orcel, Philippe. Socie, Gerard. Robin, Marie. (2010). Prospective assessment of bone turnover and clinical bone diseases after allogeneic hematopoietic stem-cell transplantation. *Transplantation. Vol. 89, No. 11, (Jun 2010), pp. 1354-1361. 1534-6080 (Electronic)*

Psihogios, Vicki, Rodda, Christine, Reid, Elizabeth, Clark, Malcolm, Clarke, Caroline, Bowden, Donald. (2002). Reproductive health in individuals with homozygous beta-thalassemia: knowledge, attitudes, and behavior. *Fertility and Sterility, Vol. 77, No. 1, (Jan 2002), pp. 119-127, 0015-0282 (Print)*

Rabinovich, C. Egla. (2004). Osteoporosis: a pediatric perspective. *Arthritis and Rheumatism. Vol. 50, No. 4, (Apr 2004), 0004-3591 (Print)*

Roodman, G David. (2004). Mechanisms of bone metastasis. *The New England Journal of Medicine. Vol. 350, No. 16, (Apr 2004), pp. 1655-1664, 1533-4406 (Electronic)*

Rund, Deborah. Rachmilewitz, Eliezer. (2005). (MEDICAL PROGRESS)Beta-thalassemia. *The New England Journal of Medicine. Vol. 353, No. 11, (Sep 2005). pp. 1135-46, 1533-4406 (Electronic)*

Salehi, S A. Koski, T. Ondra, S L.(2004). Spinal cord compression in beta-thalassemia: case report and review of the literature. *Spinal Cord. Vol. 42, No. 2, (Feb 2004), pp. 117-123, 1362-4393 (Print)*

Sankaran, VG. Nathan, DG. (2010). Thalassemia: an overview of 50 years of clinical research. *Hematology/Oncology Clinics of North America, Vol. 24, No. 4, (Dec 2010, pp. 1005-1020, 0889-8588 (Print)*

Schonau, E. (1998). Problems of bone analysis in childhood and adolescence. *Pediatric Nephrology (Berlin, Germany), Vol 12, No. 5, (Jun 1998), pp. 420-429, 0931-041X (Print)*

Schulte, Claudia M S. Beelen, Dietrich W. (2004). Bone loss following hematopoietic stem cell transplantation: a long-term follow-up. *Blood, Vol. 103, No. 10, (May 2004), pp. 3635-3643, 0006-4971 (Print)*

Soliman, Ashraf T. Khalafallah, Hany. Ashour, Rasha. (2009). Growth and factors affecting it in thalassemia major. *Hemoglobin. Vol. 33, No. Suppl 1, (2009), pp. S116-S126, 1532-432X (Electronic)*

Toumba, Meropi. Skordis, Nicos. (2010). Osteoporosis syndrome in thalassaemia major: an overview. *Journal of Osteoporosis, Vol. 2010, p. 537673, 2042-0064 (Electronic)*

Tyler, P A. Madani, G. Chaudhuri, R. Wilson, L F. Dick, E A. (2006). The radiological appearances of thalassaemia. *Clinical Radiology, Vol. 61, No. 1, (Jan 2006), pp.40-52, 0009-9260 (Print)*

van Kuijk, Cornelis. (2010). Pediatric bone densitometry. *Radiologic Clinics of North America. Vol. 48, No. 3, (May 2010), pp. 623-627, 1557-8275 (Electronic)*

Vogiatzi, Maria G. Macklin, Eric A. Fung, Ellen B. Cheung, Angela M. Vichinsky, Elliot. Olivieri, Nancy. Kirby, Melanie. Kwiatkowski, Janet L. Cunningham, Melody. Holm, Ingrid A. Lane, Joseph. Schneider, Robert. Fleisher, Martin. Grady, Robert W. Peterson, Charles C. Giardina, Patricia J. (2009). Bone disease in thalassemia: a frequent and still unresolved problem. *Journal of Bone and Mineral Research. Vol. 24, No. 3, (Mar 2009), pp. 543-557, 1523-4681 (Electronic)*

Vogiatzi, Maria G, Tsay, Jaime, Verdelis, Kostas, Rivella, Stefano. Grady, Robert W. Doty, Stephen. Giardina, Patricia J. Boskey, Adele L. (2010). Changes in bone microarchitecture and biomechanical properties in the th3 thalassemia mouse are associated with decreased bone turnover and occur during the period of bone accrual. *Calcified tissue international. Vol. 86, No. 6, (Jun 2010), pp. 484-94, 1432-0827 (Electronic)*

Vogiatzi, Maria G. Autio, Karen A. Mait, Jeffrey E. Schneider, Robert. Lesser, Martin. Giardina, Patricia J. (2005). Low bone mineral density in adolescents with beta-thalassemia. *Annals of the New York Academy of Sciences. Vol. 1054. (2005), pp. 462-466, 0077-8923 (Print)*

von Scheven, Emily. (2007). Pediatric bone density and fracture. *Current Osteoporosis Reports. Vol. 5, No. 3, (Sep 2007), pp. 128-34, 1544-1873 (Print)*

Voskaridou, Ersi. Terpos, Evangelos. (2004). New insights into the pathophysiology and management of osteoporosis in patients with beta thalassaemia. *British Journal of Haematology, Vol. 127, No. 2, (Oct 2004), pp. 127-39, 0007-1048 (Print)*

Wittrant, Y. Gorin, Y. Mohan, S. Wagner, B. Abboud-Werner, S L. (2009). Colony-stimulating factor-1 (CSF-1) directly inhibits receptor activator of nuclear factor-{kappa}B ligand (RANKL) expression by osteoblasts. *Endocrinology. Vol. 150, No. 11, (Nov 2009), pp. 4977-88, 1945-7170 (Electronic)*

Wonke, B. (1998). Bone disease in beta-thalassaemia major. *British Journal of Haematology, Vol. 103, No. 4, (Dec 1998), pp. 897-901, 0007-1048 (Print)*

12

What's BMD and What We Do in a BMD Centre?

Zohreh Hamidi
*Endocrinology and Metabolism Research Institute of
Tehran University of Medical Sciences (EMRI-TUMS),
Islamic Republic of Iran*

1. Introduction

The main parts of osteoporosis clinics are BMD (Bone Mineral Densitometry) centers. For increasing our knowledge about osteoporosis we have to increase our knowledge about BMD (Bone Mineral Density), and increasing the knowledge about BMD has a close relationship with realizing the principles and appliances of BMD machines and DXA method. For specific development in a BMD department, we need to know some historical, technical and practical points about these method and machines. In this review, the last developments in this field are suggested, also.

2. General information about BMD and BMD centres

2.1 What we do in a BMD centre?
1.   Determine patient's BMD
2.   Estimate the risk of fracture (pathologic fracture) in a patient

2.2 Some historical points about dual X-ray absorptiometry
It is very useful to know the history of BMD and DXA devices. The first marketing of this machine was in 1987 and in1994 this method described as gold standard for osteoporosis diagnosis by World Health Organisation (WHO). It means osteoporosis disease, as we know now, was described in 1994 for the first time.(Lukaski, 1993; Kanis, 1994).

2.3 Distribution of BMD devices around the world
As Kanis and Johnel reported in 2005, 9 countries from 20 countries (in Europe), had more than 10 DXA units per million of the population (the European standard). However it is unclear which percent of machines were dedicated in part or in full to clinical research. They conclude that the majority of countries are under-resourced. Inequity of geographical location, is an important problem, which is a known problem in Italy, Spain, Switzerland and the UK. (Kanis & Johnell,2005). However the distribution and utilization of these machines are increasing worldwide. This statistics seems interesting when you know there was almost 183 machines in Canada in 1998, and there was no such device in Prince Edward Island (of Canada) around 1998. In Canada there are almost 600 devices, nowadays. The European standard is 0.11 DXA machine per 10 000 population (Mithal et al., 2009).

Asian audit in 2009, show us a very different picture in Asia. DXA technology is relatively expensive and is not widely available in most developing Asian countries, especially in rural areas. There was only 450 DXA machines in China for a population of 1.3 billion. In Srilanka only 4 machines exist. (Mithal et al., 2009). In 2008, Indonesia had a total of only 34 DXA machines, half of them in Jakarta, for a population of 237 million (0.001 per 10,000 population)(IOF, 2011). One of the most extreme examples is found in India, reportedly, there was only approximately 100 DXA units, located in six cities. This inequity results in long waiting times or long distances to travel or in many cases, no access (Kanis & Johnell,2005) (Fig. 1. And Fig. 2.). With above examples about distribution of these machines around the world, we explain here the formula used for calculating standard requirement of these machines (this formula is calculated according to number of population and prevalence of risk factors in target population).

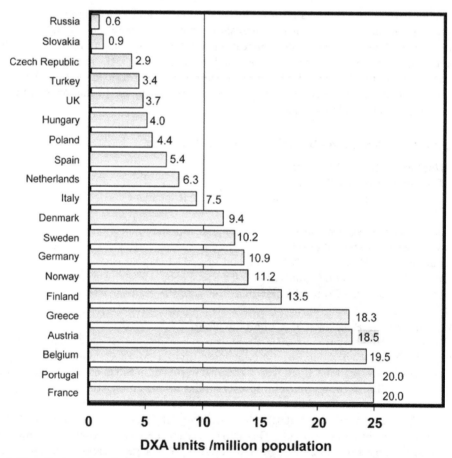

Fig. 1. Density (number / million of the population) of central DXA (spine/hip) units in different European countries in 2003 (from Kanis and Johnell, 2005).

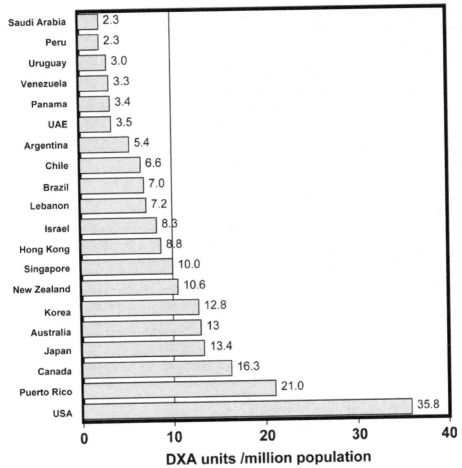

Fig. 2. Density (number / million of the population) of central DXA (spine/hip) units in non-European countries in 2003 (from Kanis and Johnell, 2005).

2.4 Requirement for DXA

Kanis and Johnel, extensively explained the method used for estimation of required number of DXA machines in Europe. As the method is interesting and contained demographic and osteoporotic statistics in Europe, we repeat their explanation as extensive as is used in their article in 2005. Repeat the explanation may be helpful, clearing a guideline for clinicians and researchers, to calculate the requirement of DXA machines in their area or countries. They suggested the requirement for three scenario and in two category, requirements of DXA for risk assessment and requirements of DXA to monitor treatment.

2.4.1 Requirements of DXA for risk assessment

From total population of Europe, it is estimated that, 4 million of them were 65 years old women. The authors assumed that individuals over the 65 years would be tested over the ensuing 10 years and repeated BMD tests would perform in patient that need treatment or those patients at high risk on the basis of the screening BMD test.

The first scenario (scenario A or screening women with BMD), proposed monitor all women with at the age of 65 years. If the main goal was to measure BMD in all 65 years old women (4.045.000, 65 years old women), this required 3231 DXA units or 4.42 DXA/ million of the total population. In this first scenario, if we assumed that people with the age 66 years and older didn't screen and if they want to screen over a 10- year period, the needs for DXA units would be 6.79/million of total population, giving a total need 11.2 units/million.

The aim of second scenario (scenario B, or clinical case finding with selective use of BMD) was to screen 65 years old women with clinical risk factor referred for DXA at 10 yearly intervals. It means that we sent 65 y/o women for BMD, only when they were high risk for fracture. Finding patients at high risk was based on clinical risk factors. Patients were high risk, when 10-year probability of hip fracture in them (calculated upon risk factors), was 4% and more (This is also called intervention threshold, and the authors considered it a cut-off that treatment is needed for patients). Screening all these patients, need 767 DXA units or 1,05 scan/million of the population. No surprising, the population that need intervention and treatment advances with age. The probability of risk fracture is about 1% at the age of 50 and 52% at the age of 80 years old. Author emphasize that the absolute population size decreases the higher the starting age for testing. They calculated that assessment of women at the older age, (during 10 years period) would require an extra need of 2301 DXA units or 3.16/million of the population (total need for women 65 y/o and older equals to 4.21/million). At younger age, small population is selected for BMD test. So the requirements are not markedly differ by screening policy that starts at age of 50 years. At this age, only nearly 1% of women are selected for treatment. It would be required that more 50,000 DXA tests do for 50 years old women (that add 40 scanning units or 0.05 units/million machines to requirement). After added screened population aged more than 50 years over a 10 year term interval, the total requirement will be 4.5 unit/million. Compare it with 4.21 unit/million required only for screening of 65 y/o women and older.

The third scenario (scenario C, or classic case finding strategy) enlisted only women with strong risk factors for fracture, to do BMD. The authors suggested a different prevalence of risk factors in different age population (29% to 46% depending on age). For testing women of 65 years, 1481 units or 2.03 units/million of the population was required. If BMD considered in women aged more than 65 years and a risk factors prevalence as 46%, 3 million/year over a 10 year interval (30 million, for 10 years) would require testing . This is equal to 3.33 units/million of the population. On the other hand, if BMD tests considered for women aged 50 years or more with one or more these risk factors, BMD testing was needed in 36.9% of the female population aged 50 years or more. Authors calculated this would need 3842 scanning units or 5.3/million of the total population (It seems it is a yearly need, when the whole 10 year need is divided by 10). When only women with incident osteoporotic fracture and aged 65 years or older sent to BMD centers, requirement was 918 scanning visits or 1.3/million of the general population.

2.4.2 Requirements of DXA to monitor treatment

When women referred for treatment, 2 BMD tests may be required. One is at the time of diagnosis, and a second at an interval of 2 years. For scenario B, BMD tests would have been done in 24% of the population at the age of 65 years, some of them do not need treatment and so don't need a further BMD test in the beginning of treatment (they did't cut the threshold for need to intervention). Additional BMD testing would be required in approximately 10% of women for the purposes of baseline investigation for treatment. If all 65-year-olds were screened, additional pre-treatment BMD tests would equal to 0.4/million scans (322 units) and approximately increase 2-fold after 2 years later. Thus, the steady state requirements would be 966 scanners or 1.33 units/million of the population. Women older than 65 years have a smaller population , but not surprisingly ,a larger proportion would cut an intervention threshold. For example, at the age of 80 years there are approximately 2.15 million women, but with the same test, 73% would be need treatment. But in 50 years old women, approximately 1% of their 5 million population would need treatment. The author emphasized that in women aged 65 years or more, approximately 35% will need treatment and require a BMD tests before and after treatment (2 years later). This gives an annual requirement for 4.6 million scans or 3686 scanning units and a requirement of 5.06/million of the general population. It means for the monitoring of treatment (in 65 y/o women and older), 6.39 uint/million is needed under scenario B. All of these, means the total number 10.6 scanning units/million of the population is needed for assessment plus monitoring of treatment in scenario B (Kanis & Johnell,2005).

2.5 Secular trend of use of DXA

The total number of all older patients performed DXA in the USA has grown up from 501,105 in 1996 to 2,195,548 in 2002. This 4 fold growth during 6 years related to increase the average of lifespan, increase public awareness of osteoporosis and development in therapeutic cares. The maximum application of DXA has been observed in central densitometry. The usage of this method maybe continued for the next few years. However, in some countries, DXA just applied for patients with certain (or specific) risk factors. There are national organization in other countries that prescribe DXA only for patients at multiple risks of osteoporosis. It cause different statistics of use of DXA in different countries (Damilakis et al., 2010).

Results show a great increase in use of bone mass densitometry in Canada. DXA-BMD tests increase 10-fold between years 1993 to 2005, and approximately 500,000 scans perform per year. In Ontario, showed an excessive use of anti-osteoporotic drugs along with the reduction rate of hip and wrist fractures with the increase in BMD test.The growth rate of BMD test appeared to be decreased to 6 to 7% per year. The increase usage rate of BMD-test occurred mainly in 65 years old people or older (Legislative Assembly of Ontario, 2006).

3. Bone densitometry instruments

3.1 Instruments

Lukaski, had a good review of instruments in dual x-ray absorptiometry. Because of its clear and good explanation about the complexity of matter, we mension it here, with almost no change. The first generation commercial dual-energy X-ray absorptiometry (DXA) system became available in 1987 after its initial progress in the late 1960s and 1970s. The three main companies, introduced three X-ray-based absorptiometry systems (approved by the Food and Drug Administration): QDR-1000W3 (Hologic Inc., Waltham, MA), DPX (Lunar Radiation Corp., Madison, WI) and XR-26 (Norland Corporation, Fort Atkinson, WI). Each system uses a source- that generates X-rays at two different energies- a detector and an interface with a computer system.

These three DXA systems operate in different ways. The QDR-1000 and QDR- 1000W systems produce two X-ray beams of different energies by using an X-ray tube alternately pulsed at 70 and 140 kVp peaks. The DPX system uses a constant potential generator and a Cerium K-edge X-ray filtration to generate photons at two energies (40 and 76 keV). The Norland XR-26 unit also employs a constant potential X-ray generator, but it operates at 100 kVp and employs a Samarium filter (K-edge = 46.8 keV). Unlike the DPX and XR-26 systems, the QDR-1000W system has an internal calibration system that consists of a rotating filter wheel composed of three sections (two sections of epoxy-resin-based material consistent with the densities of bone and soft tissue and one section of air). In the QDR system, photons of only one energy are present at any one time, and the detector measures the intensity of the transmitted photons without energy discrimination. An integral line single detector is used in the Lunar DPX system. The XR-26 detector consists of thin and thick sodium iodide crystals (low intensity X rays are stopped by the thin crystal, and high intensity photons are trans mitted and detected by the second thick crystal).

An important advantage of the DXA systems is the increased photon flux emanating from the X-ray sources in comparison to the photon flux from the radioisotope source used in dual-photon absorptiometry. The increased photon flux improves the resolution and precision of the image and reduces the time for a scan. To assess soft tissue composition, the DXA systems use different forms of external calibration. The QDR and XR-26 systems rely on external standards, which are wedges made of aluminum and ucite (polymethylmethacrylate) calibrated against stearic acid as 100% fat, and dilute saline solution as 100% fat-free mineral free tissue. The DPX systems use a plastic polyoxymethylene (Delrin), as 40% fat equivalent and water (~5% fat) as standards (Lukaski, 1993). Recently, the name of Medi-link brand is added to list of machines in FRAX software. Fan beam models are added to DXA machines family and have different beam geometry from pencil beam models. They are explained later.

BMD devices are popular machines, because they are low X-ray radiating, don't need especial preparation for patients and they are not invasive but as it mentioned before, these instruments are not widely distributed in the world, and the expensive cost of these machines is a main reason for it. Properties of these devises that make them expensive are:

- Safety
- The Hardware
- The Software

3.2 Safety

The special method used in these devices, make them low X-ray radiating. They don't need special shielding. We can evaluate the safety of DXA by the radiation dose that each patients or subjects receive. The average skin dose is 1-3 mrad per scan. The radiation dose of DXA is less than other radiologic methods, such as single-photon absorptiometry, dualphoton absorptiometry and quantitative digital radiography, conventional chest x-ray and many others. For example, skin exposures from environmental background are ~3.5 mrad/wk; from dental bite-wing posterior films, 334 mrad and from chest X-ray films, ~8-10 mrad. Thus, we can conclude; for routine measurement of human body composition and bone mineral status , DXA may be noticed a relatively safe method. Manufacturers suggest that it is safe from 1 meter (Lukaski, 1993).

3.2.1 Dose reduction techniques for patients

Damilakis et al, remind us that the system for patients protection against radiation is based on 2 principles: (a) justification and (b) optimisation. Clinically justification of all X- ray exposures used for bone densitometry is very important. Examinations that do not influence patient care, must be avoided.

Preparing patients before bone densitometry is very important. For example metallic things such as jewelry or coins can cause artifact and careful checking for the presence of these items and proper positioning of patient before bone densitometry, will optimize the imaging quality and there will be no need to repeat imaging with additional radiation exposure. In pediatric examinations, proper interaction with the children and parents is essential. All actions should be taken to avoid movement of the child during imaging and to avoid repeating measurement. The duration time of DXA should be minimize and should take into account patient's body size, if possible (Damilakis et al., 2010).

3.2.2 Occupational radiation doses and shielding

Although the annual occupational doses from DXA is very lower than standard occupational radiation dose, but for a pregnant employee that declares pregnancy, special dose reduction should be applied. As Damilakis et al. suggest, The ICRP and European Commission recommend that pregnant individual be protected by the application of a dose up to 1 mGy. Of course, as they emphasize, the exclusion of pregnant workers from DXA examinations on the basis of radiogenic risks from occupational DXA exposure cannot be justified on scientific grounds. Because the scatter radiation can increase the exposure limits for pregnant workers, especially for fan-beam systems. Radiation protection measures should always be taken to ensure that the conceptus dose will be kept below 1 mGy during the declared pregnancy. For monitoring radiation dose, it is recommended to use personal radiation meter at waist level.

Correcting design of the room in which the imaging device has been installed, can influence in limiting the risk of radiation exposure in the workplace. Measurements performed by Larkin et al. as cited in Damilakis et al., 2010, showed that the scatter from fan-beam DXA systems can increase the limits for public exposure i.e. 1 mSv/year. In these cases, additional structural shielding might be required, especially when the distance from the imaging table to the adjacent wall is less than 1 m. They say, parameters like the workload, the material of the walls, the location of the operator and the location and use of rooms that adjoin the imaging room must also be remembered as important factors (Damilakis et al., 2010).

3.3 Hardware
3.3.1 Basic principles of dual-energy X-ray absorptiometry (DXA)

The proportion of beam of X- rays weaken (attenuating) during transporting through a complex material depend on composition of material, the thickness of material and any of its components. Soft tissues, which contain principally water and organic compounds create limitation to the flux (number of X-rays per unit area) of X-rays, and of course, this limitation is lesser than the limitation creates by bone tissue. The un-weakened or un-attenuated energy, in the form of X-ray radiation, is detected by an external detector. In dual-energy X-ray system, there is a source that emits X-rays, which are collimated into a beam (there is a shutter that can turn on and turn off the beam, also). The source lies beneath the patient and the beam transports in a posterior-to-anterior direction, through the body of patient (bone and soft tissue), and goes upward to be detected by a detector, above the patient, lies in the arm of machine (Lukaski, 1993).

3.3.2 Specific technology of dual energy X-ray absorptiometers scanners (DXA)

Before using dual x-ray absorptometry (when single-photon or single-x-ray absorptiometry used), the ROI (region of interest) of scanning, should be immersed in a water bath for densitometry (Fig. 3.). By use of water bath, the water and soft tissue (with almost the same attenuation), make a single compartment of attenuation (on the other hand, the influence of soft-tissue in the measurement significantly reduces and soft tissue don't contributed to measured absorption). They make one compartment and bone makes another compartment with its specific attenuation (than is very different and very higher that other compartment). This can lead to calculating of density of bone, because the attenuation of energy of x-ray beam is related to density of tissue. The density of soft-tissue (and water) is known and constant in almost all humans. The density of bone is not constant and changes one by one. By comparing the attenuation of energy of bone compartment of anyone to attenuation of energy of his soft tissue, machine can calculate the bone density. Without water bath, there is 3 compartment (air, soft tissue and bone), that machine can't separate them exactly and so can't differ between their density, and there is not single reference for comparing density of bone. So finding the exact density of bone would be impossible. Using of water-bath was a development for bone densitometry. But some big practical problems remained. It is practically, impossible to immerse whole body in water bath to measure the bone density of e.g. Spinal region or neck of femur. Water bath was useful for testing BMD of forearm. Remember spine and femur are most important parts of densitometry, because the important or fatal pathologic fracture occurs in these regions and measuring the BMD of e.g. forearm is not a good predictor of BMD or fracture in these important parts. The creating DXA methods, came helpful in solving this big problem. Imagine, using Dual x-ray absorptiometry (using 2 different energy beams) works as water bath in creating two distinguished compartment from compartments that were previously three different compartments of air, soft tissue and bone. The DXA (Dual X-ray absorptiometry) method depends on the differential absorption of two distinct beam energies - a high and low energy beam. When measuring bone, bone will normally have air and soft tissue around it. The high and low energy photons don't change in soft tissue, but the lower energy photon will be significantly reduced by bone tissue (high energy photon don't changes significantly). This difference in reduction of low energy beam, in two different tissue-bone and soft-tissue- can be used for measurement of bone density. On the other hand, the soft tissue component becomes the reference for determining the bone component (Royal Adelaide Hospital, 2009). When two different beams, pass from body compartments, the difference between their intensity before and after passing the soft tissue (and air), don't change (so, the air and soft tissue around the bone create a single compartment). This constant difference can be considered as 1 unit of difference. When two different beams, pass from bone tissue, the low energy beam attenuates significantly after passing bone, it means there is big difference in the intensity of low energy beam before and after passing bone. So the difference between intensity of two high and low energy beams increase significantly and may be multiple times of 1 unit difference reported for soft tissue (and air). This increase in difference is a result of attenuation of low beam energy in bone tissue and relates to bone density. If we have the density of soft tissue compartment, now we can calculate the density of bone. As mentioned before, the density of soft tissue is known and constant and is used as reference for determining bone density in DXA method. It means use of DXA, makes bone densitometry possible, without need to water bath that was needed in single x-ray absorptiomtery. Dual x-ray absorptiometry, makes axial bone densitometry in the conventional form that is performing now, possible (with patient lying on a table in normal atmosphere of an imaging room with no special preparation).

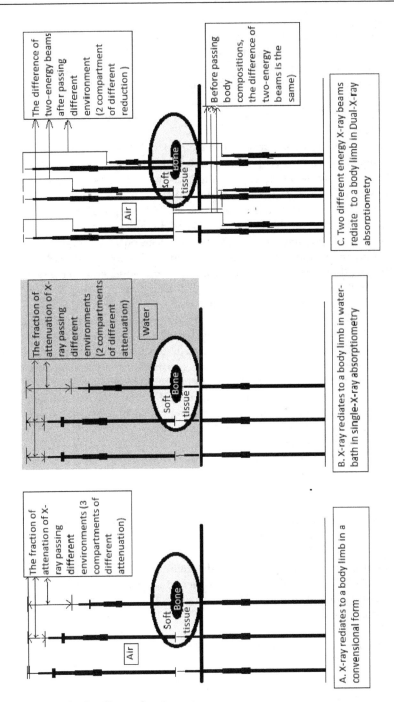

Fig. 3. Different methods of bone densitometry

3.3.3 Quality control

For diagnosing longitudinal changes, assessment of precision error in bone mineral density (BMD) testing is very important (Leslie et al., 2007). Lukaski emphasizes that one parameter of quality control in the use of DXA is the precision of the measurements. Precision is generally reported as the coefficient of variation (CV), which is the standard deviation of repeated measurements expressed as a percentage of the mean of the measurements. The precision of DXA has been assessed for short-term (in vitro and in vivo) and for long-term (in vitro) (Lukaski, 1993).

The International Society for Clinical Densitometry (ISCD) has a standardized methodology for performing an in vivo precision study and recommends that this be performed by each densitometry center. Leslie at al., explain the ISCD procedure as gaining precision error from an assessment with 30 degrees of freedom (df; e.g., 30 subjecs with 2 scans each or 15 subjects with 3 scans each) drawn from the patient of referral population and using the root mean square (RMS) approach (RMS is not explained there) (Leslie et al., 2007).

Lukaski, reports that in first studies, short-term precision and long-term Precision, in different period times and different devices studied. Wahner et al. (1988), as cited in Lukaski; 1993, reported a short-term precision (repeat measurements on the same day) of 0.2 and 0.5% for BMC and BMD, respectively, and a long-term precision (for up to 6 mo) of 0.4% for BMD in lumbar spine phantoms made of hydroxyapatite. Duplicate scans performed on the same day in patients showed a difference of <1% between scans for BMC and BMD. Kelly et al. (1988), as cited in Lukaski; 1993, also observed high reproducibility (CV = 0.23%) of BMD measurements in spine phantoms measured over 6 months. Rencken et al. (1991), as cited in Lukaski; 1993, evaluated the precision of DXA measurements using six different QDR instruments at separate locations. Nine consecutive scans were performed on a single spine phantom at each site. The investigators reported an average precision for BMC and BMD of <1% (range: 0.3-0.6%). The average of the highest and lowest mean values was 1.1% for BMC and 1.07% for BMD. Mazess et al. (1989), as cited in Lukaski; 1993, reported a long-term precision in BMD measurements of 0.6% using a DPX system in a spine phantom over 6 mo. Estimates of 1.8 and 0.9% for the measurement of total body BMC and BMD, respectively, in 12 adults were also reported with a DPX instrument (Mazess et al. 1990, as cited in Lukaski; 1993). Johnson and Dawson-Hughes (1991), as cited in Lukaski; 1993, assessed long-term precision of BMD measurements in six volunteers scanned six times initially and at the same frequency 9 mo later. The short-term precision of BMD measurements in the spine, femoral neck and whole body were 1.08, 2.08 and 0.66%, respectively. The long-term precision was 1.01, 2.07 and 0.62%, respectively. The investigators also reported the precision in determining body composition variables; thus, the precision of whole-body BMC, fat-free mass and fat mass was 0.8, 1.1 and 2.7%, at the start of the study, and 1.2, 1.0, and 1.7%, respectively, after 9 months.

Another aspect of quality control is the accuracy of the DXA measurement. The extent to which DXA measurements represent true bone mineral status has been assessed by measuring the mineral content of cadaver vertebrae of known ash weights and volumes. Ho et al. (1990), as cited in Lukaski; 1993, measured BMC and BMD in lumbar vertebrae from 11 cadavers. The ash weights of 31 lumbar vertebrae and the DXA BMC values were significantly correlated (r = 0.963, SEE = 1.01 g; P< 0.001). The slope of the regression of ash weight as the dependent variable versus QDR-BMC as the independent variable was 1.0, but the intercept was 0.59. Although the value of 0.59 was not statistically different from 0, the authors concluded that DXA under estimates ash weight (Lukaski, 1993).

Before to 2000, DXA measurements were conducted with a pencil-beam instrument (Lunar DPX, GE Lunar, Madison WI), and after that a fan-beam instrument was used. As Leslie et al suggested in 2011, instruments were cross-calibrated using anthropomorphic phantoms and 59 volunteers. They say there was no clinically significant differences (T-score differences <0.2). Densitometers showed stable long-term performance [CV<0.5%] and satisfactory in vivo precision (CV 1.7% for L1–4 and 1.1% for the total hip) (Leslie et al., 2011)

3.3.4 The long-term performance of DXA bone densitometers

Monitoring the performance of DXA after long time utilization is very important because any deterioration could change bone mineral density (BMD) measurements and affect clinical management. The importance of DXA in longitudinal trials of new osteoporosis therapies also need constant performance over years to confirm that any altration in bone density is real and not due to machine shifts or fluctuation. In this way, Wells and Ryan, assessed the performance of a 6-year-old bone densitometer (a Lunar DPX alpha), which has undertaken 1500 scans/year over this period. They concluded that the machine performs extremely well over a long period and after 6 years of Performing, measurements is very suitable to be fit for clinical use. It may be can be generalized to all main DXA devices in market (Wells & Ryan, 2000).

3.3.5 Beam geometry

At website of department of nuclear medicine, PET & bone densitometry of Royal Adelaide Hospital (Australia), at section of "Bone Densitometry Equipment", beam geometry of "DXA devices" are explained so:

3.3.5.1 Pencil beam

First generation bone densitometers (isotope and x-ray) use this beam geometry. The photon beam is tightly collimated with one photon source and one detector (some scanners have two, usually photomultiplier tubes). The source and detector are rigidly coupled and moved together in a rectilinear manner to build an image of the bone being examined line by line. The disadvantage of this technology is the relatively slow scan speed (typically 2-4 minutes per scan site). However, the direct relationship between source and detector means that calculated bone and tissue masses are less likely to be artefactual.

3.3.5.2 Fan beam

The second generation of x-ray bone densitometer has a fan geometry, with a source which fans out in the short axis plane of the patient and is measured by an array of detectors in the same plane.

The bones are imaged in one pass along the long axis of the body (as illustrated at middle) providing an immediate advantage in scan speed which is typically about 1 minute on modern scanners.

The disadvantage of fan beam DXA is that the photon flux at the edges is lower than the middle of the image (due to the inverse square law). As a result, mass calculations may have some systematic error, although bone mineral density values have been shown to be unaffected.

3.3.5.3 Narrow fan beam

This is designed to overcome some of the limitations of the fan beam geometry. A small fan beam radiation (about 4cm wide at the detector) in the long axis is detected by an array of detectors. The beam scans the bones in the short patient axis on each individual sweep along the long axis of the patient with some beam overlap. Although slightly slower than a fan beam scanner (1-2 minutes per scan), the mass results should be more accurate as the photon flux has little variability in the area being measured (due to the beam overlap). You can see the schematic figure of different beam geometries in the Fig. 4, from mentioned website (Royal Adelaide Hospital, 2009).

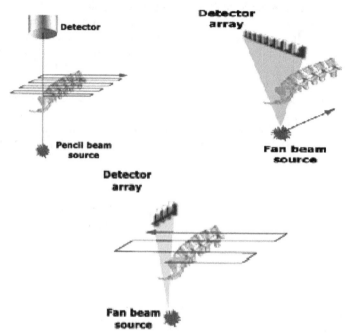

Fig. 4. Beam geometry of DXA mechines (from website of Royal Adelaide Hospital (Australia)

3.4 Software

The reference data of these machines, contain data of BMD tests of almost 5000 Caucasian white normal persons; around 20-80 y/o. Any brand of these machines has different reference data. It is clear that collecting such huge database, nowadays, seems impossible (especially due to cost and financial problems). This makes these method (DXA) and machines, unique. It seems impossible that any other method or brand can replace them in future, at least in near future.

Another ability of the software of this machines is, ability to calculate T-score and Z-score for patients (Shepherd &Blake, 2007):

$$\text{T-score} = \frac{\text{Measured BMD-Young adult mean BMD}}{\text{Young adult population SD}}$$

$$Z\text{-score} = \frac{\text{Measured BMD-Age-matched mean BMD}}{\text{Young adult population SD}}$$

It means after acquisition of absolute BMD of patients by Hardware, the software compute the difference between BMD of patient and young adult mean BMD (from reference data in the software). Then divide it on young adult population standard deviation, contained in the software, the result is T-score. When Z-score is under calculation, the software divides the difference between BMD of patient and age-matched mean BMD and divides it on age-matched population standard deviation. The ability of calculating T−score and Z-score is another interesting characteristic of software of these machines.

As the different brands, have different database, scientists tried to find ways to compare the results of deferent machines. Now we suggest some of these methods.

3.4.1 Providing sBMD

Genant et al, as inventors of sBMD, explained the methods of providing sBMD in their article, so.

We can t compare patient information between various DXA scanners, because there isn't any acceptable universal cross-calibration procedure or standard. Although operating on the same basic principles, normative databases, are specific and different for each scanner. The instruments show differences in scanner design, bone mineral calibration, and analysis algorithms. Lunar and Norland scanners rely on daily scanning of standards to provide a bone tissue equivalent calibration. Hologic uses an internal calibration system, which corrects for short-term instabilities. Also, the software used for analysis of the scans, is manufacturer specific (and unique), especially with regard to the edge detection algorithms used for separating bone and soft tissue regions. This implementation causes in variations in the defined bone area (cm2) and bone mineral content (BMC, g) and density (BMD) of the same subject on different systems. Genant et al, study was performed under the auspices of the International DXA Standardization Committee to establish appropriate cross-calibration parameters. Posteroanterior (PA) lumbar spine measurements of 100 women, ages 20-80 years (mean 52.6 ± 16, range of BMD = 0.4-1.6 g/cm2) were obtained on a Norland XR26 Mark II, a Lunar DPX-L, and a Hologic QDR 2000 densitometer using standard procedures (pencil beam mode for all three scanners). Area, BMC, and BMD results from the different scanners were compared for all patients. In addition, the European spine phantom (ESP) and the European spine phantom prototype (ESP prototype), as well as standard phantoms from all three manufacturers, were evaluated on the three systems. To reach universal scanner calibration, they used the intercept and slope of the patient's correlations and the value of the middle vertebra of the ESP as a reference point in a series of standardization formulas, and expressed the results as sBMD (mg/cm2). The correlations of the patients' spinal BMD values were excellent for each of the three scanner pairs. The average absolute difference in patient spinal BMD values (L2-L4) between Hologic and Norland was 0.012 g/cm' (1.3%); it was 0.113 g/cm' (11.7%) between Hologic and Lunar and 0.118 g/cm2 (12.2%) between Norland and Lunar. The phantoms' regression lines approximated those of the patient regression lines, and the phantoms with only one measurement point were very close to the patients' regression lines. After applying the standardization formulas, the average absolute variations for the 100 patients were 28 mg/cm2 (2.7%) for Hologich/Norland, 23 mg/cm2 (2.2%) for Hologic/Lunar, and 29 mg/cm2 (2.8%) for Norland/Lunar. Average BMD results for the patients before correction were 0.972 g/cm2 for Hologic, 1.100 g/cm2 for Lunar, and 0.969 g/cm2 for Norland. After correction, sBMD results for patients were 1045 mg/cm2 for Hologic, 1047 mg/cm2 for Lunar, and 1043 mg/cm2 for Norland. The standardization approach as performed in our study provided compatibility of DXA results obtained on different scanners. Finally the sBMD for different machines calculates as sBMD = 1.0761BMDnorland, sBMDl = 0.9522BMDlunar and sBMDh = 1.0755BMDhologic. (Genant et al., 1994).

3.4.2 Use of NHANES III

When the reference-data of different machines (the young-adult mean BMD), used for defining T-score of patient, the variability within these reference data of different brands, substantially impacts osteoporosis prevalence with using this T-score-based approach. Binkley et al, emphasize that ideally, all bone mass measurement devices would use the same population to define the young-normal mean BMD and SD, a process that cause obtaining of similar T-scores with instruments of different manufacturers. Although use of a single large sample population to develop a unique normative database for all densitometers has been suggested, this process has not been possible. To increase coordination between diagnostic classification, the International Committee for Standards in Bone Measurement (ICSBM) agreed on a universal reference database for the femur based on NHANES III, the only large standardized reference database ever published (Binkley et al., 2005). Looker et al., mention that this data were gathered from 14646 men and women aged 20 years and older, using dual-energy X-ray absorptiometry, and included bone mineral density (BMD), bone mineral content (BMC) and area of bone scanned in four selected regions of interest (ROI) in the proximal femur: femur neck, trochanter, intertrochanter and total. These variables are separated by age and sex for non-Hispanic whites (NHW), non-Hispanic blacks (NHB) and Mexican Americans (MA). They emphasize that the updated data on BMD for the total femur ROI of NHW have been selected as the reference database for femur standardization efforts by the International Committee on Standards in Bone Measurements (Looker et al., 1998). The ICSBM published formulae to convert measured BMD into standardized BMD (of total femur), thereby allowing use of the NHANES III database by other brands' densitometer. The NHANES III data were acquired using Hologic densitometers (Binkley et al., 2005).

4. General consideration in bone mineral densitometry

4.1 Recommendation about ROIs that should assess

Siminoski et al., have some recommendations about ROIs that are under measurement:

- In the lumbar spine, using a minimum of 2 valid vertebra is recommended (if there is problems in L1-L4 vertebrae that cause exclusion one or 2 of them).
- In the proximal femur, Ward's area should not be included in the report, as the small amount of bone yields measurements of poor accuracy and reproducibility.
- If either hip or spine is not valid, forearm BMD is recommended. Preferred site is 1/3 radius, 33% radius or proximal radius.
- When the final report includes a graph of the patient's BMD, it should be based on the same anatomic levels that were used for numeric results; for example if L3 and L4 were excluded from spinal analysis because of degenerative objects, the graph should be based on the combined value for L1 and L2(Siminoski et al., 2005).

4.2 What is the criteria for using other sites for densitometry? Calcaneus an example

For densitometry we can also use appendicular skeleton. Particularly the calcaneus is an excellent site for measurements by a range of techniques. So we use it as an example for describing the rules of choosing ROI for bone mineral densitometry. The calcaneus is easily accessible with little overlying soft tissue. It is not a common fracture site but remember that in the spinal region, the most susceptible sites for fracture are at T7_ T8 and T11_L1, but we measure bone mineral content to L1_L4 because of less overlying soft tissue.

The remodeling of trabecular bone is more active than cortical bone. It means trabecular bone is more active metabolically and more sensitive to metabolic bone changes. Calcaneus is made up, almost entirely of trabecular bone and may provide a more sensitive measurement site for finding early signs of diseases that affect mostly metablism. A number of studies suggested that bone mass of calcaneus may contribute to fracture risk in other sites and that its predictive power is not very different than that of spine and hip. The study by Cummings et al. as cited in Kang and speller; 1999, confirmed this in 65 years old women and over.Interestingly, many early single energy measurements of bone mineral were made in the calcaneus, because it is a peripheral site that can be immersed to water. The arrival of dual energy techniques changed the focus. Earlier studies validated a highly significant correlation between the ashed bone mass of cadaver calcanei and the measured BMC values of calcaneus by densitometry (r=0.97). Kang and Speller, describe calcaneus as a site with excellent accuracy that it's measurements can be made quickly and easily and with portable instruments. (Kang & Speller, 1999)

4.3 Operators, the heart of a BMD center

Correct positioning among other factors is very important to ensure an optimal scan. Simonoski et al., emphasize that correct and consistent positioning and labelling of hip and lumbar spine (as the main job of operators), are important when evaluating serial assessments (monitoring of patients). It is important to follow manufacturer-specific protocols to ensure appropriate comparisons with normative reference data.

Structural abnormalities and artifacts can significantly influence the results. Independent factors, like body weight, may affect BMD results. However, in interpreting the results of a scan, first of all, it must be described whether the scan is valid with regards to positioning, artifact, and analysis, or not (Siminoski et al., 2005)

Fuleihan et al, assessed the effects of the machine, operator and subjects on error of measurements of bone density. They explained their technique for this assessment as an analysis applied to data from a prospective study of BMD measurements on spine phantoms and on pre- and postmenopausal women. Scans performed on the same day or up to 4 weeks apart with DXA (QDR IOOOW, Hologic). Their model assessed (or suggested) that : operators' and subjects' variability were the most causes of errors in measurements rather than machine performance (Fuleihan et al., 1995). Subjects are not changeable or controllable, but operators job can be under quality control and its quality develops by time (and experience). These machines, are not very extensively distributed, and any machine is unique in its way (the data of a second scan of a patients, can be compared to data on the same machine that first BMD is performed, only). These make finding expert operators for these machines, not very easy. What mentioned above, is the cause that operators are called "the heart" of BMD centers. So some-ones believe in this sentence "Never change your operators (in BMD departments) and if the change is inevitable, never change them again."

4.4 Material of a standard BMD report

Shimonoseki et al, recommend that , a standard BMD report should include:

- Patient identifiers.
- DXA scanner identifier.
- BMD results expressed in absolute values (g/cm2; 3 decimal places) and T-score (1 decimal place) for lumbar spine; proximal femur (total hip, femoral neck, and trochanter); and an alternate site (forearm BMD preferred: 1/3 radius, 33% radius or proximal radius) if either hip or spine is not valid.
- A statement about any limitations due to artifacts, if present.
- The fracture risk category (low, moderate, or high). It must be included major clinical factors that modify absolute fracture risk probability (with an indication of the corresponding absolute 10-year fracture risk of <10%, 10-20%, or >20%).
- A statement as to whether the change is statistically significant or not for serial measurements. The BMD centre's least significant change for each skeletal site (in g/cm2) should be included (Siminoski et al., 2005)

4.5 Discordance

Discordance makes difficulties in diagnosis of osteoporosis and management of osteoporotic patients. Moayyeri et al, explain, discordance in diagnosis of osteoporosis that is defined as presence of different categories of diagnosis based on T-score (osteoporosis, osteopenia, and normal) in two skeletal sites of an individual patient. They mansion that discordance has been divided into two groups: major and minor . When the different sites results, are close; i.e., normal in one site and osteopenic in the other site, or, when patient is diagnosed as osteopenic in one site and osteoporotic in the other site, minor discordance happens. When patient diagnosed normal in one site and is osteoporosis in another site, major discordance happens. (Moayyeri et al., 2005). In a clinical study, BMD measurements performed at lumbar spine both for baseline risk assessment and for monitoring purposes. Leslie et al. discuss a difficulty that clinician are confronted with highly discordant measurements and at the same time lumbar spine is worse than femoral neck and about how this should be integrated into the decision-making process. They discuss about different guideline recommendations in this situation. They say under NOF guideline, if t-score in lumbar spine is in osteoporotic range without consideration to estimated risk -by special soft-wares-, treatment should be recommended. In other national guideline such as those from the UK, till a 10 year fracture risk prediction from the femoral neck does not reach the intervention threshold, don't recommend any treatment for patients with osteoporotic lumbar spine. Canadian guidelines have attempted to show the issue of site discordance (in femur) by recommending use of the minimum T-score, in femur for diagnosis and treatment of osteoporosis. However, Leslie et al. suggest that this may systematically overestimates fracture risk and does not consider site-specific differences in fractures or the way BMD declines with age. They suggest that as lumbar spine and hip measurements are both performed for clinical purposes, using a procedure that accurately reflects the contribution of each measurement site to fracture risk, is clearly preferred, so they propose a a procedure for adjusting FRAX probability, based upon the T-score difference between the lumbar spine (LS) and femoral neck (FN). This procedure is termed "offset". They furmulated following rule: "Increase/decrease FRAX estimate for a major fracture by one tenth for each rounded T-score difference between LS and FN." (Leslie et al., 2011)

4.6 Pediatric consideration
4.6.1 Low bone mass in pediatrics
New investigations show prevalence of low BMD in children is very high and it is higher than expected range. Genetic, environmental and iatrogenic factor are 3 most important factor that lead to bone disorders in children.

Bogunovic et al., name causes of pediatric osteoporosis as idiopathic juvenile osteoporosis and heritable connective tissue disorders like osteogenesis imperfect and Ehler–Danlos. They also name a long list of factors as secondary causes of pediatric osteoporosis that include neuromuscular disorders (cerebral palsy and Duchenne muscular dystrophy), childhood cancer, endocrine disorders (Turner Syndrome and juvenile diabetes mellitus), and inborn errors of metabolism (Gaucher disease) and Chronic diseases like thalassemia. Anticonvulsants, glucocorticoids, and various forms of chemotherapy may adversely affect normal skeletal maturation (Bogunovic et al., 2009).

4.6.2 Problems with DXA in pediatric
Bone mass densitometry by dual X-ray absorptiometry (DEXA) of the lumbar spine and femoral neck is recommended as one of the most reliable and non-invasive technique for the assessment of bone mass (Hamidi et al., 2008). This method is very common around the world and many pediatric studies about bone densitometry and body composition have been published by using this method. (Van Kuijk, 2010).WHO osteoporosis diagnostic criteria should not be applied to children. We can't use T-score because children have not reached PBM, yet. Instead, in children, Z-score must be noticed, that it is a comparison of BMD of child to pediatric normative data. If the z- score is below -2 , we can use the term 'low bone density for chronologic age" (Daniels et al., 2003). DXA is reliable and accurate for adult but in children there is a challenge for it. As it is known, true bone density is a result of dividing BMC(g) by volume(cm3). In DXA , BMD is determined by dividing BMC by 2 dimensional area of a three dimensional objective (bone). By the use of these criteria smaller bone appear to have a lower BMD than larger bones. (Bogunovic et al., 2009). Bone size does not change, in adults, over time. On the contrary, bone size changes in growing children in 3 dimentions. When we screen children with DXA and follow them over time, we actually measure their growth instead of measuring actual changing in BMD.(Van Kuijk, 2010). It must be remembered that wide variation of height, and bone size in children makes interpretation of BMD difficult, especially in short children. Bogunovic et al., mention that longitudinal evaluation of a given patient over time is affected by the ever-changing size of the growing skeleton and the rates of skeletal growth vary with each bony dimension (Bogunovic et al., 2009). All this problems, cause to ask a question: Is it right to use DXA for measuring bone density and fracture risk in children or not? In response we emphasize some useful points about DXA. First it has fewer radiation than other methods, that is very important in radiology of children, 2) it is not a fearful (less noisy with no tunnel) method for children densitometry, 3) It is used worldwide and many pediatric studies, have been published in the field of bone densitometry and in the field of body composition studies, by using DXA method also 4) Studies about the relationship between bone density and fractures in healthy children, suggested that bone mass may contribute to fracture risk in childhood (Van Kuijk, 2010). So may be the answer is that performing DXA for measurement bone density and fracture risk in children, is a helpful method yet. However

we should emphasize that bone fragility in children extends beyond single BMD measurement, and bone geometry and body size influence it and in the diagnosis of osteoporosis, the presence of both a clinically significant fracture history and low bone mass, must be noticed (Bogunovic et al., 2009).

4.6.3 Special consideration of comparison of normal children and children with chronic disease, some points in BMD of chronic ill children

The measurement of BMC (g/cm) and BMD (g/cm2) are not only dependent on the mineral density of cortical and spongious bone, but also depend on the bone geometry. Lower BMD or BMC in shorter children may not describe a mineral deficiency or mineralization disorder, as is often thought, because the smaller bone may show lower BMD because of properties of DXA methods (Schonau,1998). BMD measurement in children is more affected by the wide variation of age at onset and progression of puberty. This leads to a wide variation in the age at reach of peak bone mass. It is thought the presence of a chronic disease, like juvenile arthritis, cause delay in pubertal onset and development. It has been estimated that one-third to one-half of the total mineralization in the lumbar spine in adult women is occurred during the 3 years around the onset of puberty. Therefore, we can t compare the BMD of a well-grown 13-year-old girl who is in mid-puberty with that of a small pre-pubertal 13-year-old with juvenile arthritis. Rabinovich remembers us that a DXA scan is not needed to tell who has the lower BMD. The question then is, is the BMD result in this small pre-pubertal girl normal? (Rabinovich, 2004).

As van Kuijk suggests, children with chronic disorders or medication, should never be compared with age-matched reference (normal) values. They should be compared with children with the same maturation status (skeletal age) (Van Kuijk, 2010).

5. Geometry (Another use of dual x-ray absorptiometry)

Some important factors such as the shape and structure of bone and the risk of falling, affect susceptibility to fracture so BMD alone cannot exactly predict who will have fracture. As Gregory and Aspden emphasize, the geometry of the proximal femur is a vital component in determining a person's risk of hip fracture. When a trauma occurs, such as a fall, the shape and structure of the femur determines how the forces are passed through the bone from the point of impact and whether they surpass the inherent strength of the bone and result in a fracture or not. Geometry component is seen in the picture from Gregory and Aspden article (Fig. 5.)

They explained any of these components

- Hip axis length: The distance from greater trochanter to inner pelvic brim, shown between points A and C in Fig. 5
- Femoral neck axis length (FNAL):

Femoral neck axis length is the linear distance measured from the base of the greater trochanter to the apex of the femoral head. It is illustrated by points B to C in Fig. 5. Confusingly, it is also sometimes referred to in the literature as hip axis length.

- Femoral neck width (FNW):

The narrowest distance across the femoral neck, often constrained to being perpendicular to the neck axis. The distance between points F and G in Fig. 5.

- Neck-shaft angle:

Usually defined as the angle between the femoral neck axis and the shaft axis (angle at point H in Fig. 5).

- Other geometrical measures: In addition to the most common measures of geometry discussed above, a number of other measures have also been related to fracture; including a thinner femoral shaft cortex , a thinner femoral neck cortex , a smaller calcar femoral (a dense, vertically orientated bone present in the posteroemedial region of the femoral shaft under the lesser trochanter of the femur) , a narrower trochanteric width and smaller inner and outer pelvic diameters. In contrast, an increased femoral head diameter has been related to increased bone strength.

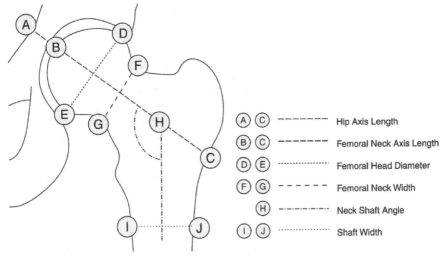

Fig. 5. Diagram illustrating some of the most common geometrical measurements made from the proximal femur (from Gregory and Aspden, 2008).

Two methods are must commonly used for assessing bone geometry, radiography and dual energy X-ray absorptiometry (DXA) (fan beam devices, more provide this service). Each of them; has its own advantages and disadvantages. Femoral geometry is important in determining both bone strength and fracture risk. The strongest associations with both outcomes appear to be a longer (Hip axis length) HAL and larger NSA (Neck-shaft angle) (Gregory & Aspden, 2008).

6. Finite element (An helpful method for better understanding of bone)

Need to a mathematical tool for solving complex mathematical problems, is answered by inventing Finite-element modeling (FEM). It helps to understand patterns of stress, strain, deflections, heat transfer, fluid flow, etc., in computer models of organic structures. Ross, emphasize that FEM provides a method for addressing a range of questions that are otherwise intractable, or very difficult to solve -in vivo or in vitro- and is potentially one of the most powerful tools in the methodological tool of vertebrate biomechanics. For example, clarifying functional consequences of the remarkable histological and morphological diversity of the vertebrae, is one of the important aims of vertebrate biomechanics. Many of researches on various disorders or diseases of the bone, are relied on this structure-function relationship. Skeletal health during long term space flight, as well as interpretation of skeletons found in the fossil and archeological records, are benefitted from these researches. Ross mentions that form-function relationships of the skeleton are therefore of concern to bioengineers, clinicians, biological anthropologists, and paleontologists, and FEM provides a method for studying them. He also suggests that the availability of increasingly powerful computers at progressively more affordable prices has made FEM an accessible tool for biomechanists and the wide use of FEM in clinical research is now imitating many basic science researches (Ross, 2005). Finite element can be helpful in femoral characteristics finding as helpful as is in spinal vertebrae and finding the mechanisms and risk factors for fracture.

7. Recent progress in bone imaging for osteoporosis research

Development in bone imaging techniques have provided tools for analyzing bone structure at the macro-, micro- and nano-level. Ito, provided a list of recent progress in bone imaging as

- High-resolution CT (HR-CT) and high-resolution magnetic resonance (HR-MR). They are in vivo quantitative techniques for assessing the microstructure of trabecular bone non-invasively and non-destructively. Compared with MR imaging, CT-based techniques have the advantage of directly visualizing the bone in the axial skeleton, with high spatial resolution (of course, disadvantage of delivering a considerable radiation dose remains).
- Micro-CT (μCT) and Synchrotron μCT (SR-CT). The farmer provides a higher resolution of the microstructure and is principally applicable in vitro, has undergone technological advances such that it is now able to elucidate the physiological skeletal change mechanisms associated with aging and determine the effects of therapeutic intervention on the bone microstructure. In particular, synchrotron μCT (SR-CT) provides a more detailed view of trabecular structure at the nano-level.
- DXA-based hip structure analysis (HSA) and CT-based HAS. DXA-based HSA is a convenient tool for analyzing biomechanical properties and for assuming cross-sectional hip geometry based on two-dimensional (2D) data. CT-based HSA provides these parameters three-dimensionally in robust relationship with biomechanical properties, at the cost of greater radiation exposure and the lengthy time required for the analytical procedure.

The author, suggests that further progress in bone imaging technology is promising to bring new aspects of bone structure in relation to bone strength to light, and to establish a means for analyzing bone structural properties in the everyday clinical setting (Ito, 2011).

8. Conclusion

Tanner in his article reminds us the Bonnick suggestion (noted in the preface of the most recent edition of the author's book on bone densitometry in clinical practice)". . . as strange as it may seem, the technology itself is in danger of becoming so devalued that improvements in accessibility and advances in applications may be lost." (Bonnick SL. as cited in Tanner, 2011 from book "Bone densitometry in clinical practice: application and interpretation"(current clinical practice series). 3rd ed. Totowa, New Jersey:Humana Press; 2010). The future of DXA bone density testing is challenged by reimbursement, complicated guidelines, and the controversy over the monitoring of treatment. Nevertheless, bone health assessment and fracture risk prediction rely on quality bone density measurement using DXA (Tanner, 2011).

9. Acknowledgement

Author must thank Dr. B. Larijani (the director of EMRI-TUMS), Dr. A. Soltani, Dr. AR. Khalili, Dr. H. Adibi, Dr.E. Rahimi, Mrs. S. Azizi , Mrs. M. Hajiloo , Miss S. Shirazi, Mrs. F.

Zare, Mrs. P. Athari, Mrs. MR. Dadras, Mrs. M. Mirzaee , Mr. D. Sadeghian and Mrs. A. Oojaghi for their valuable assistance in this study.

10. References

Binkley, Neil. Kiebzak, Gary M. Lewiecki, E Michael. Krueger, Diane. Gangnon, Ronald E. Miller, Paul D. Shepherd, John A. Drezner, Marc K. (2005). Recalculation of the NHANES database SD improves T-score agreement and reduces osteoporosis prevalence. *Journal of bone and mineral research*. *Vol.20, No. 2, (Feb 2005), pp. 195-201, 0884-0431 (Print)*

Bogunovic, Ljiljana. Doyle, Shevaun M. Vogiatzi, Maria G. (2009), Measurement of bone density in the pediatric population. *Current opinion in pediatrics, Vol. 21, No. 1, (Feb 2009), pp. 77-82, 1531-698X (Electronic)*

Damilakis, John. Adams, Judith E. Guglielmi, Giuseppe. Link, Thomas M. (2010). Radiation exposure in X-ray-based imaging techniques used in osteoporosis. *European radiology, Vol. 20, No. 11, (Nov 2010), pp 2707-2714, 1432-1084 (Electronic)*

Daniels, Mark W. Wilson, Darrell M. Paguntalan, Helen G. Hoffman, Andrew R. Bachrach, Laura K. (2003). Bone mineral density in pediatric transplant recipients. *Transplantation. Vol. 76, No. 4, (Aug 2003), pp. 673-678, 0041-1337 (Print)*

Department of nuclear medicine, PET & bone densitometry of Royal Adelaide Hospital (Australia), at section of "Bone Densitometry Equipment". (19 May 2009). Bone Densitometry Equipment, In *Royal Adelaide Hospital,* Available from: <http://www.rah.sa.gov.au/nucmed/BMD/bmd_equipment.htm#DEXA>

Fuleihan, G E. Testa, M A. Angell, J E. Porrino, N. Leboff, M S. (1995). Reproducibility of DXA absorptiometry: a model for bone loss estimates. *Journal of bone and mineral research. Vol. 10, No. 7, (Jul 1995), pp. 1004-1014, 0884-0431 (Print)*

Genant, H K. Grampp, S. Gluer, C C. Faulkner, K G. Jergas, M. Engelke, K. Hagiwara, S. Van Kuijk, C. (1994). Universal standardization for dual x-ray absorptiometry: patient and phantom cross-calibration results. *Journal of bone and mineral research, Vol. 9, No. 10, (Oct 1994), 0884-0431 (Print)*

Gregory, Jennifer S. Aspden, Richard M. (2008). Femoral geometry as a risk factor for osteoporotic hip fracture in men and women. *Medical engineering & physics, Vol. 30, No. 10, (Dec 2008), pp. 1275-1286, 1350-4533 (Print)*

Hamidi, Zohreh. Sedaghat, Mojtaba. Hejri, Soroosh Mortaz. Larijani, Bagher. (2008). Defining cut-off values for the diagnosis of osteoporosis in postmenopausal women by quantitative ultrasonography of the phalanx. *Gynecological endocrinology, Vol. 24, No. 10, (Oct 2008), pp. 546-8, 1473-0766 (Electronic)*

Health professional page of international osteoporosis foundation (IOF). (Jan 2011). Facts and statistics about osteoporosis and its impact, In : *International Osteoporosis Foundation (IOF),* Available from: < http://www.iofbonehealth.org/facts-and-statistics.html>

Ito, Masako, (2011). Recent progress in bone imaging for osteoporosis research. *Journal of bone and mineral metabolism, Vol. 29, No. 2, (Mar 2011), pp. 131-140. 1435-5604 (Electronic)*

Kang, C. Speller, R. (1999). The effect of region of interest selection on dual energy X-ray absorptiometry measurements of the calcaneus in 55 post-menopausal women. *The British journal of radiology, Vol. 72, No. 861, (Sep 1999), pp. 864-871, 0007-1285 (Print)*

Kanis, J A. (1994). Assessment of fracture risk and its application to screening for postmenopausal osteoporosis: synopsis of a WHO report. WHO Study Group. *Osteoporosis international. Vol. 4, No. 6, (Nov 1994), pp. 368-381, 0937-941X (Print)*

Kanis, J A. Johnell, O. (2005). Requirements for DXA for the management of osteoporosis in Europe. *Osteoporos International*, Vol. 16, No. 3, (Mar 2005), pp 229-238, 0937-941X (Print)

Leslie, W D. Lix, L M. Johansson, H. Oden, A. McCloskey, E. Kanis, J A. (2011). Spine-hip discordance and fracture risk assessment: a physician-friendly FRAX enhancement. *Osteoporosis international*, Vol. 22, No. 3, (Mar 2011), pp. 839-847, 1433-2965 (Electronic)

Leslie, William D. Moayyeri, Alireza. Sadatsafavi, Mohsen. Wang, Liqun. (2007). A new approach for quantifying change and test precision in bone densitometry. *Journal of clinical densitometry*. Vol. 10, No. 4, (Oct-Dec 2007), pp. 365-369, 1094-6950 (Print)

Library page of Legislative Assembly of Ontario, (November 2006). Utilization of DXA Bone Mineral Densitometry in Ontario Health Technology Literature Review, In: *Legislative Assembly of Ontario*, Available from: <http://www.ontla.on.ca/library/repository/mon/16000/272076.pdf>

Looker, A C. Wahner, H W. Dunn, W L. Calvo, M S. Harris, T B. Heyse, S P. -Johnston, C C Jr. Lindsay, R. (1998). Updated data on proximal femur bone mineral levels of US adults. *Osteoporosis international*. Vol. 8, No. 5, (1998), pp. 468-489, 0937-941X (Print)

Lukaski, H C (1993). Soft tissue composition and bone mineral status: evaluation by dual-energy X-ray absorptiometry. *The Journal of nutrition*, Vol. 123, No. 2 Suppl,(Feb 1993), pp. 438-443, 0022-3166 (Print)

Mithal, Ambrish.. Dhingra, Vibha. Lau , Edith.   (September 2009) .The Asian Audit Epidemiology, costs and burden of osteoporosis in Asia 2009, In: *International Osteoporosis Foundation*, Available from: <http://www.iofbonehealth.org/download/osteofound/filemanager/publications/pdf/Asian-audit-09/2009-Asian_Audit.pdf>

Moayyeri, A. Soltani, A. Tabari, NK. Sadatsafavi, M. Hossein-Neghad, A. Larijani, B. (2005). Discordance in diagnosis of osteoporosis using spine and hip bone densitometry. *BMC endocrine disorders*, Vol. 5, No. 1, (Mar 2005), p. 3, 1472-6823 (Electronic)

Rabinovich, C. Egla. (2004). Osteoporosis: a pediatric perspective. *Arthritis and rheumatism*. Vol. 50, No. 4,(Apr 2004), 0004-3591 (Print)

Ross, Callum F. (2005). Finite element analysis in vertebrate biomechanics. *The anatomical record*, Vol. 283, No. 2, (Apr 2005), pp. 253-258, 1552-4884 (Print)

Schonau, E. (1998). Problems of bone analysis in childhood and adolescence. *Pediatric nephrology (Berlin, Germany)*, Vol 12, No. 5, (Jun 1998), pp. 420-429, 0931-041X (Print)

Shepherd, John A. Blake, Glen M.(2007). T-scores and Z-scores. *Journal of clinical densitometry*, Vol. 10, No. 4, (Oct-Des 2007), pp. 349-350, 1094-6950 (Print)

Siminoski, Kerry. Leslie, William D. Frame, Heather. Hodsman, Anthony. Josse, Robert G. Khan, Aliya. Lentle, Brian C. Levesque, Jacques. Lyons, David J. Tarulli, Giuseppe. Brown, Jacques P. Recommendations for bone mineral density reporting in Canada. *Canadian Association of Radiologists journal*. Vol. 56, No. 3, (Jun 2005), pp. 178-188, 0846-5371 (Print)

Tanner, Simpson Bobo. (2011). Dual-energy X-ray absorptiometry in clinical practice: new guidelines and concerns. *Current opinion in rheumatology*, Vol. 23, No. 4, (Jul 2011), pp. 385-388. 1531-6963 (Electronic)

van Kuijk, Cornelis. (2010). Pediatric bone densitometry. *Radiologic clinics of North America*. Vol. 48, No. 3, (May 2010), pp. 623-627, 1557-8275 (Electronic)

Wells, J. Ryan, P J. (2000). The long-term performance of DXA bone densitometers. *The British journal of radiology*, Vol. 73, No. 871, (Jul 2000), pp. 737-739, 0007-1285 (Print)

Permissions

The contributors of this book come from diverse backgrounds, making this book a truly international effort. This book will bring forth new frontiers with its revolutionizing research information and detailed analysis of the nascent developments around the world.

We would like to thank Yannis Dionyssiotis, MD, PhD, for lending his expertise to make the book truly unique. He has played a crucial role in the development of this book. Without his invaluable contribution this book wouldn't have been possible. He has made vital efforts to compile up to date information on the varied aspects of this subject to make this book a valuable addition to the collection of many professionals and students.

This book was conceptualized with the vision of imparting up-to-date information and advanced data in this field. To ensure the same, a matchless editorial board was set up. Every individual on the board went through rigorous rounds of assessment to prove their worth. After which they invested a large part of their time researching and compiling the most relevant data for our readers. Conferences and sessions were held from time to time between the editorial board and the contributing authors to present the data in the most comprehensible form. The editorial team has worked tirelessly to provide valuable and valid information to help people across the globe.

Every chapter published in this book has been scrutinized by our experts. Their significance has been extensively debated. The topics covered herein carry significant findings which will fuel the growth of the discipline. They may even be implemented as practical applications or may be referred to as a beginning point for another development. Chapters in this book were first published by InTech; hereby published with permission under the Creative Commons Attribution License or equivalent.

The editorial board has been involved in producing this book since its inception. They have spent rigorous hours researching and exploring the diverse topics which have resulted in the successful publishing of this book. They have passed on their knowledge of decades through this book. To expedite this challenging task, the publisher supported the team at every step. A small team of assistant editors was also appointed to further simplify the editing procedure and attain best results for the readers.

Our editorial team has been hand-picked from every corner of the world. Their multi-ethnicity adds dynamic inputs to the discussions which result in innovative outcomes. These outcomes are then further discussed with the researchers and contributors who give their valuable feedback and opinion regarding the same. The feedback is then collaborated with the researches and they are edited in a comprehensive manner to aid the understanding of the subject.

Apart from the editorial board, the designing team has also invested a significant amount of their time in understanding the subject and creating the most relevant covers. They scrutinized every image to scout for the most suitable representation of the subject and create an appropriate cover for the book.

The publishing team has been involved in this book since its early stages. They were actively engaged in every process, be it collecting the data, connecting with the contributors or procuring relevant information. The team has been an ardent support to the editorial, designing and production team. Their endless efforts to recruit the best for this project, has resulted in the accomplishment of this book. They are a veteran in the field of academics and their pool of knowledge is as vast as their experience in printing. Their expertise and guidance has proved useful at every step. Their uncompromising quality standards have made this book an exceptional effort. Their encouragement from time to time has been an inspiration for everyone.

The publisher and the editorial board hope that this book will prove to be a valuable piece of knowledge for researchers, students, practitioners and scholars across the globe.

List of Contributors

Margarita Valdés-Flores, Leonora Casas-Avila, Valeria Ponce de León-Suárez and Edith Falcón-Ramírez
Instituto Nacional de Rehabilitación, Secretaría de Salud, México, D.F., México

Gholamreza Rouhi
Faculty of Biomedical Engineering, Amirkabir University of Technology, Tehran, Iran
Department of Mechanical Engineering & School of Human Kinetics, University of Ottawa, Ontario, Canada

Delphine Farlay and Georges Boivin
INSERM, UMR 1033, F-69372 Lyon, France
Université de Lyon, F-69008 Lyon, France

Naohisa Miyakoshi, Michio Hongo and Yoichi Shimada
Department of Orthopedic Surgery, Akita University Graduate School of Medicine, Japan

Tiffany K. Gill, Anne W. Taylor and Catherine L. Hill
University of Adelaide, Australia

Julie Black
Arthritis SA, Australia

Frank Bonura
St. Catherine of Siena Medical Center, Smithtown, NY, USA

Antonio Bazarra-Fernández
A Coruña University Hospital Trust, Spain

Kanika Singh
KHAN Co, Ltd, Aju-dong, Geoje-do, Republic of Korea
Pusan National University, Busan, Republic of Korea

Kyung Chun Kim
Pusan National University, Busan, Republic of Korea

H.J. Choi
Department of Family Medicine, Eulji University School of Medicine, South Korea

Tatsuro Hayashi, Xiangrong Zhou and Hiroshi Fujita
Department of Intelligent Image Information, Gifu University Graduate School of Medicine, Japan

Huayue Chen
Department of Anatomy, Gifu University Graduate School of Medicine, Japan

Minoru Onozuka
Department of Physiology and Neuroscience, Kanagawa Dental College, Japan

Kin-ya Kubo
Seijoh University Graduate School of Health Care Studies, Japan

Zohreh Hamidi
Endocrinology and Metabolism Research Institute of Tehran University of Medical Sciences (EMRI-TUMS), Islamic Republic of Iran

9 781632 423993